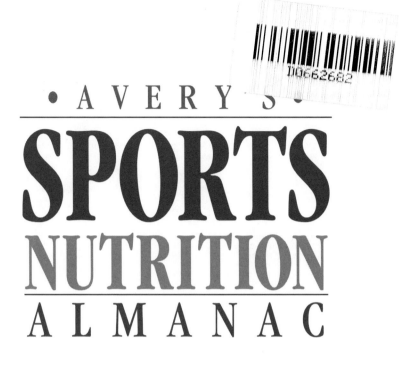

· A V E R Y ' S ·

SPORTS
NUTRITION
ALMANAC

• AVERY'S •

SPORTS

NUTRITION

ALMANAC

Edited by
EDMUND R. BURKE, Ph.D.
DANIEL GASTELU, M.S.

AVERY PUBLISHING GROUP
Garden City Park • New York

The information and procedures contained in this book are based upon the research and the personal and professional experiences of the authors. They are not intended as a substitute for consulting with your physician or other health-care provider. The publisher and authors are not responsible for any adverse effects or consequences resulting from the use of any of the suggestions, preparations, or procedures discussed in this book. All matters pertaining to your physical health should be supervised by a health-care professional. It is a sign of wisdom, not cowardice, to seek a second or third opinion.

Cover designer: Doug Brooks
In-house editor: Elaine Will Sparber
Typesetter: Gary A. Rosenberg
Printer: Paragon Press, Honesdale, PA

Avery Publishing Group
120 Old Broadway
Garden City Park, NY 11040
1–800–548–5757
www.averypublishing.com

If you have any suggestions for the next edition of this book, please send them to Avery Publishing at the address to the left.

Avery's Sports Nutrition Almanac is an ongoing project.

Permission Credits

The table on page 10 is used with the permission of the American Diabetes Association. It is adapted from *Diabetes Care,* Vol. 5 (1982).

The "Tips From Top Athletes" on pages 200 to 209 are used with the permission of Virgo Publishing, Inc. They are reprinted from *HSR—Health Supplement Retailer,* Vol. 4, No. 8 (July 1998).

Cataloging-in-Publication

Avery's sports nutrition almanac / edited by Edmund
   R. Burke, Daniel Gastelu. — 1st ed.
     p. cm.
     Includes bibliographical references and index.
     ISBN: 0-89529-885-6

     1. Athletes—Nutrition. I. Burke, Ed, 1949–
II. Gastelu, Daniel. III. Title: Sports nutrition
almanac

TX361.A8A84 1999   613.2'024796
                    QBI99-700

10   9   8   7   6   5   4   3   2   1

CONTENTS

ACKNOWLEDGMENTS

To Avery Publishing, without whose steady and professional editorial guidance this *Sports Nutrition Almanac* would never have come to fruition. In particular, my heartfelt thanks to Elaine Sparber for her ability to pull together all the edits of the manuscript.

To all the athletes with whom I have come in contact over the last twenty years, who have given me the insight to look beyond "traditional" nutritional information and research to find the truth behind sports nutritional supplementation and support. To the many scientists, nutritionists, and medical professionals who, in their laboratories and clinics, are pushing back the frontiers of our knowledge of sports nutrition and are waging the war against complacency in nutrition research and education.

E.B.

I would like to thank Rudy Shur, Norm Goldfind, Elaine Sparber, and the other hardworking people at Avery Publishing who made this *Almanac* possible, as well as my family, friends, and colleagues, whose constant support inspired me to make this *Almanac* an extremely valuable resource for all athletes to use to pick the most effective supplements and achieve the best results nutrition science has to offer.

D.G.

The editors of *Avery's Sports Nutrition Almanac* would also like to thank Ben Weider, Dr. Jim Wright, Dave Tuttle, and Jon Benninger for their help in the preparation of this book.

PREFACE

After intensive research and writing, we have produced *Avery's Sports Nutrition Almanac,* an encyclopedic resource on sports nutrition that athletes and fitness exercisers, as well as the specialists who guide them, can put to immediate use. In this *Almanac,* we present information on basic performance-nutrition factors, dietary supplements, and the latest research on sports nutrition. In writing the book, we relied both on nutritional principles that are established in the scientific literature and on those that evolved from our personal-practice experiences, the experiences of the elite athletes with whom we work, and published research. The performance-nutrition information that we present bridges the gap between theoretical research and practice. We never meant for this book to be a critical scientific overview, so we have limited ourselves to presenting useful facts, not theoretical debate. For technical and professional readers, we have included an extensive listing of our reference sources for further study.

As scientific fields go, sports nutrition is still in its infancy. In spite of this, enough has been learned over the past twenty-five years to confirm that sports nutrition is, indeed, a science, and this requires that established rules of scientific evidence be applied to the collection and distribution of information. This means that we can learn by carefully collecting data from individuals who have achieved the best in sports performance or who have shown improvement by following a particular protocol. However, the generalization of this information for use by others, given nutritional, psychological, physiological, anatomical, and motivational differences, is not easy to do. Therefore, while global generalizations on how to achieve optimum performance or health can be made, even for relatively homogeneous groups or sports teams, our strength lies in understanding and focusing on the individual.

There is still much to be learned in the area of sports nutrition, and we will all require more time to understand fully what we think we already know. The information base is increasing so rapidly that existing beliefs are constantly being questioned and re-evaluated. For example, it would be comforting to think that an increase in activity is associated with a concomitant increase in food intake, so that the increased nutrient demands of the activity are automatically met. After all, doesn't regular activity influence appetite so that physiological needs are met? In reality, however, some nutrients are used or lost at a rate faster than that at which they can easily be replaced by typical food intakes, and many athletes suffer from poor nutrition, which puts them at frank nutritional risk. This is why the use of sports supplements for improved performance is at the heart of this book.

Most often, the athletes who are led astray nutritionally are enticed into choosing their diet or dietary-supplement program by marketing slogans or similar forms of misinformation. Sidetracked by this Madison Avenue hype, these athletes are blinded to the new scientific advances being made in performance nutrition. In this book, we present and discuss proven scientific performance-nutrition techniques and will help you reach your peak physical-performance level by explaining how to apply them.

In Part One, the basics of sports nutrition, and of nutrition in general, are discussed. The macronutrients—carbohydrates, protein, lipids, and water—and the primary micronutrients—vitamins, minerals, and enzymes—are discussed and intake recommendations presented. In Part Two, the focus is sports-performance enhancers. Herbs and mushrooms, metabolites, and meal replacements, protein powders, and metabolic optimizers are explained in easy-to-understand language. The winning nutrition and training programs of several accomplished athletes are described to show how the information presented in this book can be pulled together into a program to optimize health and performance. Finally, the sports-enhancing products currently new on the market are discussed, and the trends just getting underway are assessed. Part Three is a roundup of the facts and resources that you may find yourself searching for as you put together your own training and nutrition program.

Avery's Sports Nutrition Almanac is your comprehensive resource for nutrition success. With its easy-to-use format and library of information, it will become an important part of your life. Use it as your guide to maximum performance and health.

HOW TO USE THIS BOOK

*A*very's *Sports Nutrition Almanac* is intended for everyone interested in health and fitness. Whether you're a point guard for the New York Knicks or an outfielder for your company's softball team, an Olympic gymnast training for Sydney in 2000 or a lunchtime jogger, *Avery's Sports Nutrition Almanac* will help you plan your diet and supplement program for maxiumum health and performance.

Combining a primer on basic nutrition with a review of the latest in sports nutrition, *Avery's Sports Nutrition Almanac* is divided into three parts. Part One presents the basic principles of nutrition and health. It provides both an overview of the primary nutrients that athletes need and, at the same time, an introduction to the basic terminology that scientists, nutritionists, and health professionals use to categorize and represent the many nutritional concepts covered in this book. Specifically, Chapters 1, 2, and 3 discuss carbohydrates, protein and amino acids, and lipids, respectively. Chapter 4 covers water, an often neglected nutrient, and Chapter 5 reviews vitamins and minerals. Chapter 6 explains enzymes for novices and experts alike.

Part Two of *Avery's Sports Nutrition Almanac* concentrates on the cutting-edge, high-tech supplements that have only recently become widely available. Chapter 7 focuses on herbs and mushrooms, used for centuries by Eastern health-care practitioners but only now coming into popular use in the West. Chapter 8 presents a roundup of the metabolites and other performance enhancers that are familiar to most athletes and are now either in the news again or being sold in "new and improved" forms. Meal replacements, protein powders, and metabolic optimizers are the subjects of Chapter 9, which explains what they are, what they do, and how to use them. Chapter 10 is a natural extension of everything before it, showing how a number of accomplished athletes have combined diet, nutritional supplementation, and training to attain and maintain optimum performance and health. Rounding out Part Two is an analysis, in Chapter 11, of the nutritional products new on the market this year and a look, in Chapter 12, at the trends developing for the future.

Part Three offers facts and resources to help you in your quest for personal fitness. In Chapter 13, a "Who's Really Who in Sports Nutrition" is presented to help you weed through the mass of often confusing and conflicting "expert" information and determine what may be valid and what may be nonsense. In Chapter 14, you will find a directory of names, addresses, and phone numbers of leading sports-nutrition companies, as well as websites offering in-depth information on health and sports-nutrition concerns. Chapter 15 is a dictionary of training and health terms that will help you while reading this book, when comparing nutritional regimens with your friends, or while discussing the pros and cons of the latest training techniques with your coach. Chapter 16 points you toward other books on sports nutrition and software to help you track your nutritional intake. And Chapter 17 lists the numerous reference sources used in the creation of *Avery's Sports Nutrition Almanac* that you can look up to expand your knowledge of sports nutrition even further.

Fortunately, almost daily, more and more information is becoming available on sports nutrition and supplementation. We are living through an explosion of sports nutrition information. Scientific and lay journals are publishing articles on sports nutrition, newspapers are covering sports-nutrition topics, and morning news shows are featuring sports-nutrition experts as guests. But with this increased awareness comes, unfortunately, increased *mis*information about sports nutrition as well.

Avery's Sports Nutrition Almanac is designed to give you up-to-date information about sports nutrition in clear, easy-to-understand language. It can be read cover to cover or dipped into as necessary when information is needed on a specific topic. Based upon scientific research and documentation, it will show you how good nutrition and supplements can help improve your performance and boost your recovery ability. Use this *Almanac* as your guide to your physical best, in your health and your sport.

PART ONE

SPORTS-NUTRITION BASICS

Every day, the body requires many nutrients for energy, growth, and performance. The nutrients needed for athletic performance are grouped into several categories. Most, however, fall into two main categories—macronutrients and micronutrients. Macronutrients are nutrients that are required daily in large amounts and that are thought of in quantities of ounces and grams. They include carbohydrates, protein, lipids, and water. Macronutrients are important because they supply the body with energy and serve as the building blocks for growth and repair. They are found in all foods, but they occur in each food in a different proportion. For example, meat is high in protein and fat but has almost no carbohydrates. Pasta, on the other hand, is very high in carbohydrates but has just a moderate amount of protein and a very small amount of fat.

Carbohydrates affect energy and performance according to when they are eaten and what kind they are. The two kinds of carbohydrates are the complex carbohydrates, or starches, and the simple carbohydrates, such as glucose and fructose. Starch provides the body with a slow, steady supply of glucose because it is composed of chains of glucose that must first be broken down during digestion. Glucose itself does not need to be broken down and therefore enters the bloodstream immediately, providing a quick supply of energy. Fructose gets into the bloodstream at a rate that is somewhere between starch and glucose.

Lipids are fats, oils, and other plant and animal nutrients that are insoluble in water. Triglycerides, the fatty acids that make up fat, contain the most energy of any macronutrient on a per-weight basis. Other lipids, such as cholesterol, are not important energy sources but are major components of some hormones and bile acids.

The body always uses a mixture of carbohydrates and fat, plus a little protein, for energy. This energy mixture varies depending upon the intensity and duration of the physical activity and the composition of the food from which the energy is derived. Endurance sports, such as marathon running, tend to cause the body to burn a higher proportion of fat for energy, while power sports, such as powerlifting, tend to cause the body to burn a greater amount of carbohydrates. The physical demand therefore dictates the proportion of macronutrients needed in the diet. A marathon runner generally needs a diet high in carbohydrates and moderate in fat and protein, while a sprinter needs a diet high in carbohydrates and protein and low in fat.

The way the body uses protein during and after exercise is more complicated than the way it uses carbohydrates or fat for energy. Protein supplies the body with building blocks in the form of amino acids. The body therefore tends to avoid using protein or amino acids for energy. However, during exercise, the body does use certain amino acids for energy and other metabolic functions. This cannot be prevented, but it can be counterbalanced by ingesting proteins with higher amounts of the amino acids used during exercise, such as the branched–chain amino acids. Research has shown that even while athletes rest, their highly trained muscles still use certain amino acids for energy, despite the presence of carbohydrates and fat. Athletes can use special dietary supplements that are designed to boost the efficiency and utilization of dietary protein plus supply certain vitamin and mineral cofactors that help prevent muscle breakdown and encourage muscle repair. A cofactor is a substance that must be present for another substance to perform a certain function.

Scientists have always recognized the importance of water, but recently, additional research has shown that sustaining the optimum level of hydration is important for maintaining peak performance and for achieving adequate recovery. In a sport such as soccer or basketball, an athlete can lose several pounds of water weight during just one game. This can adversely affect performance and, in the long run, can cause peaks and valleys in the athlete's performance curve.

In addition to remaining hydrated, the body also needs to maintain its electrolyte balance. The major electrolytes found in the bodily fluids are chloride, magnesium, potassium, and sodium. Water is a part of every cell. How much water a cell contains depends on the function of the cell. Likewise, specific quantities of the electrolytes are found in intracellular and extracellular fluid. These water and electrolyte concentrations are closely controlled, even under extreme temperature conditions. The same as water, the electrolytes are lost through sweat. Replenishing water and electrolyte stores during exercise and throughout the day has become an increasingly complex task for the athlete, as scientists are continually discovering new roles that these nutrients play in the body.

Even more diverse as a group than the macronutrients are the micronutrients. As the name implies, micronutrients are nutrients that are present in the diet and the body in small amounts. They are measured in milligrams and micrograms. If these nutrients are present in the body, they are called nonessential, since it is not essential that they be obtained from the diet. If they are not present and must be obtained from the diet, they are called essential. Micronutrients do not provide significant amounts of calories to the body but act as cofactors in making molecules, play various structural roles, and function as electrolytes and enzymes.

Broadly speaking, the essential and nonessential vitamins and minerals, vitaminlike substances, and other dietary substances that are important to performance and health fall into the micronutrient category.

Vitamins are organic compounds that the body needs for the maintenance of good health and for growth. By convention, the name *vitamin* is reserved for certain nutrients that the body cannot manufacture and therefore must get from food. Vitamins are further classified as fat soluble or water soluble. The fat-soluble vitamins include vitamins A, D, E, and K. Because they are soluble in fat (lipids), these vitamins tend to become stored in the body's fat tissues, fat deposits, and liver. This storage capability makes the fat-soluble vitamins potentially toxic. Care should be exercised when taking the fat-soluble vitamins.

The water-soluble vitamins include the B vitamins and vitamin C. In contrast to the fat-soluble vitamins, the water-soluble vitamins are not easily stored by the body. They are often lost from foods during cooking or are eliminated from the body.

Vitamins are not usually metabolized for energy, but some are essential for the production of energy from the macronutrients and act as cofactors. As with the macronutrients, vitamin research has only begun to illuminate how these nutrients benefit performance and health beyond the prevention of nutritional deficiencies. However, current findings give us a good picture of how vitamins are important to health and performance.

Minerals are inorganic nutrients or inorganic–organic complexes that are essential structural components in the body and necessary for many vital metabolic processes, even though they make up only about 4 percent of the body's weight. Every day, the body needs minerals such as calcium in large amounts, about 1,200 milligrams or more, while it needs other minerals, such as chromium, in smaller amounts, measured in micrograms. A microgram is one-thousandth of a milligram. Although the minerals are needed on a daily basis in a wide range of amounts, their relative importance is equal. Some minerals are found in the body in an inorganic form; examples are calcium salts in the bones and sodium chloride in the blood. Other minerals are present in organic combinations; examples are iron in hemoglobin (the oxygen carrier in red blood cells) and iodine in thyroxine (a thyroid hormone). How well the body absorbs each mineral varies greatly. Researchers are discovering that just because a mineral, or a vitamin, is present in a food does not mean that all of it will be absorbed into the body. This is another reason that dietary supplements are recommended. Supplements ensure that the body receives exact amounts of the nutrients. Additionally, the nutrients in supplements are of a high quality, unaccompanied by the fat, salt, pesticides, and other junk that is found in many foods.

All life processes consist of a complex series of chemical reactions. These reactions are collectively referred to as metabolism. Enzymes are the catalysts that make metabolism possible. Without enzymes, many of the body's chemical reactions would never take place. The body contains millions of enzymes, which continually renew, maintain, and protect it. No person, plant, or animal could exist without enzymes. Unfortunately, many athletes have never heard of enzymes and are unaware of their importance in regulating the body and maintaining health. Enzymes are responsible for synthesizing, joining together, and duplicating whole chains of amino acids. They are proteins, consisting of long chains of amino acids that differ in order and number. Enzymes are available in supplemental form to help improve metabolism and injury repair.

In Part One, we will provide an overview of the primary nutrients that athletes need and, at the same time, will introduce the basic terminology that scientists, nutritionists, and health professionals use to categorize and represent the many nutritional concepts covered in this book. In Chapters 1, 2, 3, and 4, we will discuss carbohydrates, protein and amino acids, lipids, and water, respectively. In Chapter 5, we will cover vitamins and minerals. Rounding out our discussion of the basic nutrients, we will review enzymes in Chapter 6.

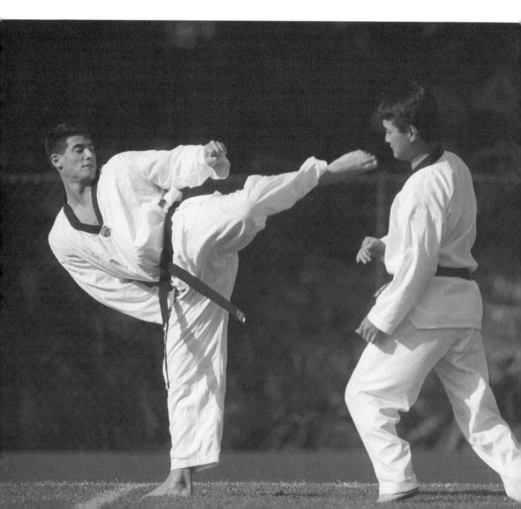

CARBOHYDRATES

THE ULTIMATE PERFORMANCE FUEL

1

In the United States, the average daily intake of carbohydrates is 287 grams for adult males and 177 grams for adult females. Approximately half of the carbohydrates that normal American adults consume are simple carbohydrates, with the other half being complex carbohydrates. This is off-balance. The National Research Council (NRC) and the Surgeon General have determined that the typical American diet is too high in fat, sodium, and sugar (simple carbohydrates), and too low in complex carbohydrates and fiber.

Most athletes eating for top performance should get at least 55 to 60 percent of their total daily calories from carbohydrates. For some kinds of athletes, the percentage should be even higher. In addition, research has shown that the type of carbohydrate eaten can affect performance.

Take the simple carbohydrate glucose as an example. Studies have shown that consuming a high-glucose food or drink approximately thirty minutes to two hours before exercising stimulates a rise in the insulin level. This rise in insulin in turn promotes the uptake of glucose by cells throughout the body and may cause hypoglycemia (low blood sugar). The net result is decreased performance and early onset of fatigue. In contrast, a glucose drink taken just prior to—that is, about five minutes before—and during exercise maintains the blood sugar, spares glycogen, and increases the time it takes the body to become exhausted. In other words, it increases performance and capacity. Complex carbohydrates eaten two to three hours before exercise also increase performance and delay fatigue in endurance activities because they enter the bloodstream at a slow, steady rate.

The most recent studies show that carbohydrates are the body's primary high-energy fuel source for all activities. Early researchers studied the effects of nutrient intake on work performance. By putting their subjects on a variety of nutritional regimens—from outright starvation to diets consisting of different proportions of fat, protein, and carbohydrates—they found a few interesting dynamics. First, when the body runs out of its stored glycogen and must turn to fatty acids as its primary source of energy, physical performance declines dramatically. The body must push much harder to keep up the work pace. Endurance athletes call this "hitting the wall." They commonly encountered this phenomenon before the importance of carbohydrate loading and ingesting carbohydrate drinks during exercise was discovered. Carbohydrate loading is a supercompensation in glycogen storage. Studies have revealed that it can be initiated by depleting the body's glycogen stores and then replenishing them using a diet high in carbohydrates.

Since all this early research, even more light has been shed on the importance of carbohydrates to performance. As well as consuming an adequate supply of carbohydrates by means of a mixed diet, athletes must consider the type of carbohydrates they eat, the time of day they eat them, and their intake of cofactors. All these elements together help increase the glycogen stores and enhance energy production during exercise.

In this chapter, we will discuss the basic types of carbohydrates that are found in food and dietary supplements. We will then examine the ways in which these basic types of carbohydrates can be used to enhance athletic performance.

TYPES OF CARBOHYDRATES

There are several types of carbohydrates, some of which are better than others. Starch, sugar, and dextrose are examples. The different types of carbohydrates can be divided into three general categories. Monosaccharides are carbohydrates that have one sugar molecule. Disaccharides are carbohydrates that have two sugar molecules. And polysaccharides are carbohydrates that have three or more sugar molecules. Monosaccharides and disaccharides are commonly called sugars, while polysaccharides are called complex carbohydrates or glucose polymers. Some of the more commonly encountered carbohydrates in these three categories include the following:

☐ *Monosaccharides*—Glucose, fructose, sorbitol, galactose, mannitol, and mannose.

☐ *Disaccharides*—Sucrose, which is made of one molecule each of glucose and fructose; maltose, made of two molecules of glucose; and lactose, made of one molecule each of glucose and galactose.

☐ *Polysaccharides*—Starch, dextrin, cellulose, and glycogen, which are all made of chains of glucose and are called glucose polymers or maltodextrins; and inulin, a unique carbohydrate made of multiple molecules of fructose.

Another kind of carbohydrate is fiber, which is composed mainly of the indigestible polysaccharides that make up a plant's cell walls. These polysaccharides include cellulose, hemicellulose, pectin, and a variety of gums, mucilages, and algal polysaccharides.

SIMPLE CARBOHYDRATES

The principal monosaccharides in food are glucose and fructose. Glucose, which is also called dextrose or grape sugar, is found commonly in fruit, sweet corn, corn syrup, certain roots, and honey. Fructose, which is also called levulose or fruit sugar, is found together with glucose and sucrose in honey and fruit.

While glucose has traditionally been a frequently encountered dietary sugar, fructose is becoming more popular due to the discovery that it does not cause the rapid rise and fall in the blood-sugar level that glucose does. Researchers realized this in 1984 when they undertook the first extensive comparisons of the different sweeteners available at the time. They found that the main reason fructose is easier on the blood-sugar level is that the body absorbs and utilizes fructose much slower than it does glucose. In fact, they discovered, the body starts absorbing glucose in the stomach. Fructose allows people to enjoy sweets without suffering a roller-coaster ride in the blood-sugar level and has therefore become a main ingredient in health foods.

As a result of all the recent attention, fructose is now used in a variety of drinks and foods in place of glucose and sucrose. It is pitched as the "healthy sugar." But while fructose may have some benefits over the other sugars, it is still a sugar and supplies raw energy without much other nutrition. Furthermore, the exact athletic benefits of fructose, other than the help it provides in controlling the appetite by maintaining the blood-sugar level, are not very apparent. In addition, remember that eating too much of any sugar can lead to tooth decay. Concern over cavities is not just for children. Adult athletes with tooth decay may end up with disrupted seasons due to root-canal surgery or tooth extractions.

Fructose does have its place, though, and is a wise choice in beverages. In addition to its less damaging effects on the blood-sugar level, it has also been found to replenish the glycogen stores in the liver over the glycogen stores in the muscles. This is important because the brain derives most of its energy supply from the liver, which is especially low in glycogen in the morning. Perhaps the desire to drink juices high in fructose in the morning is more than coincidence, since these juices provide the mental surge of energy that so many people need to start the day.

Note, however, that once fructose is mixed with food, its effect on the blood-sugar level becomes less clear.

COMPLEX CARBOHYDRATES

The two polysaccharides that are the most important energy contributors to the body are starch and glycogen. Processed forms of polysaccharides are maltodextrin and glucose polymers, which are shorter polymers of glucose than starch and are commonly used in sports drinks because they are more soluble in water than starch is. Starch occurs in various parts of plants and consists of long chains of glucose units. It is found in grains, roots, vegetables, pasta, bread, and legumes. Starch and other polysaccharides are called complex carbohydrates.

When starch is eaten, it is digested slowly in the body, releasing glucose molecules from the intestines into the bloodstream at a slow, steady rate. This is unlike most simple sugars, which are absorbed quickly from the digestive system into the bloodstream. Quick absorption leads to a high blood-sugar level and conversion of the food to fat by the liver. This is one reason why individuals on fat-reduction diets should minimize their intake of simple sugars as well as their consumption of fat. Additionally, individuals who participate in power sports should minimize their intake of simple carbohydrates and fat because their bodies obtain energy by burning primarily muscle glycogen, not the large amounts of fatty acids that endurance athletes burn.

FIBER

Fiber is another type of polysaccharide, but one that cannot be digested in the human gut and that does not provide any energy of which to speak. It does, however, play an important role as the main contributor to the roughage content of the diet. Among its protective qualities, roughage, which is also known as dietary fiber, helps promote efficient intestinal functioning and aids the absorption of sugars into the bloodstream.

Fiber is found along with simple and complex carbohydrates in various plant foods, such as fruits, leaves, stalks, and the outer coverings of grains, nuts, seeds, and legumes. Dietary fiber helps soften the stool and encourages normal elimination. Fiber-rich diets also promote satiety. In addition, research has shown that people who eat high-fiber diets experience reduced rates of cardiovascular disease, colon cancer, and diabetes. A high-fiber diet works best when it includes plenty of fluids.

How much dietary fiber do adults need to get these benefits? The NRC estimates that the average intake of fiber in the United States is 12 grams per day. This is much lower than what has been observed in other cultures, some of which boast fiber-intake levels as high as 150 grams per day. Health-care practitioners recommend that the average adult consume at least 40 to 60 grams per day. You can achieve this intake goal by eating foods high in fiber and by adding a fiber supplement to your diet.

Some experts fear that diets high in fiber interfere with mineral absorption. This interference, however, can be offset by a daily dietary supplement or even by the minerals already present in the high-fiber foods themselves.

DIGESTION OF CARBOHYDRATES

The chemical digestion of carbohydrates begins immediately in the mouth via enzymes that are present in the saliva. In the stomach, the digestive juices further break down the long chains of glucose that make up starch. The stomach has some capacity to allow glucose to enter the bloodstream, which helps endurance athletes who drink glucose drinks during exercise in an effort to promote glycogen sparing (the saving of glycogen for other functions). Once they reach the intestines, glucose and fructose are absorbed at their respective rates, with glucose taken up more quickly than fructose. When complex carbohydrates are eaten, either alone or with sugars, their short chains of glucose polymers slowly release glucose in the intestines for an hour or two. This slow release provides both a prolonged supply of glucose to the bloodstream and a supply of nutritional energy that further spares and replenishes muscle glycogen.

Carbohydrates are more quickly released from the stomach to the intestines than either protein or fat. The more protein and fat that you eat, the longer your stomach will take to empty. Logically, therefore, you should eat and drink foods that are very high in carbohydrates before and during exercise to take advantage of this process. Again, this is why special sports-nutrition drinks can help increase performance.

CARBOHYDRATES IN THE BODY—GLUCOSE AND GLYCOGEN

Glycogen is similar to the starch that is found in plants in that it consists of chains of glucose units. However, glycogen and starch differ in structure. In addition, while starch occurs only in plants, glycogen occurs only in animals. Very little glycogen is found in food, however. This is mainly because meat contains only small amounts of glycogen. Due to the human body's small storage capacity for glycogen, it needs a relatively constant supply of carbohydrates throughout the day. The body converts a portion of all ingested complex carbohydrates into glycogen, thereby replenishing its limited glycogen supply.

In the human body, glycogen is found in all the cells. However, it is present in greater percentages in the muscle fibers and liver cells. In this way, the liver and muscles act as reservoirs for glucose. The liver's glycogen supply is used to regulate the blood-sugar level. Furthermore, the glucose that is fed into the bloodstream from the liver's glycogen supply is the main source of energy for the brain. The brain can use over 400 calories per day of glucose from the liver's glycogen. Athletes and other physically active individuals sometimes have a feeling of being bogged down. Many times, this feeling is due to a low level of liver glycogen. Eating a good amount of complex carbohydrates, especially at night, will replenish the glycogen supply and restore mental alertness and physical energy. High-fructose drinks also replenish the liver glycogen. (For a discussion of how foods affect the blood-sugar level, see "The Glycemic Index" on page 10.)

Glycogen is not stored by itself in the liver. Rather, it is stored together with water. In fact, every 1 ounce of glycogen is stored with about 3 ounces of water. This means that when glycogen is used, water is also removed from the body. Many fad diets take advantage of this phenomenon by requiring a low caloric intake coupled with a high protein consumption, which causes liver and muscle glycogen to be depleted in twenty-four to forty-eight hours. This glycogen depletion can result in a loss of several pounds of water, which many dieters mistake for a loss of body fat. Moreover, because most weight-loss diets are low in calories, the body eliminates a few pounds of gastrointestinal bulk within a few days. Dieters usually mistake this, too, for a loss of body fat. So, a week or two of fad dieting may result in a loss of several pounds of water weight and gastrointestinal bulk but perhaps only a mere pound or two of body fat. This is one reason why fad dieters quickly, almost overnight, gain back the weight they lost. Understanding this is especially important for weight-conscious athletes, who typically deplete their glycogen supplies on low-calorie diets, blow up when they return to a normal diet, and then have to lose several pounds again a few days later. By keeping their caloric and carbohydrate intakes at normal levels, athletes can help their bodies work better and can maintain their glycogen supplies for better overall performance.

Glycogen is also stored along with potassium. Therefore, when dietary conditions encourage the depletion of the body's glycogen stores, potassium is also lost. The loss of potassium, which is an important electrolyte, can result in impaired performance. So, if you go through periods of glycogen depletion, make sure that

The Glycemic Index

The glycemic index is a measurement of the way the blood sugar responds two hours after a certain food is ingested in comparison to the way it responds two hours after an equivalent amount of pure glucose is ingested. The lower a food's glycemic index is, the less is the body's glycemic response to that food. By eating foods with lower glycemic indexes, you can maintain a more stable blood-sugar level. For the glycemic indexes of some common foods, see the table below.

The glycemic index is important for two primary reasons—it indicates the metabolic consequences that different foods can have, and it helps when foods with certain glycemic indexes need to be consumed at specific times. For example, it is better to consume foods with low glycemic indexes for meals and snacks, since these foods help maintain the proper blood-sugar level and ensure a sustained energy supply. Conversely, during workouts and competitions, it is better to eat foods with high glycemic indexes because these foods help spare glycogen in the body and supply quick energy to exercising muscles.

Glycemic Indexes of Selected Common Foods

Glycemic Index	Food
Rapid Inducers of Insulin Secretion	
100 percent	Glucose
80–90 percent	Corn flakes, carrots*, parsnips*, potatoes (instant mashed), maltose, honey
70–79 percent	Bread (whole-grain), millet, rice (white), Weetabix cereal, broad beans (fresh)*, potatoes (new), swede*
Moderate Inducers of Insulin Secretion	
60–69 percent	Bread (white), rice (brown), muesli, Shredded Wheat cereal, Ryvita crispbreads, water biscuits, beetroot*, bananas, raisins, Mars Bars
50–59 percent	Buckwheat, spaghetti (bleached), sweet corn, All Bran cereal, digestive biscuits, oatmeal biscuits, Rich Tea biscuits, peas (frozen), yams, sucrose, potato chips
40–49 percent	Spaghetti (whole-wheat), oatmeal, potatoes (sweet), beans (canned navy), peas (dried), oranges, orange juice
Slow Inducers of Insulin Secretion	
30–39 percent	Butter beans, haricot beans, black-eyed peas, chickpeas, apples (Golden Delicious), ice cream, milk (skim), milk (whole), yogurt, tomato soup
20–29 percent	Kidney beans, lentils, fructose
10–19 percent	Soybeans, soybeans (canned), peanuts

*This food item was tested in portions containing 25 grams of carbohydrates.

The above table is adapted from *Diabetes Care,* vol. 5 (1982). It is used with the permission of the American Diabetes Association.

ON THE CUTTING EDGE

Ingesting Carbs During Low–Intensity and Intermittent Exercise Benefits Performance

The ingestion while exercising of carbohydrates, in the form of carbohydrate-electrolyte beverages, leads to performance benefits during prolonged submaximum and variable-intensity exercise, according to a report published in *Sports Medicine* in 1998. Maintaining the blood-sugar level and the metabolism of blood sugar at high rates late in exercise, as well as a decreased rate of muscle-glycogen utilization, have been proposed as the possible mechanisms underlying the performance-enhancing effect of carbohydrate ingestion. The prevalence of one mechanism over the others depends on factors such as the type and intensity of the exercise; the amount, type, and timing of the carbohydrate ingestion; and the pre-exercise nutritional and training status of the exerciser. The ingestion of carbohydrate (except fructose) at a rate of more than 45 grams per hour, accompanied by a significant increase in the plasma-insulin level, could lead to decreased muscle-glycogen utilization during exercise. Endurance training and alterations in the pre-exercise muscle-glycogen level do not seem to affect glucose metabolism during submaximum exercise. Thus, at least during low-intensity or intermittent exercise, carbohydrate ingestion could result in reduced muscle-glycogen utilization in well-trained individuals with high resting muscle-glycogen levels. This finding is especially important for athletes who participate in extended running, cycling, or cross-country skiing events.

you maintain an adequate intake of potassium, as well as of the other essential vitamins and minerals.

Glycogen depletion followed by glycogen replenishment, which is also known as carbohydrate loading, causes the muscles to increase their water content considerably. When glycogen replenishment is complete, the increased body weight may induce the muscles to feel heavy and stiff. This can interfere with physical performance in certain athletic events, particularly in connection with sports that rely on repeated short bursts of all-out effort, such as sprinting, football, and basketball. Bodybuilders can take advantage of this phenomenon, however, and experienced bodybuilders know how to add size and hardness to their physiques on contest days for an added competitive edge.

Understanding glycogen storage and dynamics is a cornerstone of improving athletic performance nutritionally. Knowledgeable athletes recognize that they must keep their muscle and liver glycogen stores filled up. They comprehend that they must follow a daily nutrition program that encourages glycogen replenishment and spares glycogen utilization. And they know how to use carbohydrate loading to maximize their glycogen stores for endurance sports and tournaments.

CARBOHYDRATES FOR INCREASED ATHLETIC PERFORMANCE

To maintain their glycogen stores, athletes must focus on their carbohydrate intake on a twenty-four-hour basis and on a pre-event basis. This means that they must devote attention to the following important factors:

☐ Maintenance of carbohydrate balance at each meal.

☐ Increase in carbohydrate intake before athletic events
or exercise sessions.

☐ Ingestion of selected types of carbohydrates during exercise.

☐ Ingestion of carbohydrates after exercise.

☐ Methodical buildup of muscle and liver glycogen stores before events.

☐ Carbohydrate loading for events lasting more than one and a half hours
and for tournaments.

☐ Ingestion of high amounts of complex carbohydrates, with intake of
increased amounts of simple carbohydrates at breakfast, during exercise,
and directly after exercise to quickly replace depleted glycogen stores.

You can easily maintain carbohydrate balance by eating several servings of carbohydrates per day. In general, you should eat a plentiful amount of complex carbohydrates with each meal and reserve simple carbohydrates for special parts of the day. This means that you must make sure that you eat carbohydrates with every meal and with snacks.

ON THE CUTTING EDGE

Weight Lifters
Also Need Adequate Carbs

Most of us are aware that during endurance exercise, the muscle fibers become depleted of glycogen. This is why endurance athletes need to ingest adequate carbohydrate. If they don't, they become fatigued very quickly. According to an article in the *Journal of Strength and Conditioning Research* in 1998, Dr. Per Tesch showed that glycogen loss in both the fast- and slow-twitch muscle fibers also occurs during weight training. Muscle-glycogen depletion in the fibers of a thigh muscle was determined by muscle biopsies before and after five sets of ten repetitions of knee-extension exercises. The sets were completed using 30, 45, and 60 percent of a one-repetition maximum. Significant glycogen loss in both the fast- and slow-twitch fibers was shown after all three workouts, but was the greatest after the sets at 60 percent.

Carbohydrates Before, During, and After Exercise

When consuming carbohydrates before, during, or after exercise, you also need to take in fluids and the electrolytes. Before exercise, your meal should be high in carbohydrates, moderate in protein, and low in fat. You should eat this meal about three hours before beginning the exercise. This is important because it will take this long for your stomach to empty and for the glucose to enter your bloodstream. If you eat too much protein or fat before exercising, you will lengthen the time it will take for your stomach to empty. You should also drink several glasses of water after finishing your pre-exercise meal and again thirty minutes before beginning the exercise session. Studies have shown that drinking fluids with glucose and some electrolytes several minutes before beginning to exercise is the best way to spare the body's supply of glycogen.

During exercise, you should drink water or a sports beverage containing water plus 70 to 100 calories of carbohydrates per serving and a supply of the electrolytes. However, if the carbohydrate or electrolyte content of the sports drink is too high, your stomach will take longer to empty. For practice sessions and events lasting more than two hours, you must consume a drink containing adequate amounts of carbohydrates and the electrolytes. Preferably, the drink should consist of glucose or sucrose mixed with a complex carbohydrate such as maltodextrin. For events less than two hours long, you should still try to drink at least water to rehydrate your body. The benefits of drinking beverages containing carbohydrates and the electrolytes are less clear for exercise sessions lasting less than two hours. But while sports drinks might not supply immediate benefits, they could help preserve glycogen stores and prevent glycogen depletion on a day-to-day basis. Research indicates that many athletes suffer from chronic glycogen depletion, with decreased performance and increased recovery time.

After exercise—any exercise—you must replenish your body with water, carbohydrates, the B-complex vitamins, vitamin C, and protein. You can do this by consuming a supplement drink designed especially for this purpose followed by a full meal. If you trained after your last evening meal, you should consume a high-carbohydrate, multinutrient supplement drink containing 300 to 600 calories about one to two hours after finishing the session. In addition, you should drink two or more glasses of water.

The practice of drinking carbohydrate beverages before, during, and after exercise may be new to you. Give it a try and see how your system responds. If you find that your stomach cannot tolerate a carbohydrate beverage before or during exercise, eat extra amounts of carbohydrates before and directly after exercise instead. In addition, drink plain water while exercising. Before giving up on the practice completely, however, experiment with different brands of beverages and different caloric totals. Your problem may not be with carbohydrate beverages in general but just with a certain brand or formula. Generally, carbohydrate solutions that are pure glucose and contain about 50 calories in every 8 ounces are the easiest to stomach. As the amount of carbohydrates goes up and more electrolytes and other nutrients are added in, the rate at which the stomach empties slows down and the feeling of being bloated may become more pronounced.

ON THE CUTTING EDGE

Amount of Carbs, Not Their Form, Is Important

Recently, it was shown that carbohydrate content, not form, is the important factor in exercise performance, according to a report published in the *Journal of Conditioning Research* in 1998. Scientists from the Ball State University Exercise Physiology Laboratory evaluated exercise performance after the consumption of carbohydrates in various forms, from semi-liquids to sports bars, in 460-calorie servings. The carbohydrates were consumed two hours prior to the exercise, which consisted of a sixty-minute exercise trial on a bicycle ergometer. The trials were randomized, and the oxygen consumption and heart rate of the subjects were checked every fifteen minutes. No significant differences were observed in any of the cardiovascular measurements, including blood glucose. The authors concluded that what is important is the amount of carbohydrate taken before exercise, not the form in which it is taken.

High-Carbohydrate Diet May Keep Cortisol Levels Low

A team of researchers led by Michael Gleesen, PhD, from the University of Birmingham, England, examined the effects of a low-carbohydrate diet on the plasma-glutamine and circulating-leukocyte responses to prolonged strenuous exercise. According to an article published in the *International Journal of Sports Nutrition* in 1998, twelve untrained male subjects cycled for sixty minutes at 70 percent of their maximum exercise capacity on two separate occasions three days apart. All of the subjects performed the first exercise task after consuming a normal diet and the second after three days on either a high (75-percent) carbohydrate diet or low (7-percent) carbohydrate diet. The subjects who consumed the low-carbohydrate diet experienced a greater rise in their plasma-cortisol levels during the exercise and a greater fall in their plasma-glutamine concentrations during recovery. The subjects who consumed the high-carbohydrate diet did not experience any effects on their levels of plasma glutamine and circulating leukocytes. The authors concluded that carbohydrate availability can influence the plasma-glutamine and circulating-leukocyte responses during recovery from intense prolonged exercise. This may be another case made for the consumption of a higher-carbohydrate (60 to 70 percent) diet during hard training.

FOOD AND SUPPLEMENT SOURCES OF CARBOHYDRATES

Carbohydrates tend to be the least expensive of the macronutrients. You can buy several pounds of potatoes for only a few dollars and have a week's supply of high-quality complex carbohydrates. Other foods that are high in carbohydrates—that is, over 60 percent of their calories come from carbohydrates—are ready-to-serve and cooked cereals, whole-grain bread, crackers, popcorn, rice, pasta, corn, winter squash, and yams.

Supplement sources of carbohydrates include sports drinks, which vary in caloric content and carbohydrate type. The caloric content of sports drinks generally runs from 90 to 400 calories per 8-ounce serving. Many different types of sports drinks are available, but most are based either on a simple-carbohydrate source or on a complex formulation that contains a mixture of simple carbohydrates, glucose polymers, and micronutrients. Some research has indicated that while foods alone can be used for glycogen sparing and carbohydrate loading, these special supplement products are slightly better for improving performance. However, they are also more expensive. Most athletes on tight budgets use these special products just during the season or during the week preceding an important competition.

It is interesting that carbohydrates, such a seemingly simple group of macronutrients, are utilized by the body in such a diversity of ways. It is equally fascinating that they have such profound effects on performance. Keeping close track of your carbohydrate intake, however, is just one ingredient in your performance-nutrition formula.

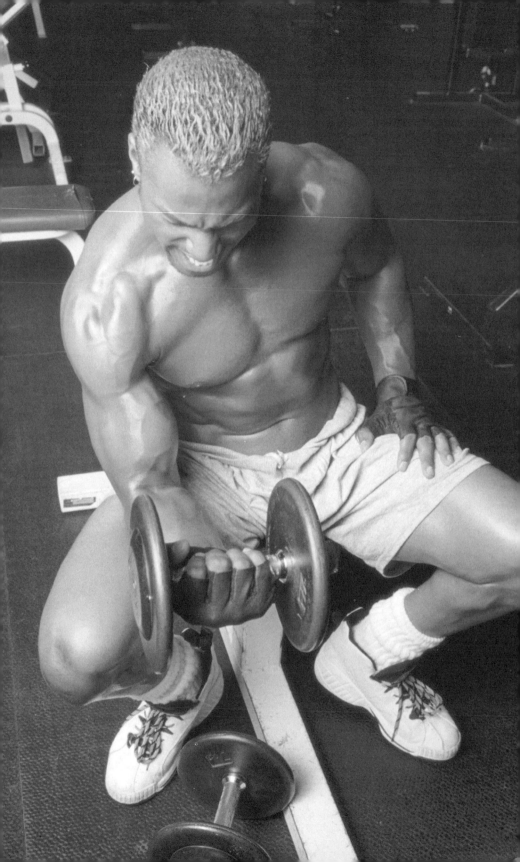

PROTEIN AND AMINO ACIDS

2 MUSCLE BUILDERS AND MORE

The relationship between protein and the athlete has become legendary. As already mentioned, one of the earliest recorded athletic nutritional practices was that of consuming large amounts of protein to improve strength and performance. The most recent research confirms protein's role as a vital component of health and performance. However, studies have also established that diets that are too high in protein can be as counterproductive as diets that are too low in protein. One thing is certain—athletes require at least twice as much protein as nonathletes do.

Protein is an essential part of the diet and plays many roles in the body. Protein's roles are primarily structural, but it is also sacrificed by the body for energy during intensive exercise or when nutrition is inadequate. In these situations, to meet its metabolic needs, the body breaks down precious muscle tissue, which is a setback for an athlete who has been training hard to make gains. In addition, athletes need to eat just the right amount of protein to minimize the formation of metabolic waste products. When too much protein is consumed, the body converts the excess to fat and increases the blood levels of ammonia and uric acid. Ammonia and uric acid are toxic metabolic waste products. The athlete's goal therefore is to maintain proper protein intake.

In this chapter, we will discuss protein and its special relationship with the athlete. We will learn about the various methods used to rate the quality of proteins and how to estimate individual daily requirements. We will also look in detail at the amino acids, which are the building blocks of protein.

WHAT IS PROTEIN?

Protein is a large molecule called a macromolecule or supermolecule. It is a polypeptide, a compound containing from ten to one hundred amino-acid molecules. The amino acids are linked together by a chemical bond called a peptide bond.

When we talk about protein, we are really discussing these amino-acid subunits. There are about twenty-two amino acids that are considered biologically important, but many more exist in nature, including in the body. Amino acids are important not only for being the building blocks of protein, however, but also for the individual roles that they play in the body. For example, some amino acids are used by the body in metabolic processes such as the urea cycle. Others act as neurotransmitters, the chemical substances that help transmit nerve impulses.

Protein is needed for the growth, maintenance, and repair of cells, including muscle cells, and for the production of enzymes, hormones, and deoxyribonucleic acid (DNA). It occurs in various sizes and shapes and is divided into two main categories—simple proteins and conjugated proteins. Simple proteins consist only of amino acids, while conjugated proteins also have nonprotein molecules as part of their structures. Some simple proteins are serum albumin, which is present in blood; lactalbumin, which is present in milk; ovalbumin, which is present in eggs; myosin, present in muscle; collagen, present in connective tissue; and keratin, present in hair. Examples of conjugated proteins are nucleic acid, found in chromosomes; lipoprotein, found in cell membranes; glycoprotein, chromoprotein, and metaloprotein, all found in blood; and phosphoprotein, found in casein (milk protein). Protein constitutes about 74 percent of the dry weight of most body cells.

PROTEIN AND ENERGY

In addition to the functions discussed above, protein—the same as fat and carbohydrates—can also be used for energy. Under conditions of both outright and training-induced starvation, the body releases amino acids from muscle tissue for use as energy or in energy cycles. This catabolism (breakdown) of protein occurs during exercise—especially during intensive workouts, in particular power exercises and prolonged endurance activities—or when the body runs out of carbohydrates from the diet or glycogen from its muscle and liver stores. Even though the body can depend on the fat that it has stored, it still uses muscle protein, unless it is fed protein as food. When dietary circumstances cause the body to use amino acids as a source of energy, it cannot also use these amino acids for building muscle tissue or for performing their other metabolic functions. This is why a proper protein intake is essential every hour of the day.

Even if you do consume a proper diet, your body will still use certain amino acids as fuel during grueling exercise bouts. The muscles use the branched-chain amino acids (BCAAs)—isoleucine, leucine, and valine—to supply a limited amount of energy during strenuous exercise. (For a discussion of these special amino acids, see "The Branched-Chain Amino Acids" on page 33.) However, research has shown that although the body can utilize all three BCAAs for energy during exercise, it uses leucine the most. As demonstrated by studies, a trained person's muscles use leucine even while that person is at rest. This disproportionate use of leucine, as well as of the other BCAAs, affects the body's overall use of amino acids for growth. Here, the BCAAs, especially leucine, are limiting nutrients—that is, nutrients that, through their absence or presence, restrict the utilization of other nutrients or the functioning of the body.

For optimum muscle growth, cellular growth, metabolism, and recovery, the body needs to receive the amino acids in the proper proportions. Merely eating amino-acid sources, such as meat and eggs, does not ensure that the amino acids they supply will be available for muscle growth or for the formation of other proteins. For example, suppose you consume a total of 100 grams of protein, with all the essential amino acids present in equal amounts. How will your body use these amino acids? To begin, it will utilize a considerable percentage of the leucine for energy for exercising muscles. This means that only a small amount of leucine will be available for growth and repair purposes. When your leucine supply runs out, your protein formation will be negatively affected because leucine is an essential amino acid—that is, your body cannot manufacture it. The result is that perhaps only 15 grams of the original 100 grams of protein will be available for growth and repair.

On a similar note, a trend in some circles of athletes—bodybuilders in particular—has been to ingest pure-protein meals or supplements. This practice is counterproductive because the body also needs carbohydrates to rebuild its glycogen stores. When it does not receive carbohydrates, it must break down some of the protein and convert it to glucose and fatty acids in the liver. Therefore, you should always consume at least some carbohydrates, and even a modicum of fat, to prevent the undesirable destruction of ingested protein for energy.

RATING PROTEINS

Just as there are differences among the carbohydrates, the various proteins are not created equal. Some proteins have more-complete amino-acid contents than others and are therefore better suited for growth purposes. Scientists are currently using a number of methods to rate proteins. Most of these rating methods do not take into account the extra protein and the specific amino acids that are required by athletes. However, as more research is conducted using athletes, methods for rating proteins for athletic purposes will hopefully result.

Complete Versus Incomplete Proteins

Due to the fact that an adequate protein intake is essential for optimum growth in children, the World Health Organization (WHO) has conducted significant research on protein requirements. What the WHO researchers determined was that not all proteins supply the proper amounts and proportions of the amino acids necessary for adequate growth and development. Complete proteins are proteins that contain the essential amino acids in amounts that are sufficient for the maintenance of normal growth rate and body weight. Complete proteins are therefore said to have a high biological value. Most animal products have complete proteins.

Incomplete proteins are usually deficient in one or more of the essential amino acids. This amino-acid deficiency creates a limiting-amino-acid condition, which adversely affects growth and development rates. Most plant proteins are incomplete. However, considering the dynamics of amino acids in the body, even high-quality proteins can be incomplete for athletes' needs. Furthermore, research indicates that the proper proportions of both the essential and nonessential amino acids are required for optimum growth and recovery. This means that athletes should consume protein supplements as well as high-quality food protein sources. Their dietary goals should be to eat a diet fortified with the amino acids that are used for energy and nongrowth functions and to ensure an adequate intake of the amino acids that are necessary for growth and recovery—but not to eat so much protein that there will be an excess that is converted to fat.

Protein Efficiency Ratio

Another method of determining the quality of protein is the protein efficiency ratio (PER). The PER is calculated using laboratory animals. It refers to the amount of weight gained versus the amount of protein ingested. For example, casein has a PER of 2.86, which means that 2.86 grams of body weight are gained for every 1 gram of casein eaten. Table 2.1, below, provides a sampling of foods and their PER values.

One criticism of the PER system as a method for determining the quality of proteins for human consumption is that the values were derived through testing on animals, mostly rats. Does a rat's growth rate correlate to a human's? Perhaps not. Additionally, rats and other laboratory animals have a large amount of fur all over their bodies. This places an extra demand on amino acids such as methionine, which is used in fur growth and which is a common limiting amino acid in plant protein sources. Moreover, we now realize that athletes need higher amounts of certain amino acids, such as the BCAAs. Therefore, the PER and other similar data should be used only as guidelines for determining minimum intakes of protein for nonathletes. Additionally, different proteins can be combined to improve the quality of the individual proteins. This is commonly done to increase the PER of plant proteins. Many powder supplements now include a mixture of two or more of the less-expensive lesser-quality proteins, such as soy and casein, which boost each other's PERs when used together, instead of using one of the more-expensive high-quality protein sources, such as egg white.

An interesting note is that WHO suggests that newborns need complete dietary proteins containing about 37 percent of the protein's weight in essential amino acids. Adults, on the other hand, require complete dietary proteins containing just 15 percent of the protein's weight in essential amino acids. This demonstrates that the proportion of essential to nonessential amino acids is an important factor in growth and development. Athletes training to develop stronger and bigger muscles should try to maintain higher proportions of the essential amino acids in their diets.

Table 2.1. Selected Foods and Their Protein Efficiency Ratios

FOOD	PER	FOOD	PER
Eggs	3.92	Casein	2.86
Whey	3.6–3.9	Soy flour	2.30
Fish	3.55	Beef	2.30
Lactalbumin	3.43	Oatmeal	2.25
Whole milk	3.09	Rice	2.18

Net Protein Utilization

Net protein utilization (NPU) is a way of determining the digestibility of a protein. It does this by measuring the percentage of nitrogen that is absorbed from a protein's amino acids. Generally, the more nitrogen that is absorbed from a protein, the more digestible the protein is.

The NPU of a protein is calculated by measuring an individual's intake of nitrogen from amino acids, comparing that amount to the amount of nitrogen that the individual excretes, and determining how much of the protein in question is needed to balance out the two amounts. If a protein has a low NPU, more of it is needed to achieve nitrogen balance. (For a more complete discussion of this, see "Nitrogen Balance," below.) Therefore, proteins with high NPU values, such as egg and milk proteins, are more desirable for athletes.

Biological Value

While the methods used to determine a protein's biological value (BV) are not entirely standardized, the one that most scientists prefer is described as "the efficiency with which that protein furnishes the proper proportions and amounts of

Nitrogen Balance

Nitrogen balance is a topic that is frequently encountered when reading articles about athletes' protein and amino-acid requirements. In addition to carbon and hydrogen, amino acids also contain nitrogen as part of their molecular structure. This is a unique characteristic, one that we can use to our advantage, since it allows us to determine if our protein intake is adequate. Specifically, nitrogen balance refers to the condition in which the amount of dietary nitrogen taken in is equal to the amount of nitrogen excreted. A nitrogen balance that is positive indicates a possible net growth in body tissues. A nitrogen balance that is negative indicates an inadequate protein intake and the possibility that the body is cannibalizing its muscle tissue. During the season, athletes who want to maintain their body weight should strive to equalize their nitrogen intake and excretion. Athletes who want to increase their muscle mass should aim for a positive nitrogen balance.

Determining nitrogen balance is not an easy task, however. Because nitrogen from broken-down amino acids can be excreted in both the urine and the feces, and because some is lost as sweat, all these excretions must be collected and analyzed. In addition, all the nitrogen ingested from protein must be accurately measured. This is impractical for most individuals. However, some companies have now developed methods that enable athletes to get a rough idea of their nitrogen balance by taking measurements using just their urine and measuring their nitrogen ingested as protein. This approach makes assumptions about the relative amount of nitrogen lost in feces and sweat. Although you would have to spend time making calculations every day, you would probably find it interesting to learn what your nitrogen balance is to give you an approximate guideline for what your daily protein intake should be. You could then experiment with combining different food and supplement protein sources to tailor-make an efficient protein-intake program for yourself.

the essential or indispensable amino acids needed for the synthesis of body proteins in humans or animals."

The general formula for determining BV is as follows:

$$BV = \text{nitrogen retained} \div \text{nitrogen absorbed} \times 100$$

When applying mathematical data, the breakdown of the above equation is as follows:

$$\text{Nitrogen retained} = (\text{dietary } N) - (F - Fm) + (U - Ue)$$
$$\text{Nitrogen absorbed} = (\text{dietary } N) + (F - Fm)$$

In the above breakdown, **dietary *N*** represents dietary nitrogen, – equals the fecal nitrogen excreted during the testing of a protein, *Fm* equals the fecal nitrogen excreted on a protein-free diet (endogenous fecal nitrogen), *U* equals the urinary nitrogen excreted during the testing of a protein, and *U* equals the urinary nitrogen excreted on a protein-free diet (endogenous urinary nitrogen). The highest BV that can be obtained using this method is 100. By substituting your mathematical readings for these factors listed in the general formula, you can determine the BV of a food.

No matter what method is used to determine BV, the score does not indicate the ultimate fate of the amino acids in the body—that is, it does not show whether they will be used for muscle growth or enzyme synthesis. In addition, BV measurements vary for the same protein according to the animal species tested. For example, chickens have different amino-acid needs than do rats due to, among other things, the fact that chickens have feathers and rats have fur. Because feathers require different amino acids than fur does, the two animals need different proportions of the amino acids. Therefore, unless the BV for a particular type or brand of protein was determined specifically for humans, that protein may not offer any advantages to humans, even though it may have a high BV according to the testing done with animals.

Amino-Acid Score

The amino-acid score is one additional method of determining the quality of proteins that is worth mentioning, since sports-nutrition advertisers are using more and more scientific jargon to sell their products. The amino-acid score of a food protein is determined by comparing its content of essential amino acids with a reference pattern. This is a crude method, however, because the reference pattern does not relate to athletes' needs. It does not account for the digestibility of the protein, the availability of the amino acids, or the utilization of the amino acids by the body.

Ideally, more research needs to be conducted on athletes to determine protein scores for athletic purposes. In 1990, a group of inventors led by Robert Fritz developed the first effective home testing tool for measuring urinary nitrogen. Called NitroStix, these diagnostic sticks are available commercially and give athletes, as well as nonathletes, a tool for monitoring their nitrogen balance on a daily basis to determine if their protein intake is sufficient. Use of these diagnostic sticks can also help athletes determine how other factors, such as training and nutrient intake, affect their nitrogen balance.

THE FUTURE FOR PROTEIN PRODUCTS

The future for protein and amino-acid sports science lies in designing an amino-acid source that brings about nitrogen balance using a minimum amount of protein. This goal can be reached in several ways, and manufacturers have already developed pioneering ingredients and products that accomplish it. Creating an amino-acid profile that has all the essential amino acids with extra BCAAs and the nonessential amino acids is a start. Products with a variety of amino-acid combinations are available. Among their benefits are growth-hormone (GH) stimulation, blood-ammonia detoxification, increased mental alertness, and mental relaxation.

Absorption is also an important factor. Some protein manufacturers are inventing better ways to purify the protein from milk and other sources. One manufacturer even combined medium-chain triglycerides with high-quality protein to increase utilization; the resulting product is marketed under the brand name SuperProtein. Adding nonprotein ingredients can further improve utilization, as well as supply other growth factors, such as glucosamine for connective tissue. (For a discussion of glucosamine, see page 168.)

The diversity of amino-acid combinations possible and the benefits that they offer make protein and amino acids a very interesting field of research and a very important part of the athlete's nutrition program.

FREE-FORM AND PEPTIDE-BONDED AMINO ACIDS

When referring to the amino-acid content of food or supplements, the terms *free form* and *peptide bonded* are used. In fact, the debate seems to be constant over which supplement form is better. Free-form amino acids are amino acids that are in their free state, or single. When protein is digested, some of its amino acids are eventually broken down into their free forms for transport and use in the body. Peptide-bonded amino acids are amino acids that are linked together. Di-peptides are two amino acids linked together, tri-peptides are three amino acids linked together, and polypeptides are four or more amino acids linked together. Interestingly, the intestines can absorb free-form, di-peptide, and tri-peptide amino acids but not polypeptides.

Because the body has the capacity to digest protein, it can make use of whole-protein supplement sources. However, many supplements now contain free-form amino acids or combinations of free-form and peptide-bonded amino acids. Some also contain hydrolyzed proteins. Hydrolyzed proteins are already broken down, usually by enzymes, and are a mixture of free-form, di-peptide, and tri-peptide amino acids. Many people consider them better than nonhydrolyzed proteins because their partial digestion possibly makes them more easily absorbed by the body. Preliminary research, however, is unclear regarding the benefits of hydrolyzed proteins in healthy individuals.

The benefits of using a multi-amino-acid supplement that is composed of just free-form amino acids are even less clear. The trend apparently got its start in early nutrition studies that attempted to chemically create a balanced protein by using free-form amino acids, along with other nutrients. In the United States, the use of free-form L-tryptophan was banned a number of years ago. Any multi-amino-acid supplement that consists of free-form essential amino acids minus L-tryptophan is basically useless. Make sure that your multi-amino-acid formulation is full spectrum—that is, has all the essential amino acids in addition to nonessential amino acids.

The use of free-form amino acids is still common in clinical applications when intravenous solutions are used to supply amino acids directly into the bloodstream. Free-form amino acids can also be used to fortify food proteins. Taking the BCAAs with meals can be useful for compensating for the amino acids already used for energy. Additionally, when you just want to take extra amounts of one or several amino acids, a free-form amino-acid formulation makes perfect sense. Concerning multi-amino-acid and powder supplements, however, whole-protein or hydrolyzed-protein sources are the best.

Another reason why a mixture of free-form and peptide-bonded amino acids is better than free-form amino acids alone is that the intestines can better absorb mixtures for transport into the bloodstream. While it might seem logical that free-form amino acids could be absorbed more quickly, the upper part of the small intestine is better able to absorb amino acids in twos and threes. Furthermore, free-form amino acids are manufactured, and ingestion of large amounts of these synthetics for long periods of time can cause problems in the stomach and intestines. If you choose to up your protein intake, you should use whole proteins or hydrolyzed proteins from foods and supplements as your primary sources of protein. Limit your use of free-form amino acids to supplementing your meals with the BCAAs, ammonia-detoxifying agents, or single amino acids for precursor therapy, as is done with L-tyrosine.

D-, L-, AND DL-FORMS OF AMINO ACIDS

Most amino acids come in two forms. The two forms are isomers, mirror images of each other, and are denoted by the letter "D" or "L" placed in front of the name of the amino acid. Scientists can identify which isomer an amino acid is by the direction of the rotation of the spiral that is the chemical structure of the molecule—L-form amino acids rotate to the left and D-form amino acids rotate to the right. "L" stands for *levo,* which is Latin for "left," and "D" stands for *dextro,* which is Latin for "right." In general, the L-form is more compatible with human biochemistry and the only form that should be ingested. Never use a supplement that contains only the D-form.

A third form in which some amino acids can be found is the DL-form, a mixture of the D- and L-forms. However, the only two amino acids whose DL-forms have been observed to have metabolic advantages are phenylalanine and methionine. The D-forms of these two amino acids can apparently be converted to the L-forms in the liver. This seems to produce a positive effect in some cases.

THE COMMONLY ENCOUNTERED AMINO ACIDS

The following amino acids are the major ones that are important to the body and commonly encountered in supplements. (For a quick listing of these essential and nonessential amino acids, see Table 2.2, below.) In addition to being a part of proteins, many amino acids have specific metabolic functions. For example, arginine stimulates the release of GH. However, please note that while the following information is comprehensive, many of the amino acids have uses that are not included. These uses are mainly in the treatment of clinical and metabolic disorders, which are beyond the scope of this book.

A word of caution: Although amino acids have been used for years by the medical profession and have been taken as supplements by all types of individuals, our intention in this book is not to recommend the use of isolated amino acids or free-form amino-acid combinations. While many studies have used amino acids safely, some reports have documented side effects. If you wish to use any amino-acid supplements, seek the guidance of your health-care practitioner and make sure that you exercise caution.

If you do choose to take an amino-acid supplement, the best way is on an empty stomach or as directed on the label. This allows the amino acid to enter the body in a pure form and prevents competition with other amino acids and nutrients. For specific dosing recommendations, see the individual amino acids.

Alanine Alanine is found in high concentrations in most muscle tissue and is grouped with the nonessential amino acids because it can be manufactured by the body. Alanine is involved in an important biochemical process that occurs during exercise—the glucose-alanine cycle. In the muscles, glycogen stores are broken down to glucose and then to a three-carbon-atom molecule called pyruvate. Some of the pyruvate is used directly for energy by the muscles. Some of it, however, is converted to alanine, which is transported through the bloodstream to the liver, where it is converted once again into glucose. The glucose is then transported back to a muscle and again used for energy.

Table 2.2. Important Amino Acids Commonly Used in Supplements

Essential		Nonessential	
L-valine	L- or DL-phenylalanine	Glycine	L-proline
L-lysine	plus L-tyrosine[1]	L-alanine	L-hydroxyproline
L-threonine	L- or DL-methionine	L-serine	L-citrulline
L-leucine	plus L-cystine[1]	L-cystine	L-arginine
L-isoleucine	L-histidine[2]	L-tyrosine	L-ornithine
L-tryptophan		L-aspartic acid	L-glutamic acid[3]

[1] Because tyrosine can replace about 50 percent of the phenylalanine that is required and cystine can replace about 30 percent of the methionine that is required, these amino acids must also be considered in association with the traditional essential amino acids.

[2] Essential for infants and athletes only.

[3] Conditionally essential, particularly during intensive weight training, when it is useful in combating the catabolic effects of cortisol.

The glucose-alanine cycle serves to conserve energy in the form of glycogen. Sports physiologists believe that this helps maintain the glucose level during prolonged exercise. In this way, supplementing with L-alanine can be useful in the same way that supplementing with the BCAAs is—the supplemental L-alanine helps to spare muscle tissue, as well as liver glycogen.

Arginine

Arginine is another nonessential amino acid that influences several metabolic factors that are important to athletes. Arginine is most famous for its role in stimulating the release of human GH (somatotropin). Several studies have measured the ability of supplemental L-arginine, both alone and in combination with other amino acids, to increase the GH level in a resting individual. Potential benefits of an increased GH level include reduction in body fat, improved healing and recovery, and increased muscle mass. The exact benefits, though, are still in question and awaiting more research.

Research has also been conducted on supplementation with different forms of L-arginine, such as L-arginine-pyroglutamate combined with L-lysine hydrochloride. One study used 1,200 milligrams of each and reported significant elevations of GH levels over what were achieved using either compound alone. However, this particular study has been criticized by other scientists, who have been unable to replicate its findings, so the safety of these particular combinations has not yet been clearly determined. The exact benefits for athletes have not been determined either.

A second important function of arginine is its role as a precursor in creatine production. Creatine combines with phosphate and is an important energy source during power activities, such as weightlifting and sprinting. Daily ingestion of 4,000 milligrams each of L-arginine and L-glycine has been shown to cause a small increase in body creatine stores. This can help improve performance for power athletes.

A third function of arginine that may benefit athletes is its role in ammonia detoxification. Arginine is an intermediary in the urea cycle. It converts ammonia to the waste product urea, which can then be excreted from the body. Ammonia is toxic, and its level increases with exercise. Any ammonia-lowering effects of supplemental L-arginine would therefore be beneficial to athletes.

Even though more studies are needed to determine its specific effectiveness, supplemental L-arginine can benefit athletes because of its ability to reduce ammonia, increase GH, and increase creatine. L-arginine supplementation can especially help athletes involved in strenuous sports or training. Furthermore, L-arginine has been found to improve wound healing and to play a role in the immune system. More studies are also needed to determine L-arginine's exact safety and dosage levels, but 1,000 to about 3,000 milligrams per day have been successfully used in research to date.

Asparagine

Asparagine is a nonessential amino acid that is manufactured in the body from aspartic acid. Asparagine appears to be involved in the proper functioning of the central nervous system because it helps prevent both extreme nervousness and extreme calmness. L-asparagine supplementation by athletes has not yet been evaluated.

Aspartic Acid
Aspartic acid is a nonessential amino acid that has been shown to help reduce the blood-ammonia level after exercise. Aspartic acid is metabolized from glutamic acid in the body. It is involved in the urea cycle and in the Krebs cycle. In the Krebs cycle, energy is released from glucose, fatty-acid, or protein molecules and used to form adenosine-triphosphate (ATP) molecules, which are the form of energy that the body can utilize.

Researchers have studied potassium and magnesium-L-aspartates for their possible effects on athletic performance, which include reducing blood ammonia, sparing glycogen, and increasing free fatty acids. A total of 8,400 milligrams per day of potassium and magnesium-L-aspartates ingested in two to three dosages during the twenty-four-hour period before exercise has been shown to increase capacity in unconditioned individuals (recreational athletes). The exact benefits for conditioned individuals in active training have not been proven at this time.

Aspartic acid is an excitatory neurotransmitter in the brain. Long-term supplemental use is not recommended. Doses of 4,000 to 8,000 milligrams before an event can benefit performance in unconditioned individuals and may benefit conditioned athletes if taken before competitions and tournaments.

Citrulline
Citrulline is a nonessential amino acid and one of the two amino acids that do not occur in proteins. Both citrulline and ornithine, the other amino acid that does not occur in proteins, are important in the urea cycle for the removal of ammonia from the blood. Citrulline is made from the essential amino acid lysine. The benefits of L-citrulline supplementation have not been established at this time.

Cysteine
Cysteine is a sulfur-bearing nonessential amino acid. The body manufactures it from methionine. Cysteine is important in the formation of hair and insulin. Besides its major role as a component of proteins, it functions as an antioxidant and detoxifying agent, helping rid the body of carcinogens and dangerous chemicals. In addition, it helps form glutathione, which is another important antioxidant and detoxifying agent. Cysteine also plays a role in energy production. Like other amino acids, it can be converted to glucose and either used for energy or stored as glycogen.

Dosages of L-cysteine of around 250 to 500 milligrams, taken once or twice a day, have been used as part of an antioxidant regimen. Higher dosages taken without medical supervision are not recommended. Some reports indicate that L-cysteine works better when taken along with vitamin B_6, vitamin C, vitamin E, calcium, and selenium. Individuals with the metabolic disorder cystinuria should not take supplemental L-cysteine due to an increased risk of cysteine-gallstone formation.

Cystine
Cystine is another sulfur-bearing nonessential amino acid. It is made from two molecules of cysteine.

Cystine plays a vital role in helping many protein molecules hold their shape as they are carried around the body. It is generally poorly absorbed when taken in supplemental form and is more effectively derived by formation from cysteine. The same as cysteine, cystine is important in the formation of hair and skin. It is also a detoxifying agent. The athletic benefits of supplementation with free-form L-cystine have not yet been clearly defined.

Gamma-Aminobutyric Acid
Gamma-aminobutyric acid (GABA) is a nonessential amino acid that functions primarily as an inhibitory neurotransmitter in the central nervous system. In other words, GABA is calming to the brain. This calming effect can be beneficial for athletes who require concentration or steadiness. It can also help athletes who are affected by stress. GABA works by decreasing neuron activity.

GABA is generally taken in one of two ways—either by holding about 40 to 100 milligrams under the tongue and letting it be absorbed by the tiny capillaries in the mouth or by swallowing from 500 to 2,000 milligrams. GABA may also play a role in appetite control, so athletes taking it should make sure that they eat their prescribed amount of food each day. Supplemental vitamin B_6, manganese, L-taurine, and L-lysine can increase GABA synthesis in the body. Supplemental L-aspartic acid and L-glutamic acid may inhibit the action of GABA.

A word of caution: Some individuals who have taken GABA on an empty stomach have noted a nervous-system reaction beginning about fifteen minutes after ingestion. Among the symptoms are anxiety, increased rate of breathing, headache, and nausea. These individuals also noted that the effects lasted for up to two hours.

Glutamic Acid
Glutamic acid, also known as glutamate, is a nonessential amino acid occurring in proteins. It acts as an intermediary in the Krebs cycle and is therefore important for the proper metabolism of carbohydrates. It is also involved in the removal of ammonia from the muscles. It does this by combining with the ammonia to form glutamine, which is then removed. Glutamic acid is also needed for the production of energy from the BCAAs. In fact, some research has indicated that the amount of energy produced from the BCAAs depends upon the supply of glutamic acid that is available. The same as glucose, glutamic acid can pass readily through the blood-brain barrier, a semipermeable membrane that keeps the blood that is circulating in the brain away from the tissue fluids surrounding the brain cells.

Free-form L-glutamic acid can be used to supplement food proteins and can also be taken along with the BCAAs during exercise in dosages ranging from 500 to 2,000 milligrams per day. Ideally, L-glutamic acid (as well as vitamin B_6) should be part of all BCAA formulations and should be included in high amounts in all full-spectrum amino-acid formulations.

Glutamine
Glutamine is a nonessential amino acid found in proteins. It is formed from glutamic acid by the addition of ammonia and vitamin B_6. Gluta-

mine is a neurotransmitter in the brain, where it can be converted back to glutamic acid. It is essential for the proper functioning of the brain. It is an energy source in the brain and a mediator of glutamic-acid and GABA activity. Glutamine is also vital to immune functioning. New studies show that glutamine is required for cellular replication in the immune system. However, the majority of glutamine is made in the muscles, so the muscles have to supply a large amount of glutamine to the immune system.

Oversupplementation with L-glutamine can contribute to the ammonia load; the use of glutamine alphaketoglutarate is recommended as an alternative. Use of supplemental free-form L-glutamine by athletes is known to produce a strong anticatabolic effect, which neutralizes the cortisol that accompanies strenuous exercise. Cortisol is a steroid hormone and highly catabolic. L-glutamine's anticatabolic action allows more efficient anabolism (formation of tissue). Glutamine is also active in recovery and healing.

Supplemental glutamine has reportedly been taken in dosages ranging from 500 to over 20,000 milligrams per day during periods of high stress. Glutamine is now also commonly added to protein drinks.

(For a special report on glutamine and the athlete, see page 30.)

Glutathione   Glutathione is a tri-peptide that as a supplement is commonly thought of as a free-form amino acid. It is a sulfur-bearing tri-peptide consisting of glutamic acid, cysteine, and glycine. Glutathione occurs in plant and ani-

ON THE CUTTING EDGE

Glutamine Fights Infection During Hard Training

There is evidence that moderate regular exercise helps reduce the level of infection in normal individuals, according to an article published in the *British Journal of Sports Medicine* in 1998. However, intensive heavy exercise increases the incidence of infection. Upper respiratory tract infections have been shown to be more likely with higher training mileage and after a marathon. A number of factors probably contribute to this apparent immunosuppression. These include raised cortisol levels, reduced salivary immunoglobulin levels, and low glutamine levels. Glutamine is an essential amino acid for rapidly dividing cells such as lymphocytes (white blood cells). Low levels of glutamine have been found in overtrained athletes, and these levels are known to be even lower after hard training. Glutamine intervention studies have been carried out, and there is some evidence that the incidence of infection after prolonged exercise in endurance athletes taking glutamine is lower than in endurance athletes taking a placebo. Therefore, to help protect yourself against infection during periods of hard training, make sure you supplement your diet with 6 to 10 grams of glutamine per day.

SPECIAL REPORT

Glutamine and the Athlete

In the scientific community, interest is growing in the amino acid glutamine and its ability to increase nitrogen retention and preserve skeletal-muscle mass. A high glutamine level in a muscle cell stimulates the entry of other amino acids into the cell. Thus, glutamine is anticatabolic and can be considered an anabolic amino acid.

Glutamine is normally classified as a nonessential amino acid. It is linked to the energy-providing citric-acid cycle through glutamic acid and alphaketoglutarate. Glutamine is synthesized from glutamate by the addition of ammonia to the amino-acid side chain due to the action of glutamine synthetase. About 60 percent of the total free-amino-acid content of the body is glutamine. The muscles are its major storehouses. The lung and brain cells are regular glutamine producers, while the cells of the gut, kidneys, and immune system are regular consumers. The muscles and the liver both produce and consume glutamine.

During stress, major changes occur in the glutamine levels. The muscle concentration decreases sharply, whereas the immune and gut cells show an increase in demand. The plasma-glutamine level may drop below the physiological level, resulting in a situation of imbalance and increased vulnerability to infections. In this condition, the body needs an extra supply of glutamine from the diet. This extra demand cannot be fulfilled by consuming extra glutamate because the body's ability to synthesize glutamine from glutamate is insufficient. This is why glutamine is called a "conditionally essential" amino acid.

Dr. Eric Newsholme and his associates at Oxford University in Great Britain were the first to hypothesize that amino-acid imbalances may result from strenuous exercise and, as a consequence, induce a number of phenomena that are collectively referred to as the "overtraining syndrome." Decreased performance, depressed mood, and increased incidence of infections are among the many stress symptoms that are related to this syndrome and have been described for runners, cyclists, swimmers, skiers, ballet dancers, rowers, and even racehorses.

Glutamine from the diet may play a role in counteracting these phenomena because, as has been shown repeatedly, endurance exercise decreases the plasma-glutamine level, suggesting that the muscles cannot provide enough glutamine. Blood samples taken during the postexercise period of a high-intensity interval-training session have shown that exercise at intensities of 90-percent and 120-percent of maximum exercise capacity brought about a transient but significant decrease in the plasma-glutamine concentration. The same study also showed that a ten-day period of overload training resulted in a significant reduction in the resting plasma-glutamine concentration after only five days of training.

These data from Dr. Newsholme may provide a link between the chronic exercise stress that athletes place themselves under during prolonged periods of training and the observation of permanently low plasma-glutamine concentrations in overtrained athletes. Studies reporting depressed glutamine concentrations after exercise, particularly after high-intensity exercise, take on greater significance for athletes suffering from overtraining. Similar postexercise losses of glutamine in these athletes, who start with low resting levels, could play a significant role, particularly in immunosuppression, after exercise. Therefore, glutamine-containing products may help to maintain the plasma-glutamine level, ensuring that enough glutamine is provided to the gut and immune cells to enable the adequate performance of these tissues. In support of this, a recent placebo-controlled study reported a 32-percent reduction in the infection rate over seven days when 5 grams of glutamine were consumed within two hours after running a marathon.

Glutamine has been shown to be a key nutrient for the cells of the immune system and is considered particularly essential for the immune response, both as a precursor for nucleotide biosynthesis and as a major energy source by means of partial oxidation. Inadequate amounts of circulating glutamine may lead to impaired immune function and increased susceptibility to infection among athletes suffering from overtraining syndrome. In addition, glutamine consumption by the small intestine has been found to occur at a very high rate and would appear to be essential for the maintenance of the mucosal cells' structure. Observations of gastrointestinal disorders, particularly of diarrhea and food allergies, may be due, at least in part, to low concentrations of circulating glutamine.

Recently, it was also shown that glycogen storage in the muscles occurred significantly faster when cyclists, the subjects used in the study, consumed protein together with carbohydrates, as compared to carbohydrates alone. The responsible agent for this faster glycogen recovery may have been glutamine. After their muscle-glycogen stores were depleted during exercise, the cyclists were infused with either glutamine, a combination of alanine and glycine, or saline. The muscle-glutamine levels remained steady in the saline group, increased by 16 percent in the glutamine group, but decreased by 19 percent in the alanine-glycine group. Two hours after exercising, the increase in the muscle-glycogen levels was about three times more in the glutamine group than in the other groups.

Most manufacturers of sports-nutrition products are aware of glutamine's benefits, and it has become fashionable to add the substance to everything from protein powders to meal replacements. The problem is that glutamine is expensive, so many of these "enhanced" products contain only small amounts of the nutrient. Some manufacturers would like you to believe that a few hundred milligrams per day are adequate. They aren't.

The suggested dosage for supplemental glutamine is somewhere between 8 and 20 grams per day depending on your dietary intake, health, and intensity and frequency of exercise. It seems logical that taking 3 to 6 grams of supplemental glutamine two to four times a day would elicit a positive response without stimulating the excretion of glutamine, which has been shown to occur with large dosages because of liver-glutamine removal.

mal tissues and is a vital component of the body's defense mechanism against the effects of oxygen and free radicals. It also acts as a detoxifying agent, aids immune functioning, helps protect the integrity of red blood cells, and functions as a neurotransmitter.

Glutathione tends to decrease with age, making supplementation particularly important for adult athletes. In addition, supplemental L-cysteine raises the level of glutathione in the body, as do supplemental L- and DL-methionine. Supplemental intake of L-glutathione along with L-cysteine can be effective in reducing free-radical damage. Exercise can reduce the glutathione level.

Glycine

Glycine is a nonessential amino acid that is synthesized from serine, with folate acting as a coenzyme (enzyme cofactor). Glycine gets its name from the Greek word meaning "sweet." It is a sweet-tasting substance.

Glycine is an important precursor of many substances, including protein, DNA, phospholipids, collagen, and creatine. It is also a precursor in the release of energy. Glycine is used by the liver in the elimination of phenols, which are toxic, and in the formation of bile salts. It is necessary for the proper functioning of the central nervous system and is an inhibitory neurotransmitter. Too much supplemental glycine can displace glucose in the metabolic-energy chain and cause fatigue, but just enough can help produce more energy. During rapid growth, the body's demand for glycine increases.

Studies have shown that the use of 7,000 milligrams of glycine per day causes an increase in the GH level. Some studies have also noted that glycine ingestion causes an increase in strength, possibly due in part to its elevation of the GH level. Supplemental glycine has additionally been shown to increase the creatine level.

The long-term effects of glycine supplementation are not known, although headaches have been reported. The use of supplemental glycine is still in the experimental stage. However, 3,000 to 6,000 milligrams per day may be beneficial for power athletes, and glycine should be part of all full-spectrum amino-acid supplements. Use free-form glycine supplements with caution.

Histidine
Histidine is recognized as an essential amino acid for infants but not for adults. It is extremely important in the growth and repair of human tissue. Because of this, however, histidine is an essential amino acid for athletes, who experience high rates of growth and repair. Histidine is also important in the formation of white and red blood cells. In addition, it has a history of use as a free-form amino acid in the management of arthritis due to its anti-inflammatory properties.

L-histidine has been used as a supplement in dosages of 1,000 to 5,000 milligrams per day. It should be included in multi-amino-acid formulations. The benefits of prolonged use of supplemental free-form L-histidine by athletes are not yet clear. However, benefits may be derived in the preseason and during injury recovery.

Isoleucine
Isoleucine is an essential amino acid that, along with leucine and valine, is one of the BCAAs. Isoleucine is found in proteins and is needed for the formation of hemoglobin. It is involved in the regulation of blood sugar and is metabolized for energy in muscle tissue during exercise.

Supplemental intake of L-isoleucine, along with the other BCAAs, has been shown to help spare muscle tissue, maintain nitrogen balance, and promote muscle growth and healing. For dosage recommendations, see "The Branched-Chain Amino Acids" on page 33.

Leucine
Leucine is an essential amino acid found in proteins that is, like the other BCAAs, important in energy production during exercise. For many years, the three BCAAs were assumed to contribute equally to energy. Recent studies, however, have shown that both exercising and resting muscle tissue uses far more

The Branched-Chain Amino Acids

The branched-chain amino acids (BCAAs) are the essential amino acids isoleucine, leucine, and valine. Together, these three amino acids make up about 35 percent of the amino-acid content of muscle tissue. Each of these amino acids is also used by the body for energy. Studies confirm that under conditions of stress, injury, or exercise, the body uses a disproportionately high amount of the BCAAs to maintain nitrogen balance. (For a discussion of nitrogen balance, see page 21.) Studies also indicate that leucine is used at a rate two or more times greater than those of isoleucine and valine. Many amino-acid formulations on the market therefore have about twice as much L-leucine as the other two BCAAs.

The BCAAs have a history of use in hospital situations for patients in stressed states, such as burn victims, surgical and trauma patients, and starvation cases. These patients are fed intravenously to stimulate their protein synthesis and nitrogen balance. During the 1980s, sports-nutrition companies picked up on these clinical practices and sponsored research using animals and athletes that revealed that the BCAAs are used for energy. The researchers hypothesized that taking supplemental BCAAs would compensate for the BCAAs used for energy, promote muscle growth, and restore nitrogen balance. Additionally, leucine was found to have other growth-related metabolic effects including releasing GH and insulin.

The amounts of the BCAAs supplied vary with the different products available. Some products contain just the BCAAs, others have the BCAAs as well as a few additional ingredients, and still others contain the full spectrum of eighteen amino acids with extra amounts of the BCAAs plus cofactors. Athletes, especially bodybuilders, report muscle growth and strength benefits from *effective* BCAA formulations. However, the BCAAs are not just for power athletes. Endurance athletes can also benefit from BCAA supplementation. Research has determined that endurance athletes use as much as 90 percent of their total daily leucine for energy purposes. This means that endurance athletes might need to eat several times the normally recommended amount of protein to maintain nitrogen balance. An alternative method these athletes can use is to fortify their base diet of food proteins with a BCAA-type supplement.

HOW MUCH OF THE BCAAS IS NEEDED?

Exactly how much of each of the BCAAs is needed by the body has not yet been determined, but we have developed the following guidelines from available research and experience. If you wish to take a BCAA supplement, you can take either a combination formulation consisting of just the BCAAs and a few cofactors, a full-spectrum amino-acid formulation that includes the BCAAs, or a full-spectrum amino-acid supplement that contains extra BCAAs. Formulations that have the BCAAs, vitamin B$_6$, and L-glutamic acid are the best. Supplemental amounts of the BCAAs should range from 1,500 to 6,000 milligrams for L-leucine and 800 to 3,000 milligrams each for L-isoleucine and L-valine. Divide the dosage between two servings a day. Take the two servings thirty to sixty minutes before exercising and directly after exercising on training days, or along with meals on nontraining days, to fortify the base proteins.

The BCAAs compete for absorption with other amino acids, such as L-tyrosine, L- and DL-phenylalanine, and L- and DL-methionine. If you take supplemental amounts of these other amino acids, do so in the evening or morning, at least three hours after taking your BCAA supplement.

leucine for energy than either of the other two BCAAs. According to estimates, up to 90 percent of dietary leucine may be used for energy in exercising muscles. This makes leucine a very limiting amino acid if supplemental amounts are not taken to compensate for the loss. Leucine may also stimulate the release of insulin, which increases protein synthesis and inhibits protein breakdown.

For supplemental L-leucine dosage recommendations, see "The Branched-Chain Amino Acids" on page 33.

Lysine

Lysine is an essential amino acid that is found in large quantities in muscle tissue. It is needed for proper growth and bone development, and it aids in calcium absorption. Lysine has the ability to fight cold sores and herpes viruses. It is required for the formation of collagen, enzymes, antibodies, and other compounds. Together with methionine, iron, and vitamins B_1, B_6, and C, it helps form carnitine, a compound that the body needs in the production of energy from fatty acids. Lysine deficiency can limit protein synthesis and the growth and repair of tissues, in particular the connective tissues. It can become depleted in the brain by excess intake of L-arginine and L-ornithine.

L-lysine should be part of all full-spectrum amino-acid supplements. The effects of the use of supplemental free-form L-lysine by athletes have not yet been determined.

Methionine

Methionine is an essential sulfur-bearing amino acid. It is involved in transmethylation, a metabolic process that is vital to the manufacture of several compounds and important in muscle performance. In transmethylation, an amino acid donates a methyl group to another compound. These methyl donors often function as intermediaries in many biochemical processes. Methionine is the major methyl donor in the body.

Methionine is a limiting amino acid in many proteins, especially in plant pro-

---

ON THE CUTTING EDGE

Do You Exercise in Heat? Try BCAAs

According to an article published in *Medicine and Science in Sports Exercise* in 1998, a study was conducted to "evaluate the influence of BCAA supplementation on the onset of fatigue during prolonged exercise in the heat." In this small trial, six women and seven men bicycled to exhaustion under normal conditions and then again when the temperature was very warm. While exercising, they drank water spiked with the BCAAs or a placebo. The length of time the athletes could exercise before feeling exhausted was longer during the sessions in which they drank the BCAA-spiked drink. These results suggested that "supplementation of BCAA during prolonged, moderate exercise in the heat resulted in a modest improvement in performance in healthy, active men and women."

teins. It functions in the removal of metabolic waste products from the liver and assists in the breakdown of fat and the prevention of fatty buildup in the liver and arteries. It is used to make choline, which makes taking supplemental choline a mandatory practice for athletes to spare methionine for its other functions.

DL-methionine is commonly added to meal-replacement drinks and other nutrient beverages containing soy protein because it increases the quality of the protein. L-methionine, in supplemental dosages ranging from 500 to 2,000 milligrams per day, may be of benefit to athletes, especially those looking to reduce body fat.

Ornithine
Ornithine is a nonessential amino acid that does not occur in proteins. Ornithine's primary role in the body is in the urea cycle, which makes it important in the removal of ammonia. It is formed from arginine in the urea cycle. Like arginine, ornithine has been proven to be an effective GH releaser. It is this role that has brought it widespread recognition among athletes in recent years.

Supplementation with L-ornithine in various dosages, ranging from 2,000 to 4,000 milligrams per day, has been studied. Research using L-ornithine with other amino acids has also been conducted. Recently, a study using 1,000 milligrams of L-ornithine and 1,000 milligrams of L-arginine per day along with five weeks of weight training showed a decrease in body fat and an increase in muscle mass. However, indications are that the effective dose of L-ornithine may be as high as 5,000 to 15,000 milligrams per day. More research needs to be conducted to determine the exact dosage, as well as the specific benefits. L-ornithine may be particularly beneficial for bodybuilders, power lifters, and sprinters.

Ornithine is also an important component of ornithine alphaketoglutarate, a compound that is gaining popularity among bodybuilders and power athletes.

Phenylalanine
Phenylalanine is an essential amino acid and a precursor of the nonessential amino acid tyrosine. Ingestion of supplemental L-tyrosine therefore spares phenylalanine for its other duties.

Phenylalanine has many functions in the body and is a precursor of several important metabolites, such as the skin pigment melanin, and several catecholamine neurotransmitters, such as epinephrine and norepinephrine. The catecholamines are important in memory and learning, locomotion, sex drive, tissue growth and repair, immune-system functioning, and appetite control. Phenylalanine inhibits appetite by increasing the brain's production of norepinephrine and cholecystokinin (CCK). CCK is the hormone that is thought to be responsible for sending out the "I am full" message. These functions of phenylalanine can be of tremendous value to athletes, especially those who need to stimulate mental alertness or who need to lose weight or maintain low levels of body fat.

Dosages of supplemental L-phenylalanine ranging from 100 to 500 milligrams, taken once or twice a day, have been reported to produce no side effects. Take L-phenylalanine on an empty stomach in the morning and in the evening. However, note that dosages of over 4,000 milligrams have been shown to cause headaches. Cofactors that appear to be necessary in phenylalanine metabolism include vitamin B_3, vitamin B_6, vitamin C, copper, and iron.

DL-phenylalanine (DLPA) has been shown to be useful in combating pain. This can be beneficial for athletes who suffer from acute or chronic pain from injury. Dosages of 500 to 1,500 milligrams of DLPA per day have been reported to be effective for this purpose. The theorized mechanism is that DLPA "protects" the endorphins in the body from destruction, thereby allowing them to distribute their morphinelike pain relief. Endorphins are a thousand times more powerful than morphine. Remember, however, that more is not always better. If you experience just partial pain relief, contact your health-care practitioner to evaluate your condition. Do not take megadoses of DLPA, especially without medical supervision.

A word of caution: The artificial sweetener aspartame is a di-peptide made up of phenylalanine and aspartic acid. Soft drinks containing aspartame carry warnings that are aimed at people with phenylketonuria (PKU), a disease in which phenylalanine is not properly metabolized and can be very damaging. People with phenylketonuria should not take any supplemental L- or DL-phenylalanine.

On the other hand, people who drink a lot of caffeine-containing beverages or take energy supplements with caffeine-containing herbs, such as guarana, may need more phenylalanine. Caffeine tends to cause some of the neurotransmitters that are made with phenylalanine to become depleted in the central nervous system. This is why people sometimes feel mentally fuzzy after drinking a lot of coffee. Taking supplemental L- or DL-phenylalanine can help offset the depletion. Better yet, cut down on your caffeine consumption.

Proline

Proline is a nonessential amino acid. It occurs in high amounts in collagen tissue. It can be synthesized from ornithine or glutamic acid. Hydroproline, which is also abundant in collagen, is synthesized in the body from proline. Proline may be important in the maintenance and healing of collagen tissues such as the skin, tendons, and cartilage.

Current knowledge of L-proline and hydroproline supplementation is limited. Therefore, no reliable recommendations are possible at this time.

Serine

Serine is a nonessential amino acid found in proteins and derived from glycine. Its metabolism leads to the formation of many important substances, such as choline and phospholipids, which are essential in the formation of some neurotransmitters and are used to stabilize membranes. Serine is important in the metabolism of fat and the preservation of a healthy immune system. However, dosage guidelines for L-serine supplementation still need to be established.

Taurine

The nonessential amino acid taurine is one of the sulfur-bearing amino acids and occurs in the body only in its free form because it is not a component of proteins. Taurine plays a major role in brain tissue and in nervous-system functioning. It is involved in blood-pressure regulation and in the transportation of the electrolytes across cell membranes. It is found in the heart, muscles, central nervous system, and brain. It is also an inhibitory neurotransmitter—that is, calming to the brain—just like GABA. Taurine is also found in the eye and may be important for maintaining good vision and eye functioning.

Taurine is made from cysteine, with vitamin B_6 as a cofactor. The use of supplemental amounts of L-taurine ranging from 500 to 5,000 milligrams per day has been reported, but no research has yet been done to determine exactly how L-taurine can be used as part of an athlete's nutrition program.

Threonine
Threonine is an essential amino acid found in proteins. It is an important component of collagen, tooth enamel, protein, and elastic tissue. It can also function as a lipotropic agent, a substance that prevents fatty buildup in the liver. Supplemental L-threonine has a reported use in the treatment of depression in patients with low threonine levels. Generally, dosages of 1,000 milligrams per day are used in these depression cases. Studies still need to be undertaken to determine the exact benefits of L-threonine supplementation for athletes.

Tryptophan
Tryptophan is an essential amino acid that has recently been shrouded in controversy due to its suspected link to a rare blood disorder. Tryptophan is necessary for the production of vitamin B_3. Therefore, taking supplemental vitamin B_3 can help conserve tryptophan for its other functions. Supplemental L-tryptophan has been taken for years by millions of people for its pronounced calming effects, which include the promotion of sleep and the treatment of depression. Tryptophan is the precursor of the neurotransmitter serotonin. Serotonin helps control the sleep cycle, causing a feeling of drowsiness. L-tryptophan taken in dosages of 500 to 2,000 milligrams has been reported to correct sleep disorders.

L-tryptophan has also been reported to increase the GH level. One interesting study examined the effect of taking 1,200 milligrams of L-tryptophan twenty-four hours before exercising. The researchers found that treadmill performance (total exercise capacity and total exercise time) was greatly increased. However, due to the ban on L-tryptophan, use of this amino acid by athletes is not currently possible.

Tryptophan is one of the least abundant amino acids in food, which makes it one of the limiting essential amino acids. Some foods that are high in tryptophan are cottage cheese, pork, wild game, duck, and avocado. Eating these foods along with vitamin B_3 and the cofactors vitamin B_6 and magnesium may help athletes derive some of the benefits that tryptophan offers.

Tyrosine
Tyrosine is a nonessential amino acid that is made from the essential amino acid phenylalanine. Supplementation with L-tyrosine can have a sparing effect on phenylalanine, leaving phenylalanine available for functions not associated with tyrosine formation.

Tyrosine plays many roles in the body. It is a precursor of the catecholamines dopamine and norepinephrine, regulates appetite, and aids in melanin production. These functions are similar to the ones with which phenylalanine is associated as a precursor of tyrosine. However, tyrosine is believed to be better at stimulating these effects because it is one step closer as a precursor. An antidepressant effect and an increased sex drive in men have also been observed with tyrosine supplementation.

Supplemental L-tyrosine may be useful for athletes who are undergoing stress, who need to lose body fat, or who wish to maintain peak alertness. Dosages ranging from 100 milligrams to several thousand milligrams per day have been reported. *A word of caution:* L-tyrosine may trigger migraine headaches when it is broken down into a product called tyramine.

Valine Valine is an essential amino acid and a member of the branched-chain amino acids. The same as the other BCAAs, isoleucine and leucine, valine is an integral part of muscle tissue and may be used for energy by exercising muscles. It is involved in tissue repair, nitrogen balance, and muscle metabolism. For supplemental L-valine dosage recommendations, see "The Branched-Chain Amino Acids" on page 33.

DIGESTION OF PROTEIN AND AMINO ACIDS

The mechanical digestion of protein begins in the mouth during chewing. In the stomach, the enzyme pepsin joins in, breaking down the protein into shorter peptides. The partially digested protein then passes into the intestines, where the free-form, di-peptide, and tri-peptide amino acids are absorbed, beginning immediately.

ON THE CUTTING EDGE

BCAAs Help Increase Training Strength and Lean Body Mass

A study reported in *Medicina Dello Sport* in 1997 looked at the effect of taking supplemental BCAAs on bodybuilding progress. The study involved thirty-one male bodybuilders between the ages of eighteen and thirty-four, all of whom were drug-free, or "natural," bodybuilders. All had at least two years of training experience. The subjects were divided into two groups—sixteen took a placebo and fifteen took 0.2 gram of a BCAA supplement per kilogram (2.2 pounds) of body weight thirty minutes before training and then again thirty minutes after training. The results showed that while both groups experienced increases in body weight, the BCAA group had greater weight gains. An analysis of the weight gain in the BCAA group showed increases in the lean body mass in both the legs and arms, with no changes in the trunk area of the body. In contrast, the group taking the placebo showed no lean-mass gains in these areas. The BCAA group also showed strength gains in both the squat and bench-press exercises, while the placebo group gained strength only in the squat exercise. In addition, the BCAA group showed improvements in measures of exercise intensity.

Enzymes continue to digest any polypeptides as they travel down the intestines.

Once the free-form, di-peptide, and tri-peptide amino acids enter the bloodstream, they are transported to the liver, where a few things may happen to them. They may be converted into other amino acids; they may be used to make other proteins; they may be further broken down and either used for energy or excreted; or they may be placed into circulation and continue on to the rest of the body.

Proteins empty from the stomach in two to three hours, depending on how much fat is present. This means that you should keep the protein content of precompetition meals low to enable your stomach to pass food into your bloodstream and cells before you begin exercising.

SPECIAL PROTEIN AND AMINO-ACID NEEDS OF THE ATHLETE

In Chapter 1, we credited carbohydrates with having a protein-sparing effect. This protein-sparing effect is a function of carbohydrates providing enough energy to minimize the body's use of amino acids for energy. Calories, however, are not the only factor involved in the sparing of muscle tissue, which is extremely important to the athlete who has been working hard to build up or maintain muscle mass. For example, if you ate a whopping 10,000 calories a day from only carbohydrate and fat sources, your body still would have to break down muscle tissue to get the supply of amino acids it needed to carry on metabolism. Looking at it this way, you can see that an adequate supply of protein (amino acids) is essential to the maintenance of existing muscle tissue.

To derive optimum protein, you must achieve the proper protein-to-calorie ratio. You can accomplish this by eating enough carbohydrates and fat to meet your energy requirements and enough protein to get the amino acids your body needs for growth, energy, and other metabolic demands. But, as is evident from the material discussed so far in this chapter, adequate amount is not the only requirement for optimum protein intake. What type the protein is affects how it is used by the body, and fortification with certain amino acids and other cofactors influences how efficiently food-source proteins are used. At the very least, protein intake, especially by athletes, is a sophisticated science. Just how much protein an athlete requires depends on body weight, the quality of the protein, and the intensity and duration of the exercise.

The Recommended Dietary Allowances (RDAs) for protein can provide a baseline for athletes' protein requirements. However, the protein allowances were determined according to body weight, plus they assume normal body weight. Therefore, if you have more than the average amount of body fat, you may end up overcalculating your protein need.

According to the RDAs, an adult male between the ages of twenty-five and fifty requires 63 grams of protein per day, which can be obtained by eating about 6 ounces of chicken. However, research has shown that athletes engaged in daily exercise have difficulty maintaining nitrogen balance when their dietary-protein intake is less than 1.5 grams for each 1 kilogram (2.2 pounds) of body weight. This is about 50-percent higher than the RDA. In fact, researchers estimate that, depending on the type of sport, the requirement for protein is about 1.5 to 2.5

grams per 1 kilogram of ideal body weight. Furthermore, in some special in-stances—for example, if you are a bodybuilder preparing for a contest—the requirement may exceed 3 grams for every 1 kilogram of body weight. How much food does this translate into? For an athlete weighing 174 pounds, protein intake should be between 118 to 198 grams per day. This is two to three times the RDA and a lot of protein to eat (about 14 to 22 ounces of chicken per day). Remember that excess protein is not converted to muscle. Rather, it is either bro-ken down and used as energy in the liver or converted to fat. Because protein is also one of the most expensive nutrients, you should take special care to eat just the right amount for your sport, lean body mass, and activity level.

Another consideration in protein consumption is efficiency. You can make the proteins you eat more efficient by fortifying them with a multi-amino-acid sup-plement that includes the BCAAs. By providing your body with potentially lim-iting amino acids from supplement sources, you may be able to maintain nitrogen balance with a lower protein intake. While we offer protein-supplement guidelines in this book, the only way you can determine your nitrogen balance for sure is to monitor how it varies with different levels of protein intake and supplement use.

Additionally, protein cofactors are required for the proper metabolism of the amino acids. Vitamin B_6 is the most important cofactor because it is necessary in the functioning of the enzymes that aid this metabolism. Vitamin B_3 is an impor-tant vitamin because it spares tryptophan, which is converted to vitamin B_3 in the body. However, do not take large amounts of vitamin B_3 during exercise, as stud-ies have shown that a large intake of vitamin B_3 can increase glycogen use, which results in early onset of fatigue. Researchers have also determined that increased protein intake leads to an increase in calcium excretion. Increasing phosphorus intake seems to minimize this effect, however, as does increasing calcium intake by individuals on high-protein diets. All the essential vitamins and minerals are important in some way in the body's optimum use of the amino acids.

FOOD AND SUPPLEMENT SOURCES OF PROTEIN

Protein is found in animals, in plants, and in supplement form. Animal proteins tend to be of higher quality than plant proteins because they contain the proper proportions of the essential amino acids. Most plant protein sources, such as beans and peas, are incomplete in their essential-amino-acid contents. Therefore, it is necessary to combine different plant proteins to get an adequate balance of the amino acids. Two popular combinations are peas with corn and kidney beans with brown rice. If you are a vegetarian, you need to know how to combine legumes with grains to formulate complete proteins. Check your local library or bookstore for a book that explains how to do this. (For a special report on vegetarian ath-letes, see page 43.)

Protein is ususaly found together with fat in foods, especially in animal prod-ucts. Some good low-fat sources of protein are low-fat milk, skim milk, and other low-fat dairy products; most fishes, including cod, sole, halibut, tuna, sardines, and salmon; most shellfishes, including scallops, lobster, crab, shrimp, and mussels; lean red meat from which the fat has been trimmed; and skinless poultry.

As supplements, protein and amino acids are available in tablet, capsule, liquid, and powder forms. In tablet form, they are generally used to fortify meals or to get extra amino acids before or during exercise or before going to bed. One or several amino acids can be delivered by tablets and capsules. Liquid and powder protein supplements can be eaten between meals or with meals. The ingredients range from just a few amino acids, such as the BCAAs, to the full spectrum of eighteen amino acids with extra amounts of the BCAAs as well as cofactors. If you shop carefully, you should be able to find economical sources of protein in supplement form. The best are high in both protein and carbohydrates. Protein drinks should have whey or whey and egg as the primary sources of protein.

DECIPHERING LABELS

Proteins and amino acids come not only in several forms but also in many combinations. When purchasing a supplement formulation that supplies one or several amino acids, you must know how to determine how much of the actual amino acids you are getting. For example, the ingredient list of a supplement containing L-arginine and L-ornithine may read:

Each capsule supplies:
L-arginine . . . . 500 milligrams
L-ornithine . . . . 500 milligrams

This label is reporting the molecular amounts of L-arginine and L-ornithine.

Some products contain amino acids combined with other molecules. The ingredient list of this type of supplement may read:

Each capsule supplies:
L-arginine hydrochloride . . . . 500 milligrams
L-ornithine hydrochloride . . . . 500 milligrams

This label is reporting that each capsule has 500 milligrams of the entire molecule of L-arginine hydrochloride, of which L-arginine may make up only 60 percent, or 300 milligrams; and 500 milligrams of the entire molecule of L-ornithine hydrochloride, of which L-ornithine may make up only 60 percent, or 300 milligrams. Since the capsules in the first example actually have 500 milligrams each of L-arginine and L-ornithine, they are a better choice.

Another product may have a label that reads:

Each capsule supplies:
L-arginine (hydrochloride) . . . . 500 milligrams
L-ornithine (hydrochloride) . . . . 500 milligrams

The parentheses around the *hydrochloride,* which is sometimes abbreviated as *HCl,* indicate that this product supplies, per capsule, 500 milligrams each of L-arginine and L-ornithine in the form of hydrochloride. This is the same amount as the product in the first example.

SPECIAL REPORT

Exercising on Veggies— The Benefits and Risks

Research has shown that vegetarians are generally healthier than their meat-eating friends. They have lower rates of heart disease, high blood pressure, diabetes, and certain types of cancer, and better levels of cholesterol and body fat.

Scientists attribute much of this difference to the vegetarian's low-fat, high-fiber diet. For this reason, many health-conscious individuals have become interested in adopting a vegetarian style of eating. Even people who continue to eat meat are choosing to eat less of it and have several meatless meals each week. Lastly, some athletes swear by a vegetarian diet.

There are basically two types of vegetarians—lacto-ovo vegetarians and vegans. Lacto-ovo vegetarians consume dairy products and eggs as well as all foods of plant origin, such as vegetables, fruits, breads and cereals, dried beans and peas, nuts and nut butters, and seeds. They refrain from eating meat, chicken, and fish. A variation is the lacto vegetarian, who also avoids eggs. Vegans consume only foods of plant origin and avoid all foods of animal origin, including dairy products, eggs, meat, fish, and poultry. People who avoid only red meat but consume chicken and/or fish are not true vegetarians.

The misconception that athletes and people who exercise need to eat large amounts of meat for protein is one of the most persistent of the diet-exercise myths. In reality, vegetarian athletes can easily consume high-quality protein in ample amounts to meet the extra demands of exercise without jeopardizing their performance or health.

Everyone needs protein. A proper supply and balance of the amino acids, the building blocks of protein, are necessary for the cells to make antibodies, the hemoglobin in red blood cells, the specialized proteins in muscle cells, enzymes, hormones, and other essential protein-containing compounds. Most of the amino acids can be made by the body,

but eight to ten of them must be supplied by the diet and are called essential amino acids. Meat, chicken, fish, dairy products, and eggs contain all of the essential amino acids and are called high-quality proteins. Grains, dried beans and peas, nuts, seeds, and vegetables contain some of the essential amino acids but not all of them. Therefore, these foods are called incomplete proteins.

However, nature, in her infinite wisdom, has balanced the amino acids in grains and legumes, so when these two foods are combined, the end product is a high-quality protein. For example, grains are low in the amino acid lysine and high in methionine, whereas cooked dried beans and peas are high in lysine and low in methionine. A meal that combines grains and legumes, such as chili beans and cornbread, supplies all of the essential amino acids. Combining two foods with incomplete proteins to create a high-quality protein or combining a high-quality protein food (such as milk or eggs) with an incomplete protein food (such as oatmeal or cooked dried beans) is called complementing proteins.

In the past, it was believed that complementary proteins had to be consumed at the same meal for optimum protein production. This belief has been proven false. The body maintains a fluctuating, temporary source of amino acids called the amino-acid pool, and as long as complementary proteins are consumed sometime during the day or even every few days, normal protein synthesis and tissue functioning are maintained.

For lacto-ovo vegetarians, complementing proteins is a minor issue, since their diets contain the high-quality protein foods of milk and eggs. But, lacto-ovo vegetarians still need to watch their nutrition, since they often rely solely on milk products for their protein, thus increasing their risk of developing deficiencies of iron and the other trace minerals not supplied by dairy foods. It is important to include at least two servings of cooked dried beans or peas, nuts, or seeds in the daily diet to avoid these deficiencies.

THE VEGETARIAN EXERCISER'S NEEDS

Can vegetarian exercisers and athletes consume enough protein to meet the extra demands of their workouts or sports? Yes. People who engage in moderate exercise (less than two hours per day) can easily meet their protein needs by consuming the RDA of 44 grams for women or 56 grams for men. For example, the daily protein allowance for a moderately active woman can be met by consuming 1 cup of split pea soup, four slices of whole-grain bread, 2 tablespoons of peanut butter, a spinach salad, and two whole-wheat muffins. Additional servings of eggs, milk, or cheese would add about another 8 grams of protein each, and additional servings of grains or vegetables would add another 2 to 3 grams each. A well-balanced lacto-ovo vegetarian diet supplying at least 2,000 calories contains more than the RDA for protein.

The protein requirement might be slightly greater than the RDA for people who engage in vigorous exercise (more than two hours per day) and for people beginning a muscle-building program, such as weightlifting. However, in all cases, the increased need can be easily supplied by a vegetarian diet.

Protein is usually the new vegetarian's first concern. Although vegetarians, even vegans, get plenty of protein from foods such as legumes, seeds, and grains, many people believe that the quality of plant protein is inferior to that of animal protein. Nutritionists use the word *quality* to refer to the amino-acid composition of protein.

By eating a variety of foods, it is easy to obtain enough quality amino acids from plant sources. Each day, the vegan should select foods from at least two of the following three groups:

1. Legumes—all kinds of dried peas and beans, soybeans, tofu, peanuts.

2. Grains—cereals, breads, pasta, corn, rice, wheat.

3. Nuts and seeds—sesame and sunflower seeds.

Rice and beans, and peanut butter and bread are two common examples of high-quality protein meals.

Most of the extra calories needed by exercisers can be supplied by additional servings of basic foods, especially carbohydrates. How much dietary carbohydrate is enough? The recommendations vary from 55 percent to 70 percent of total calories. Vegetarian diets automatically meet this recommendation, since they are based on carbohydrate-rich foods, such as grains, legumes, vegetables, and fruits. For good nutrition, vegetarians, like meat-eaters, should avoid consuming more than 30 percent of their calories from fat.

A high calorie consumption requires additional amounts of the nutrients needed to process energy, including several of the B vitamins. Intake of these nutrients will automatically increase in the lacto-ovo vegetarian diet if additional foods from the basic food categories (for example, whole grains, legumes, vegetables, and fruits) are consumed.

The vegan is more susceptible to vitamin and mineral deficiencies, in particular of vitamins B_2, B_{12}, and D, and of calcium, iron, and zinc, which must all be eaten each day. Also, fortified foods, such as soymilk fortified with vitamin B_{12}, may be consumed, and a multi-vitamin-and-mineral supplement may be added to the diet.

Research is limited, but some studies suggest that people who engage in vigorous training need certain vitamins in amounts greater than the RDAs. One study showed that female athletes have an increased requirement for vitamin B_2 and that as much as 1.16 milligrams per 1,000 calories (versus the 0.6 milligram per 1,000 calories proposed by the RDA) are necessary to maintain the normal tissue levels of this vitamin. Several studies have suggested that the needs for vitamins B_5 and E are increased as a result of intensive exercise. Since exercise increases destructive free-radical production, antioxidant nutrients are important for athletes. Except for vitamin E, the vitamins and minerals are consumed in sufficient amounts in a well-balanced lacto-ovo vegetarian diet of at least 2,000 calories.

The nutrients to which vegans must pay particular attention include vitamins B_2, B_{12}, and D, and calcium and iron. Vitamin B_2 is commonly obtained from dairy products, which vegans avoid. However, it is also found in dark green vegetables, which are usually abundant in the vegan diet. Vitamin B_{12} is found only in animal products. Because of this, vegans must get their B_{12} from some form of supplement, such as B_{12}-fortified soymilk. Of particular concern is deficiency of vitamin B_{12} in growing children, pregnant or lactating women, and people who have followed a strict vegan diet for several years. The body stores only up to four years' worth of B_{12}. Vitamin D is found in milk fortified with vitamin D and made by the body when skin is exposed to the sun. A deficiency of vitamin D would be of concern to vegans who don't get much sun.

Calcium is another nutrient usually obtained from dairy products. Since vegans do not consume dairy products, they must be sure to get calcium from other food sources, such as sesame seeds, almonds, legumes, and calcium-fortified soymilk. Iron is found in legumes, whole grains, and some vegetables. Nutritional yeast is also a good source. Vitamin C triples iron absorption.

Another nutrient that vegetarian exercisers must watch is creatine. The body gets most of the creatine it needs from dietary sources. Not surprisingly, the foods that contain the greatest amounts of creatine are those derived from skeletal muscle—beef, pork, and fish such as salmon, cod, tuna, and herring. It is unclear whether poultry contains significant amounts of creatine. But while these foods are certainly good sources of creatine, there are reasons why they may not be the best sources. First, cooking destroys some of the creatine in meat. Second, vegans who do not eat meat or poultry obtain almost no creatine. Creatine supplements, therefore, are recommended. For the supplementation recommendations for active individuals, see page 165.

VEGETARIANISM AND ATHLETIC PERFORMANCE

While there is a substantial amount of information on the nutritional adequacy of vegetarian diets, little is known about the effects of vegetarianism on athletic performance. A vegan diet should not be attempted by any athlete without previous experience with this type of diet or without consultation with a dietitian or physician. Such a diet should be considered only if the athlete is willing to devote time and effort to learning the proper combinations and amounts of foods necessary to achieve a balanced diet.

For female athletes and active women who wish to consume a vegetarian diet, a sound recommendation would be to include dairy products and eggs, and occasionally (weekly) a small portion of fish or chicken. Such a diet requires bulkier or more frequent meals and careful attention to variety and food combinations. You should also consider supplementing your diet with a "power powder" or "metabolic optimizer" powder drink to ensure that you get enough quality protein and amino acids. (For a discussion of protein powders and metabolic optimizers, see Chapter 9, "Scientific Nutrition: Meal Replacements, Protein Powders, and Metabolic Optimizers."

Although a diet low in fat and high in carbohydrates can lower the risk of certain diseases in sedentary individuals, a poorly planned vegetarian diet in a very active person can lead to metabolic, endocrine, and nutritional changes that impair health and performance. Therefore, gathering as much information as possible on vegetarianism and meal-planning is a must. Good information sources include the Vegetarian Resource Group, PO Box 1463, Baltimore, MD 21203, 410–366–8343; Vegetarian Times, 1140 West Lake Street, Suite 500, Oak Park, IL 60301, 708–848–8100; and the American Vegan Society, 501 Old Harding Highway, Malaga, NJ 08328, 609–694–2887.

Always be wary of products that do not give the amounts of the amino acids they supply. Some products list only the names of the amino acids, not the quantities. This limited information is worthless, since there is no way you can figure out how much of the product to consume.

The importance of proper protein intake to maximum performance is obvious. Choosing high-quality food protein sources and properly using protein and amino-acid supplements is essential. Ingesting the correct amount of protein for your body size and activity level can help maintain your desirable body weight and improve your healing and recovery abilities.

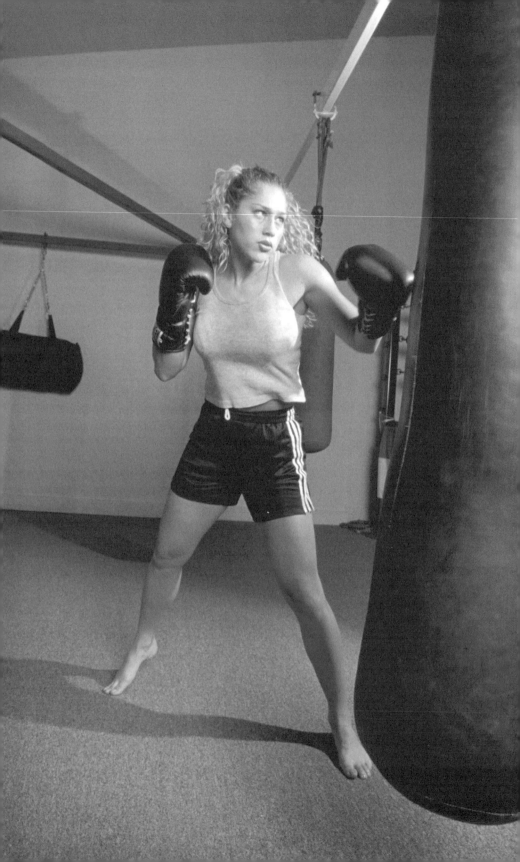

LIPIDS

UNDERESTIMATED ENERGY AND GROWTH FACTORS

3

The third major macronutrient category, along with carbohydrates and protein, is lipids. The same as carbohydrates, lipids are composed of carbon, hydrogen, and oxygen. Lipids are necessary in the human body for numerous reasons. They contain the fat-soluble vitamins A, D, E, and K. They are a source of the essential fatty acids, which play many vital roles in maintaining the functioning and integrity of cell membranes. They serve as concentrated sources of energy. They add palatability to meals. And they are important in biochemical and biophysical functions such as steroid-hormone synthesis.

The most prevalent type of lipid is the triglyceride. As an energy source, the triglyceride varies in importance according to the type of exercise performed. For endurance sports, such as marathon running, triglycerides are the primary source of energy. For power sports, such as sprinting, glycogen is the primary fuel, but some triglycerides are also used. It is important to understand that the body is constantly metabolizing triglycerides for energy; the only thing that changes is the degree to which it does this.

Power athletes are prone to becoming fat because of this differential use of energy sources—that is, because their bodies use mostly glycogen for energy and just a minor portion of body fat. These athletes must therefore follow nutrition programs that are low in fat and high in fat-metabolizing nutrients. But even though endurance athletes, such as marathon runners, can get away with eating high-fat diets, they will definitely find their performance impeded and health negatively affected if their diets are *too* high in fat.

In this chapter, we will take a look at the different kinds of lipids that exist. We will also discuss ways of cutting down on the bad lipids in the diet without reducing our intake of the beneficial nutrients such as protein.

LIPIDS—THE MOST MISUNDERSTOOD MACRONUTRIENT

In recent years, dietary lipids have gained a bad reputation. Medical research has linked a diet high in lipids to many diseases. Certain lipids are essential to health, however. Rather than cut lipids out of your diet completely, you should learn how to balance the good lipids with the bad lipids in your diet and how to trim total lipid intake.

Lipids serve many essential functions in the body. Their main functions are:

☐ To provide fuel.

☐ To provide insulation.

☐ To aid in the absorption of the fat-soluble vitamins.

☐ To act as energy storehouses.

☐ To supply the essential fatty acids.

☐ To provide protective padding for body structures and organs.

☐ To serve as components of all cell membranes and other cellular structures.

☐ To supply building blocks for other molecules.

The main problem with lipids in the diet is simple—we consume too much total lipid, too much of the wrong lipids, and not enough of the good lipids. While lipids are necessary for health, too much of the wrong kinds of lipids can have negative effects on the body and can lead to certain cancers and cardiovascular diseases. The common culprits are saturated fats and cholesterol. Of course, too much of any lipid can cause obesity. Most experts recommend a total dietary-lipid intake of less than 30 percent of total daily calories; some recommend keeping lipids under 20 percent. Because athletes generally consume over 4,000 calories a day, they can easily get an overdose of lipids in their diets. Keeping total lipid intake down, maximizing the good lipids, and minimizing the bad lipids are therefore the major focus of sports nutrition.

THE MAJOR LIPIDS

Lipids occur in both plants and animals, but plant lipids vary slightly in chemical composition from animal lipids. By definition, lipids are compounds that are soluble in organic solvents but not in water. Mammal fats tend to be more saturated than fish oils or plant oils. Beef tends to be more saturated than pork or poultry. The degree of hardness that a fat displays at room temperature is an indication of how saturated it is. Compare hard beef fat, soft fish fat, and vegetable oil. Vegetable oil has a low amount of saturated fat and a high amount of polyunsaturated fat.

The major lipids found in the diet and body are cholesterol, triglycerides and fatty acids, and phospholipids.

Cholesterol

Cholesterol is a member of a group of fats called sterols. It is made by the body and occurs naturally in foods only of animal origin. The highest concentrations of cholesterol are found in liver and egg yolks, although high levels are also present in red meat, poultry (especially the skin), whole milk, and cheese.

Cholesterol has many important functions in the body. It is a component of every cell; a precursor of bile acids, various sex and adrenal hormones, and vitamin D; and an important aid in brain and nervous-system tissues. The body needs a constant supply of cholesterol for proper health and performance. However, a high cholesterol level has been linked to a variety of cardiovascular diseases.

For good health, doctors recommend keeping cholesterol intake to under 300 milligrams per day. Since most meats contain about 90 milligrams of cholesterol in every 3 ounces, this is an almost impossible task for athletes, who generally need to consume high levels of protein. To meet both these needs, athletes must take special care to include plant protein sources, egg whites, and other high-protein, low-fat, low-cholesterol foods and supplements in their diets.

Triglycerides and Fatty Acids

Triglycerides are the major class of lipids in the diet and body. They are the lipids that make up the fats and oils in the diet and the fat that is stored by the body. They include about 98 percent of all the dietary fats.

The difference between fat and oil is simple—fat is solid at room temperature and oil is liquid. This difference in solidity gives an indication of composition. Triglycerides are composed of three fatty acids attached to a three-carbon-atom glycerol molecule. There are hundreds of different fatty acids, and they come in various lengths, from four to twenty-four carbon atoms long. A short-chain fatty acid has four to five carbon atoms; a medium-chain fatty acid has six to twelve carbon atoms; a long-chain fatty acid has thirteen to nineteen carbon atoms; and a very long chain fatty acid has twenty or more carbon atoms.

Fatty acids are also rated according to the hydrogen atoms that are attached to their carbon chains. Saturated fatty acids have the maximum number of hydrogen atoms that they can hold, with no unsaturated carbon molecules. This is why saturated fatty acids are more solid. Hydrogenation is the process of taking unsaturated fatty acids and saturating them with hydrogen atoms to make them more solid. An example is margarine, which is made of vegetable oil, a liquid fatty acid. Monounsaturated fatty acids have one unsaturated carbon molecule, and polyunsaturated fatty acids have more than one unsaturated carbon molecule.

Saturated fatty acids tend to be solid at room temperature. Therefore, fats are high in saturated fatty acids. Polyunsaturated fatty acids tend to be liquid at room temperature. Oils are high in polyunsaturated fatty acids. Saturated fatty acids are always either used for energy or stored as body fat, as are fatty acids containing sixteen or fewer carbon atoms. The fewer carbon atoms a fatty acid has, the easier it is to use that fatty acid for energy. The longer fatty acids can also be used for energy or stored as body fat, but they have other functions as well. For example, they serve as components in the structure of cell membranes, which is important for growth.

Among the fatty acids, the most important ones are the essential fatty acids, the omega-3 fatty acids, gamma linolenic acid, and medium-chain triglycerides.

The Essential Fatty Acids Of the many fatty acids that exist, only
two are essential and only one is conditionally essential. Linoleic acid is a primary essential fatty acid. It is necessary for normal growth and health. Therefore, since

the body cannot manufacture it, it must be obtained from the diet. Another fatty acid, arachidonic acid, is made in the body from linoleic acid. Arachidonic acid only becomes essential when a linoleic-acid deficiency exists. However, because arachidonic acid has to be made from linoleic acid and because it is a polyunsaturated fatty acid, arachidonic acid has a linoleic-sparing effect when it is present in the diet. This may be beneficial to athletes because arachidonic acid is also an important structural fatty acid that is present in cell membranes.

Alpha-linolenic acid is the other essential fatty acid. Alpha-linolenic acid is similar to linoleic acid in structure. Among its functions, it is important in growth and is the precursor of two other important fatty acids, eicosapentaenoic acid (EPA) and docosahexaenoic acid (DHA). As with protein and the amino acids, the body would rather use the essential fatty acids for growth and functional needs than for fuel needs. A diet that is high in the essential fatty acids and low in the nonessential fatty acids therefore increases metabolism and discourages increased body-fat formation, assuming that overeating is not a factor. Remember, excess carbohydrates and amino acids can be converted to body fat.

The essential fatty acids are important to existence and performance. Some of their specific functions are:

☐ Presence in phospholipids, which are important in maintaining the structure and the functioning of cellular and subcellular membranes.

☐ Service as precursors of eicosanoids, which are important in regulating a wide diversity of physiological processes.

☐ Involvement in the transfer of oxygen from the lungs to the bloodstream.

☐ Formation of a structural part of all cells.

☐ Reduction of the time required for recovery by fatigued muscles after exercise by helping clear away lactic acid.

☐ Maintenance of proper brain and nervous-system functioning.

☐ Production of prostaglandins, a group of hormones important in metabolism.

☐ Formation of healthy skin and hair.

☐ Assistance in wound healing.

☐ Growth enhancement.

Linoleic acid and alpha-linolenic acid are both unsaturated fatty acids and eighteen carbon atoms long. While scientists recognize that the body requires these two fatty acids for health, they have not yet established RDAs for them for adults because deficiencies in the essential fatty acids are rare.

(For a special report on a type of linoleic acid called conjugated linoleic acid, see page 52.)

The Omega-3 Fatty Acids
During the 1980s, there was a resurgence of attention focused on two fatty acids belonging to the omega-3 family—eicosapentaenoic acid (EPA) and docosahexaenoic acid (DHA). Researchers in the 1950s had documented the cholesterol-lowering effects of EPA and DHA. However, it was not until the 1970s, when the low rates of cardiovascular diseases were documented among the fish-eating Greenland Eskimos, that conclusive results were proven.

EPA and DHA can be made in the body from linoleic acid, also a fatty acid, and are found in human tissue as normal components. Despite this, when they are obtained from food sources that are part of a diet that is low in saturated fatty acids, they have beneficial effects. They have the tendency to disperse fatty acids and cholesterol in the bloodstream, which seems to be how their presence helps prevent arteries from clogging. They have a blood-thinning effect and discourage excessive blood clotting. They lower the blood-triglyceride level and raise the level of high-density lipoproteins (HDLs), the good lipoproteins that help prevent cholesterol buildup in the arteries. In addition, EPA and DHA have an anti-inflammatory effect and work by competing with arachidonic acid, which forms pro-inflammatory compounds.

Besides all their known health benefits, EPA and DHA have also been documented to improve athletic performance. Recent studies using 2,000 to 4,000 milligrams per day of EPA and DHA from supplements and fish have reported significant increases in strength and aerobic (with oxygen) performance. The improvements included increased bench-press repetitions, faster running times, reduced muscular inflammation, and longer jumping distances. Scientists believe that these improvements were due to the combined effects that EPA and DHA have on the body, including improved GH production, anti-inflammatory action, enhanced oxygen metabolism, lowered blood viscosity (thickness) leading to better oxygen and nutrient delivery to the muscles, and improved recovery.

EPA and DHA are found in high amounts in cold-water fishes such as cod, salmon, sardines, trout, and mackerel, and in lower amounts in tuna. They are also available in supplemental form, specifically as gelatin capsules and liquid supplements. Aim for a combined intake of 2,000 to 4,000 milligrams of EPA and DHA per day from supplement and food sources.

Gamma Linolenic Acid
Gamma linolenic acid (GLA) is another important fatty acid that can be made in the body from the main essential fatty acid, linoleic acid. GLA is an important precursor of the series-1 prostaglandins, a group of hormones that regulate many cellular activities. The series-1 prostaglandins keep blood platelets from sticking together, control cholesterol formation, reduce inflammation, make insulin work better, improve nerve functioning, regulate calcium metabolism, and function in the immune system. While studies on athletes have not confirmed any performance-enhancing effects, the ingestion of foods and supplements high in GLA does benefit overall health.

Foods containing GLA are not that easy to find, however. GLA is not present

SPECIAL REPORT

Conjugated Linoleic Acid Is an Essential Fatty Acid for Athletes

One very interesting bodybuilding supplement that has gained popularity of late is CLA, or conjugated linoleic acid. CLA is a very different type of dietary supplement. It is actually a fatty acid. This product takes sports supplementation in a whole new direction. The use of certain components of fat, such as key fatty acids like CLA, may not only be essential for health and muscle growth but may also enhance them.

The fatty acid CLA occurs naturally in a number of foods, primarily beef and dairy products. Its commercial form is derived from sunflower oil. The word "conjugated" in its name refers to the variation in chemical structure that sets it apart from the linoleic acid present in borage oil and flaxseed oil. Linoleic acid belongs to a family of essential fatty acids called the omega-6 fatty acids and performs a number of important metabolic functions in the body. A slight change in the double bonds that hold its atoms together transforms it from linoleic acid to CLA. This small molecular reconfiguration has profound effects on its function and bestows upon CLA nutritional benefits different from those of regular linoleic acid.

CLA's rising popularity among athletes stems from its ability to augment muscle mass and burn body fat. Scientists foresee broader applications for human health. So far, lab tests have shown that CLA acts as a powerful antioxidant, benefits the immune system, and possesses anticarcinogenic properties.

The scientists who made these discoveries have received patents for using CLA in livestock feed to improve the feed efficiency, promote animal growth, and prevent muscle wasting due to the administration of steroids. Indeed, animal studies indicate that CLA can increase lean muscle tissue and burn body fat. More recent studies with humans suggesting that CLA can work as a muscle-

building supplement and thermogenic aid have attracted the attention of athletes and weight-conscious adults.

At the 1997 Federation for Applied Science and Experimental Biology national meeting in New Orleans, Louisiana, two studies that were presented showed that CLA may help in the reduction of body fat and pointed to possible mechanisms for how it works. In the first study, scientists from the University of Wisconsin found that mice supplemented with CLA over a six-week period gained substantially less body fat (between 65 and 73 percent) than the control group of mice. The dose, 2.5 milligrams per calorie of food intake, translates into about 6,000 milligrams for a human consuming 2,500 calories per day. One explanation for the fat reduction is that the animals lowered their voluntary food intake by 9 percent to 13 percent. This calorie cut did not appear to affect the energy expenditure of the mice. On the contrary, the CLA-fed mice actually maintained a higher level of energy expenditure than did the control mice.

The second study, conducted by Michael Pariza, PhD, at the University of Wisconsin in Madison, looked at the effect of CLA on fat metabolism. He found that the effects of CLA on body composition in vitro appear to be partially due to reduced fat deposition and increased fat breakdown in the muscle cells.

In 1997, the first two studies of CLA supplementation by humans were reported. At the National Strength and Conditioning Association conference in Las Vegas, Richard Kreider, PhD, of Memphis State University, presented the findings of a study on the effects of CLA supplementation on catabolism, body composition, and strength during resistance training. In a double-blind manner, Dr. Kreider and his associates randomly assigned twenty-seven resistance-trained males to supplement their diets with capsules containing either an olive-oil placebo or CLA for twenty-eight days. Fasting blood samples, total body mass, and dual-energy X-ray absorptiometry (DEXA) determined body composition. Bench-press and leg-press tests on days zero and twenty-eight measured strength.

After the twenty-eight-day supplementation period, the researchers found no differences between the two groups in gross measures such as body weight, fat mass, and fat-free mass. However, analysis of the subjects' strength showed that the subjects in the CLA group had increased their overall strength by almost 30 pounds in both lifts, while the placebo group had improved by only 9.5 pounds. Though not statistically significant, these changes could indicate a trend. In addition, differences in the ratio of blood urea nitrogen to creatinine, a marker of tissue building versus tissue breakdown, suggested a potential net tissue-building effect. A longer supplementation period might lead to statistically significant differences.

Indeed, another researcher, Erling Thom, PhD, of Medatat Research Ltd, Lillestrom, Norway, conducted a longer study. This randomized, placebo-controlled, double-blind trial that involved twenty healthy people was three months long. Researchers measured the subjects' body weight and percent body fat at baseline and then again every four weeks. Each day, the treatment group consumed an amount of slightly more than 1,000 milligrams of CLA at breakfast, lunch, and dinner. The other half took a placebo. The average weight of the ten who took the CLA dropped by only about 5 pounds (not enough to be statistically significant), but their body-fat percentage dropped by a whopping 15 to 20 percent, or from an average of 21.3-percent body fat to about 17-percent body fat. Meanwhile, the group taking the placebo had little change. Half of the people in the study were men and half were women. Two dropped out because of unpleasant gastrointestinal upsets. Of these two, one came from the placebo group and the other from the CLA group.

The positive results from these two human studies laid the groundwork for future research on larger patient populations. In addition to looking at athletes, it would be interesting to study the effects of CLA on people who are obese.

Although scientists are not completely sure how CLA works, they've developed at least three theories. In one, CLA is believed to directly affect fat metabolism. By encouraging the body to preferentially burn fat and spare muscle glycogen, it could help muscle mass to be preserved at the expense of fat stores during exercise and fasting. In another theory, CLA is believed to somehow negate or counteract the adverse effects of hormones such as the corticosteroids. With overtraining, severe illness, and other stresses, the cortisol level rises. This adrenal-gland hormone then elevates the blood-sugar level, breaks down muscle protein, and increases fat deposition. In the third theory, CLA is thought to have the ability to increase the production of "good" prostaglandin E_1. Increased production of prostaglandin E_1 due to the supplemental intake of CLA (or, for that matter, of linoleic acid or preformed gamma-linolenic acid) offers an advantage for athletic performance. It has the unique ability to increase the brain level of the hormone somatotropin. Especially convenient for strength and power athletes, somatotropin increases GH output and thus increases the production of insulin-like growth factor I (IGF-I), which increases muscle growth. Relevant for endurance athletes is that prostaglandin E_1 also increases the blood flow to the muscles, brain, and other organs.

However it works, CLA, according to the preliminary data, may have value for people who need to burn fat while preserving muscle mass, particularly athletes. Based upon the research to date, the recommended daily dose of CLA ranges anywhere from .01 percent to 2 percent or more of daily caloric intake. One study proposes that, for a 165-pound person, a 3,500-milligram-per-day dose might be effective, with the range being 3,000 to 5,000 milligrams per day.

Daily intake goals of this magnitude require supplementation. Most people ingest less than 1,000 milligrams per day from food sources, which are largely limited to meat and dairy products. For example, cheese averages between 2.9 milligrams and 7.1 milligrams of CLA per gram of fat. To reach a 3,000-milligram CLA dose, you'd have to eat several pounds of cheese a day. That's a lot of unwanted dietary fat. For people want-

ing therapeutic results, it makes much more sense to consume CLA supplements.

Before the health conscious begin stocking up on CLA, however, more research needs to be done with people, including athletes and the overweight. Nevertheless, the message from the early studies is that CLA may hold health benefits.

in many foods. In fact, the major sources are evening primrose oil, borage oil, and black currant oil, which are also high in linoleic acid. GLA taken in dosages of 100 to 400 milligrams per day, in association with the essential fatty acids and omega-3 fatty acids, may benefit physical performance and health, especially during the season.

Medium-Chain Triglycerides

Medium-chain triglyceride (MCT) formulations were first made in the 1950s using coconut oil. MCTs contain saturated fatty acids with chains of six to twelve carbon atoms. They occur in milk fat and especially in coconut oil and palm oil. MCT formulations are high in caprylic acid and capric acid, which are saturated fatty acids. They are just now coming to the attention of athletes because they are relatively new on the market.

MCT formulations were originally developed as calorie sources for individuals who have certain pathologic conditions that do not allow normal digestion and utilization of long-chain fatty acids. MCTs tend to behave differently in the body than long-chain triglycerides (LCTs) do. They are more soluble in water, and they can pass from the intestines directly into the bloodstream. Fatty acids usually pass from the intestines first into the lymphatic system, then into the bloodstream. Because MCTs get into the bloodstream quicker than LCTs do, they are more easily and quickly digested. In addition, it has been reported in the medical literature that although MCTs can be converted to body fat, they are not readily stored in fat deposits and are quickly used for energy in the liver. They can also pass freely, without the aid of carnitine, into the mitochondria of cells. MCTs are therefore a potentially quick source of high energy for the body. MCTs reportedly also have a thermogenic effect, estimated to be 10- to 15-percent higher than their caloric value, but only when the MCTs in the diet exceed 30 percent of the total calories. Thermogenesis is the process by which the body generates heat, or energy, by increasing the metabolic rate to above normal.

These features of MCTs have recently attracted the attention of athletes, especially bodybuilders. Bodybuilders feel that these features benefit their restricted contest-preparation diets, which are aimed at reducing body fat and sparing muscle tissue. The implications of the use of large amounts of MCTs by athletes on restricted diets are not clearly evident, though. Some bodybuilders report that they are able to get "super lean" when they eat about 400 calories per day of

MCTs as part of a 2,000-calorie-a-day contest-preparation diet. Remember, though, that bodybuilders are not concerned with physical performance. In body-building contests, physique is judged.

MCTs may also have a place in the diets of endurance athletes, as part of the precompetition meal. Scientists hypothesize that this quick fuel source may be a better fuel than body stores of fatty acids and can perhaps spare muscle glycogen. Studies on athletes need to be performed to verify this. A major drawback of MCTs is their conversion to ketones during their metabolism by the body. Ketones are produced during the incomplete metabolism of fatty acids. They are acidic and can upset an individual's physiology. Although trained endurance ath-letes have developed the metabolic pathways (sequences of reactions) to better utilize ketones than untrained individuals, athletes experimenting with MCTs should do so several weeks before a major event to avoid an impaired perform-ance due to an elevated blood-ketone level.

Do MCTs have a place in every athlete's diet? More research is needed to determine the exact benefits of MCTs for athletes in general. While bodybuilders appear to derive certain benefits, some people can suffer side effects from eating too much MCT. The most common complaints are abdominal cramping and diarrhea. Prolonged use may also be harmful. MCTs are saturated fatty acids, and consuming more than 10 percent of total daily calories from saturated fatty acids is not recommended because of the link to various diseases. Additionally, in recent research, individuals who ingested only moderate amounts of MCTs developed elevated triglyceride and cholesterol blood levels. If you plan to experiment with MCTs, you should use formulations that also contain the essential fatty acids and the omega-3 fatty acids.

Phospholipids

Phospholipids are a second major class of lipids. Phospholipids are manufactured by the body. They are a major structural lipid in all organisms, a part of every liv-ing cell. In combination with proteins, they are constituents of cell membranes and the membranes of subcellular particles.

Phospholipids consist of two fatty acids attached to a three-carbon-atom glyc-erol molecule, with a phosphate-containing compound attached to the third car-bon atom. Their main function is maintaining the structural integrity of cell membranes. They also act as emulsifiers in the body—that is, during digestion, they help disperse fats in water mediums. They are important structural compo-nents of brain and nervous-system tissue and of lipoproteins, the conjugated pro-teins that transport cholesterol and fats in the blood.

Phospholipids are generally contained in the "invisible" fat of plants and ani-mals, not in the visible fat. Lecithin is the most well known phospholipid. Studies have also been conducted on the inositol-containing phospholipids, the phospho-inositides. The phosphoinositides' primary role is as a precursor of messenger mol-ecules. In this capacity, they have a profound effect on cellular functioning and on metabolism, particularly the metabolism of fats. The research into the phospho-inositides was prompted by observations made about choline- and inositol-deficient diets. Choline and inositol are nutrients that are important in fatty-acid metabolism and are said to help defat the liver. Nutrients that have this defatting action on the liver are called lipotropic agents. Choline also functions in memory, with diets deficient in choline associated with memory impairment. For the athlete, all of these important structural, metabolic, memory, and lipotropic roles of phospholipids are vital for peak performance.

Of the many phospholipids that exist, lecithin and phosphatidylserine are currently sharing the spotlight regarding supplemental use.

Lecithin

Lecithin (phosphatidylcholine) is a type of phospholipid that has choline attached to the phosphate molecule. Lecithin supplies the body with choline, which is essential for liver and brain functioning. Lecithin is also high in linoleic acid. Egg yolks, liver, and soybeans are rich in lecithin. In addition, lecithin is manufactured by the body.

The use of lecithin supplements came into vogue when researchers made the connection between choline and memory functioning. Lecithin's emulsifying properties are also thought to help keep the blood system clean of fatty deposits. Researchers have documented reduced choline levels in athletes running in the Boston Marathon and have speculated that a low choline level may adversely affect performance as well as have detrimental long-term effects on the nervous system. Choline is important in creatine synthesis and is therefore suspected of playing a role as a strength builder. Studies on athletes using dosages of 20,000 to 30,000 milligrams of lecithin have produced mixed results; some have reported beneficial effects on muscular power, performance, and endurance.

Phosphatidylserine

Recently, attention has turned to another phospholipid, phosphatidylserine (PS). In PS, serine is attached to the phosphate molecule. Serine is a nonessential amino acid whose metabolism leads to the synthesis of PS. Serine functions in fat metabolism and is vital to the health of the immune system. Intake of 200 to 300 milligrams of PS has been associated with improved memory and learning. Intake of 400 to 800 milligrams has been linked to a reduced level of cortisol, which is a catabolic hormone, as well as improved muscle growth and recovery after exercise.

DIGESTION OF LIPIDS

Lipids take the most time and effort to be digested by the human body because of their insolubility in water and their complex structures. As lipids pass through the mouth and stomach, they are treated mechanically and chemically in preparation for the main digestive processes, which take place in the intestines. Lipids take longer than the other macronutrients to empty from the stomach, about three to four hours or more, depending on the size of the meal. Their digestion takes place chiefly in the small intestine, where bile from the liver helps to bring them into contact with fat-splitting enzymes from the pancreas and the intestinal wall. In the intestines, the fatty acids are separated from the glycerol molecules; these components are then reassembled after they pass through the intestinal walls. Along the

ON THE CUTTING EDGE

Phosphatidylserine Proves Beneficial During Intensive Weight Training

A double-blind, crossover study measured the effects of 800 milligrams a day of phosphatidylserine (PS) compared to a placebo on the serum-hormone level of cortisol, the perception of well-being, and muscle soreness during two-week intensive training sessions. According to an abstract presented by Dr. Tom Fahey at the 1998 meeting of the American College of Sports Medicine, eleven trained male athletes participated in the study. The subjects were given either a PS supplement or a lecithin placebo for the first two-week session, then the opposite for the second two-week session. The subjects rested for three weeks in between the two sessions. During both of the two-week sessions, the subjects did five sets of exercises, each set consisting of ten repetitions of thirteen exercises, four times a week. For both sessions, resting venous blood samples were taken six mornings and a postexercise sample was taken fifteen minutes after the last workout. Well-being and muscle soreness were estimated using a ten-point scale. The cortisol levels of the subjects taking the PS decreased between the final resting blood sample and the postexercise sample. Well-being was perceived as greater by the subjects receiving the PS than those receiving the placebo. In the placebo groups, well-being was markedly depressed midweek. Muscle soreness increased in both groups of subjects but was 61 percent greater early in the first week and 55 percent greater later in the subjects receiving the placebo. Without exception, every subject was able to correctly identify when he was taking the PS. The subjects receiving the placebo reported a strong degree of debilitation during the study.

way, they are coated with protein. They then pass into the lymphatic system. Under normal conditions, about 60 to 70 percent of ingested fat is absorbed into the portal circulation via the lymphatic system. Medium- and short-chain fatty acids are absorbed directly from the intestines into the bloodstream.

Once in the bloodstream, fats and cholesterol are transported to the liver in conjunction with lipoproteins. The liver is the main processing center for lipids. In the liver, lipids may be converted for energy use or they may be modified—for example, the carbon chains of fatty acids may be shortened or lengthened or the degree of saturation may be increased or decreased. Any lipids that are not immediately needed by the body are converted into fat stores. The liver also synthesizes triglycerides, lipoproteins, cholesterol, and phospholipids.

Lipids are constantly being broken down, resynthesized, and used for energy in the body. They are in equilibrium when caloric intake is in balance with energy needs. However, when caloric intake from lipids, proteins, and carbohydrates exceeds energy needs, body-fat stores are increased.

YOU ARE WHAT YOU EAT

The type of lipid that you eat actually affects your body's fatty-acid composition. All cell membranes contain fatty acids. However, comparisons between vegetarians and meat eaters have revealed that a vegetarian's body is composed of more unsaturated fatty acids and a meat eater's body is composed of more saturated fatty acids. Also revealed was that people who consume diets high in saturated fat have bodies composed of more saturated than unsaturated fatty acids.

Saturated fatty acids tend to be less stable than unsaturated fatty acids and are therefore more susceptible to damage from free radicals and toxic metabolic waste products. This means that a body made of more unsaturated than saturated fatty acids may be more resistant to certain cellular damage. Since athletes are subject to high amounts of free radicals and metabolic toxins, they may be able to reduce muscle damage and increase recovery rates by consuming diets that have more unsaturated than saturated fats.

SPECIAL LIPID NEEDS OF THE ATHLETE

The NRC recommends that people of average health keep their total lipid intake below 30 percent of their total daily caloric intake and their saturated fat intake below 10 percent of their total daily caloric intake. This assumes that these people eat only the recommended total daily calories for their age and body size. Combined intake of linoleic and alpha-linolenic acids should be kept to 1 to 2 percent of total daily calories, which works out roughly to 3,000 to 6,000 milligrams. However, some health professionals estimate that males require three times this amount of these two essential fatty acids because of hormonal differences from females.

As far as athletes are concerned, the total amount of fat that should be consumed varies with the sport. In general, endurance athletes need to maintain higher levels of fat intake than do power athletes. The specific level is directly related to the energetics of the sport. Additionally, since the number of calories consumed daily by athletes is two to three times greater than the "average" total daily calories used by the NRC to determine its RDA values, using a rule of thumb can result in overestimation of fat intake.

Most athletes should concentrate on reducing their total lipid intake as well as their saturated-fat intake while at the same time increasing their essential fatty acid intake. Because athletes maintain such a high total intake of calories, they should not obtain over 25 percent of their total daily calories from lipids. In fact, most athletes should maintain a total fat intake of under 20 percent. Weight-conscious athletes should try to maintain a fat intake of about 15 percent. Furthermore, an athlete's essential fatty acid intake should be at least 9,000 or more milligrams per day of linoleic and alpha-linolenic acids. (For a discussion of lipids in the diet, see "Too Much Lipid in Our Diets" on page 59.)

FOOD SOURCES OF LIPIDS

Lipids from plant sources tend to be healthier than lipids from animal sources. At the same time, though, most plant proteins are incomplete and low in quality,

Too Much Lipid in Our Diets

Most of us consume too much lipid in our diets. Typical Americans get 45 percent of their total daily calories from lipids. When you consider that each gram of lipid contains more than twice the number of calories contained by a gram of carbohydrates or protein, you can easily see why fats and oils are such villains.

Furthermore, the very latest scientific studies reveal that fats and oils may be even more villainous than their caloric value suggests. In direct comparisons of high-fat and low-fat diets, even when the number of calories in each diet was identical, the high-fat diet caused much more fat to be stored.

So how much lipid should you consume in your diet? The American Heart Association recommends 30 percent of your total daily calories as the absolute maximum. But the closer you can get to 20 percent, or the more you can go below it, the easier it will be for you to attain your fat-loss or weight-maintenance goals. See the following table for what this means in calories.

Fat Calories Consumed on Different Diets

Total Daily Calories	Total Daily Fat Calories	
	20%-Fat Diet	30%-Fat Diet
2,400 calories	480 calories < 4 tablespoons fat	720 calories < 6 tablespoons fat
3,000 calories	600 calories < 5 tablespoons fat	900 calories < 8 tablespoons fat

The symbol < means "less than."

When calculating your own fat intake, keep in mind that 1 teaspoon of fat equals 5 grams, which equals 45 calories; and 1 tablespoon of fat equals 15 grams, which equals 135 calories.

while animal proteins are complete and high in quality. When planning your meals and snacks, you must try to strike a balance between these foods to minimize your intake of saturated fats and cholesterol but still benefit from complete proteins.

As a general rule, the foods you should avoid or eat infrequently include kidney, liver, egg yolks, custard, coconut oil, butter, palm oil, cream cheese, whole-milk products, and fatty meats, especially bacon, pork sausage, hot dogs, bologna, and hamburgers. These foods are high in saturated fatty acids and cholesterol. Instead, eat lean meats such as fish, chicken, and turkey; egg whites; skim-milk products; a combination of plant proteins that form a complete protein; and protein formulations. It is especially important for bodybuilders following a high-protein diet to monitor their lipid intake. Supplement formulations of pure proteins and amino acids can be extremely helpful.

Regarding sources of pure fat, such as oils, food sources high in polyunsaturated fats should be substituted for food sources high in saturated fats. Some fat sources that are low in saturated fats and cholesterol are margarine, corn oil, olive oil, peanut oil, cottonseed oil, safflower oil, sunflower oil, flaxseed oil, canola oil, wheat germ oil, evening primrose oil, sesame oil, soy oil, hemp oil, pumpkin seed oil, grape seed oil, fish oils, and most nuts. Nuts also supply protein. Fat sources to avoid include butter, bacon fat, cream, mayonnaise, and mayonnaise-based salad dressings.

As this chapter has made evident, you must always be on the lookout for fat, which so easily sneaks into the diet. Choose foods such as low-fat salad oil, then spoon it on rather than pour it on.

As you strive to reduce your fat intake, keep the following good news in mind: Each gram of fat that you replace with a gram of either protein or carbohydrate cuts your calories by more than half. As a result, you may be able to eat more food and lose body fat at the same time.

Why do our bodies store fat so readily when this can be so harmful to our health? The answer is that it was not always harmful. Before food became as plentiful as it is today, the body was able to pack away fat as an energy reserve for lean times. However, now that supermarkets and refrigerators make food plentiful all year long, our fat-storage capability has outlived its usefulness. Rather than serve as energy reserves, fat stores are now energy and health drains.

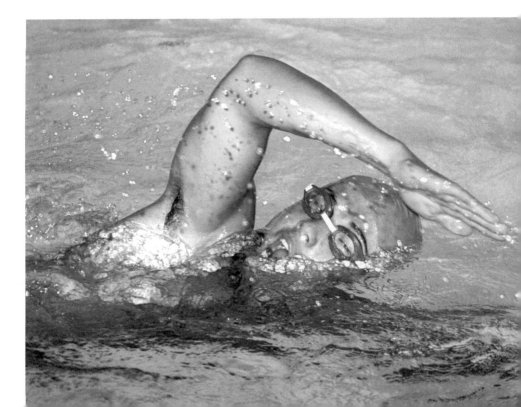

WATER
THE NEGLECTED NUTRIENT

4

ater is one of the most important nutrients for health and performance. Studies have verified that even minute fluctuations in the body's
water balance can, and often do, adversely affect performance. In spite
of this, many people take water for granted or neglect it. This is equally true for
athletes and nonathletes.

In this chapter, we will take an in-depth look at water. We will review its
functions and discuss how to optimize its intake for maximum performance.

WATER AND THE ATHLETE

Water, whimsically called H_2O by many people, consists of two hydrogen atoms
and one oxygen atom. It is the aqueous medium used for transporting the body's
food materials and the place where the body's biochemical reactions occur. Water
is found throughout the body, and depending on an individual's body fat, it can
vary in content from about 45 percent in very obese individuals to 70 percent in
very lean individuals. The different parts of the body also vary in water content.
For example, blood normally has the highest water content, at about 83 percent;
muscle tissue has a water content of about 75 percent; bone is about 22-percent
water; and fat tissue is only about 10-percent water.

A body's degree of hydration is affected by the person's rate of water intake in
relationship to his or her rate of water loss. Water loss is less under resting conditions than under conditions of high-intensity exercising. Water is obtained from
fluids that are ingested as liquids, from fluids that are present in more solid foods,
and as a result of metabolic activity within the body. It is estimated that the aver-
age-sized man, weighing about 170 pounds and performing moderate nonathletic activities, requires about 80 ounces of water per day to match his water loss.

The major sources of water for the human body are the following:

☐ *Liquids.* Liquids are by far the most abundant source of water for the body,
accounting for about two-thirds of a person's water intake per day. Liquids can
be readily taken in by the body without much digestive effort. Pure water is
taken in the fastest. As the carbohydrate and electrolyte contents of a liquid
increase, the length of time that it takes the liquid to empty from the stomach

increases. The exact concentration of carbohydrates and electrolytes that an athlete needs depends upon the sport and the level of physical activity.

☐ *Food.* All foods consist of water and solids. The amount of water that a food contains depends on what the food is. For example, fruits, vegetables, cooked cereals, and milk are 80- to 95-percent water. Meat cooked rare is about 75-percent water, while meat cooked well done is about 45-percent or less water. Ready-to-serve cereals are about 3- to 5-percent water. Generally, approximately one-third of daily water intake is from food.

☐ *Metabolic water.* Metabolic water is the water that is produced in the body as a result of energy production. Often overlooked, it totals approximately 10 ounces per day, depending on how many calories are burned. Metabolic water is produced from oxygen and hydrogen atoms. The oxygen atoms are obtained from the atmosphere and brought into the body via the lungs during breathing. The hydrogen atoms are obtained from carbohydrates, fatty acids, and other carbon molecules that are broken down in the body for energy.

☐ *Glycogen-bound water.* Glycogen-bound water is stored in the muscles along with glycogen. About 3 ounces of water are stored along with every 1 ounce of glycogen. Glycogen-bound water becomes important when the glycogen supply is in the process of being depleted for energy use. This occurs during training and endurance events lasting more than one hour and during periods of calorie restriction. During intensive endurance activities, about 16 fluid ounces of water may be released per hour. However, this water will be released only for as long as the glycogen to which it is bound remains stored in the body. Glycogen-bound water must be replenished when it is used. Altogether, approximately 3 to 4 pints of glycogen-bound water can be stored. For endurance athletes and athletes performing in day-long tournaments, glycogen-bound water is an important source of hydration during physical activity. It can be maximized through carbohydrate loading.

Water intake varies with the size of the individual, the duration and intensity of the activity, and the weather. Water loss is affected by factors such as the weather, the ability to acclimate to the temperature, the duration and intensity of the activity, the rate of sweating, the weight of the clothing worn, health, gastrointestinal problems, alcohol and caffeine consumption, the use of diuretics and other medications, and body fat.

EFFECTS OF DEHYDRATION ON PERFORMANCE

Dehydration can and does affect athletic performance. As the body loses water, its core temperature rises. This affects all the metabolic pathways, interferes with cardiovascular functioning, and reduces total exercise capacity. When the water losses reach 1 to 4 percent of the body weight, athletic performance is reduced. During a race, marathon runners can lose several quarts of water, representing 6 to 10 percent of their body weight. If they do not properly rehydrate during the race, they will find that this amount of water loss can significantly impair their performance and possibly even put their well-being at risk. Nonendurance sports such as football, basketball, hockey, and soccer can cause similar water losses. During tournaments, no matter what the sport is, athletes must make sure they increase their water intake to compensate for the prolonged exercise over the one or two days of competition.

Sports in which participants must meet weight-class requirements—boxing and wrestling, for example—are also associated with dehydration. Wrestlers typically dehydrate themselves to make a lower weight class. This type of chronic dehydration decreases performance and adversely affects health.

Chronic dehydration will develop in any athlete who does not make an effort to remain adequately hydrated. The thirst response in humans is not as finely tuned as it should be. This means that the body can enter a state of dehydration and the person may not feel the sensation of thirst for several hours. Therefore, you should not rely solely on your thirst response but should, instead, make a point to keep rehydrating your body all day long.

SPECIAL WATER NEEDS OF THE ATHLETE

The amount of water you need varies greatly according to your initial level of hydration, the climate, and the duration and intensity of your activity. As a general rule, measure your water intake by your water loss—namely, your frequency of

ON THE CUTTING EDGE

Skip Carbonated Beverages After Exercise

Drinking carbonated beverages following exercise may not be a good idea, according to a study conducted by the Gatorade Sports Science Institute and published in the *Penn State Sports Medicine Newsletter* in 1998. The problem is not that carbonation is bad for you but that it negatively affects "drink acceptability" and voluntary fluid intake. In the study, fifty-two adults participated in thirty minutes of aerobic activity two to four times a week and consumed one of five test drinks after each session. Altogether, five drinks were tested, one with no carbonation and the others with varying levels of carbonation. The amount of these drinks that the exercisers drank was voluntary and monitored for fifteen minutes. After drinking the drinks, the subjects evaluated them on the basis of factors such as throat burn, filling sensation, sweetness, and thirst quenching, which are all part of the definition of "drink acceptability." As a group, the exercisers drank less of the drinks with the two highest levels of carbonation and were less inclined to perceive those drinks as palatable. The levels of carbonation in both of these drinks fell within the range of commercially produced drinks. The authors concluded that carbonated beverages should not be the fluid-replacement choice following physical activity. Drinking a carbonated beverage might limit the consumption of fluids when they are most needed.

urination. If you are well hydrated, you should be urinating about once every one and a half to two hours. If you urinate only a few times per day, you probably need to increase your water intake. Because thirst is not a good indicator of hydration level, you should get in the habit of drinking water or other fluids frequently through the day.

Daily hydration guidelines are important for all athletes to follow. Studies have shown that endurance athletes who compete for periods longer than thirty minutes improve their performance by drinking fluids during the activity. Athletes competing in shorter events need to be properly hydrated from the start to achieve peak performance.

Daily Hydration Guidelines

Daily hydration is vital for everyone—endurance athletes, power athletes, and even nonathletes. Table 4.1 on page 65 presents water-intake guidelines for healthy, active individuals who exercise on a regular basis. Researchers have found that the best way to determine the recommended daily water intake is to look at daily energy expenditure. Table 4.1 provides a minimum daily water-intake range to accommodate individual differences as well as climatic differences. As the temperature climbs above 70° Fahrenheit (F) and the humidity above 70 percent, water loss will be increased due to increased sweating, especially during exercise.

Hydration Guidelines for Optimum Athletic Performance

Attaining and maintaining a peak hydration level starts by following the daily hydration guidelines discussed above. For athletes competing in endurance events lasting more than thirty minutes, hydration supercompensation (water loading) before an event as well as hydration maintenance during the event have been shown to increase athletic performance. (For a description of hydration super-compensation, see "Pre-event" on page 65.) Other athletes should make sure that they properly maintain their hydration levels leading up to the event, but they do

ON THE CUTTING EDGE

Go for the Sports Drink You Like

If you've ever tried to figure out which sports drink works the best, relax. Just go with the one you like. According to an article in *Medicine and Science in Sports and Exercise* in 1998, researchers in Australia had fifteen men run for ninety minutes on three different occasions. Each time, they provided the men with an unlimited amount of a particular beverage—either water or one of two different types of sports drinks. Overall, the men consumed much more of the sports drinks than they did of the water. Also, of the two sports drinks, the men drank more of the particular drink they thought tasted the best. In summary, drinking 8 to 10 ounces of *any* sports drink every fifteen to twenty minutes during exercise will help you stay hydrated and maintain your blood-glucose levels.

not necessarily need to concern themselves with drinking water during their events. One exception is athletes competing in tournaments that require participation in several events per day or several events over several days.

Specific guidelines for optimum athletic performance to be observed every day plus before, during, and after athletic events are as follows:

□ *Every day.* During your athletic season, keep track of your water intake on a daily basis. In addition, weigh yourself in the morning and after practice to keep track of your daily body-weight fluctuations. In general, the human body can lose only a maximum of a half pound of fat per day, so if you find yourself losing several pounds of body weight on a particular day, it is most likely from water loss. If you frequently perspire profusely, you should also take a multi-vitamin-and-mineral supplement every day.

□ *Pre-event.* Whether you are participating in an endurance or nonendurance event, you should load up on water about two hours before your competition. Depending on your body weight, you should consume between 18 and 24 ounces of water. This will allow you to "top off" your body with water and still give yourself enough time to urinate the excess before your event. Fifteen to twenty minutes before your event, drink another 12 to 20 ounces of water. Do not drink any alcohol, coffee, or other beverages that tend to act as diuretics. Also avoid taking any dehydrating medications.

□ *During endurance events.* Remember that the main reason for drinking water during endurance events is to replace sweat. Sweating is essential for cooling the body. If your body temperature increases too much during your event, your performance will suffer. To prevent this, you need to encourage sweating and make sure that the sweat evaporates from your body. Take special care on hot, humid days, which are the worst for athletic activities because they cause the most sweating with the least amount of evaporation. Ideally, during your event, drink 6 to 9 ounces of cool water every fifteen to twenty minutes.

□ *Postevent.* Give your body a chance to cool down and your heart rate a chance to normalize, then start drinking a sports rehydration drink. (For a discussion of sports rehydration drinks, see "Food and Supplement Sources of Water" on page 66.) Make sure to eat a meal within one to two hours after your event and consume the appropriate supplements for your sport.

Table 4.1. Daily Hydration Guidelines

Daily Energy Expenditure	Minimum Daily Water Intake
2,000 calories	64–80 ounces
3,000 calories	102–118 ounces
4,000 calories	138–154 ounces
5,000 calories	170–186 ounces
6,000 calories	204–220 ounces

Please note that if you follow these hydration guidelines during events, you should also follow them during practice. This way, your body will have a chance to adjust to ingesting the recommended amounts of water before the day of competition.

In addition, athletes participating in ultra-endurance events—that is, events lasting more than two hours—should consume fluids that contain glucose and the electrolytes. The solution should be hypotonic (diluted) because the more hypertonic (concentrated) a beverage is, the longer it takes to empty from the stomach.

FOOD AND SUPPLEMENT SOURCES OF WATER

Since water is the most abundant and most important nutrient in the body, we cannot live without it. For an athlete who trains regularly, water is even more important. Athletes who participate in endurance events must make sure to drink extra fluids. Some power athletes also perspire a lot and need fluids to replace those lost as sweat.

In recent years, however, the quality of water and other beverages has become a major concern for many people. Reports abound about the harmful effects of contaminants in drinking water and of chemicals in beverages. Because athletes consume far greater amounts of beverages than nonathletes do, their exposure to impurities in these products is greater. Try drinking pure water instead of soft drinks, juices, and other calorie-containing beverages.

Some time ago, scientists discovered that not just water is lost through sweating. Valuable minerals are lost, too. This discovery led to the development of sports rehydration drinks. The solutions that make up these drinks replace not only water but also the electrolytes—and they throw in some sugar for energy.

If you are an endurance athlete, you may find that drinking plain water for fluid replacement results in a low blood-sugar level. Low blood sugar produces early onset of fatigue and reduces endurance. Because the small intestine absorbs fluids from glucose-sodium solutions quite rapidly, sports rehydration drinks containing these two minerals are the best choice. Glucose stimulates sodium uptake in the small intestine, which markedly increases fluid absorption.

There are many different kinds of sports rehydration drinks available. In general, they fall into two broad categories—carbohydrate drinks and carbohydrate-protein drinks. Most of the drinks in both these categories are laced with minerals and/or vitamins. Calorie-wise, carbohydrate drinks range from 90 calories to over 400 calories per 16 fluid ounces of beverage, while carbohydrate-protein drinks have from 200 calories to over 500 calories per 16 fluid ounces. Carbohydrate-protein drinks also have up to 150 grams of carbohydrate and 32 grams of protein per 16 fluid ounces of beverage.

The lower-calorie carbohydrate drinks designed to rehydrate plus replenish the energy supply definitely improve performance for endurance athletes in events lasting more than one and a half hours. The performance benefits of carbohydrate drinks are less clear in athletic events and practice sessions of shorter duration. However, studies indicate that carbohydrate drinks containing a mid-range number of calories do help preserve the glycogen level during workouts lasting less than one and a half hours. Most of the research has shown that carbohydrate drinks work best when they are consumed just before and during exercise.

Carbohydrate-protein drinks can be consumed as a pretraining or precompetition meal about two to three hours before the start of an activity. They also make a convenient meal one hour after the completion of training or competition, plus they replace the protein and carbohydrates that were lost during the activity. They may also offer other benefits during workouts. Some research has indicated that consuming carbohydrate-protein drinks during weight-training sessions helps promote an overall increase in the GH level. GH is an important hormone involved in the mobilization of fatty acids, sparing of muscle glycogen, and promotion of positive nitrogen balance. Increasing the GH level is particularly important for athletes who train intensively, such as power athletes.

No matter what you choose to drink or when, remember that liquids intended to rehydrate the body work best when they are chilled. Both plain water and sports drinks are most effective when consumed at around 40°F. Remember, too, that if you plan to drink water or a sports drink during competition, you should also do so during training. The same way that your body needs to become accustomed to the physical demands of your activity, it also needs to adjust to the ingestion of liquids. The fewer surprises your body has to deal with during competition, the better your performance will be and the fewer gastrointestinal problems you will be rewarded with.

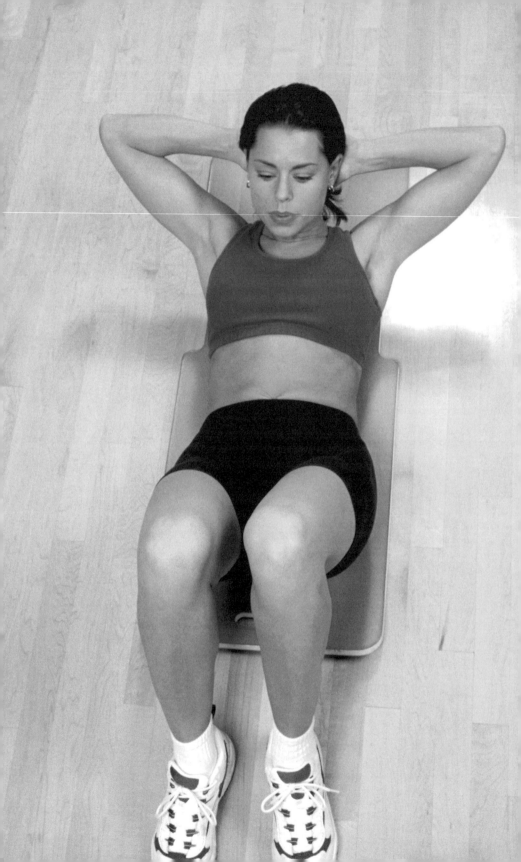

Vitamins and Minerals

5 Micronutrients for Optimum Performance

Athletes need to be especially careful about their diets. Although they may spend a good deal of time designing and following the "perfect" training program, they may also be surprisingly blasé about taking the nutrients their bodies need for increased activity and proper recovery. To do their best—and to stay healthy and injury-free—athletes must be mindful about what they eat. They also need to take vitamin and mineral supplements, which are an integral part of any carefully crafted dietary program.

A sensible starting place for any athlete would be to take one of the many multi-vitamin-and-mineral supplements commonly available for active people, such as General Nutrition Center's Mega Man or Mega Woman Formula, Twin-Lab's Sports Fuel, or Universal's Nutrition Genesis Formula. Since these formulas were specifically designed to deliver a broad range of vitamins and minerals, they can serve as an "insurance policy" against inadequate vitamin and mineral intake.

If your multivitamin supplement does not include minerals, you should take a multimineral supplement as well. While recommended intake levels have been established for calcium, iodine, iron, magnesium, phosphorus, selenium, and zinc, there are additional minerals that athletes, as well as nonathletes, require for proper functioning, even if only in trace (tiny) amounts. Vitamins and minerals tend to work in conjunction with each other, so it's vital that the necessary minerals be present to ensure that all the nutrients work properly in the body. To give just one example, zinc is required for the liver to release vitamin A from storage for use by the body as an antioxidant to protect against free-radical production. If you have no zinc, you will get no benefits from your vitamin A, even if your liver is bursting with it.

It's important to be aware of the recommended dosages, benefits, and possible side effects of all the vitamins and minerals you take. No one should take a nutritional supplement indiscriminately or without guidance, even if that guidance is only the label on the supplement bottle or a book about the nutrient. This is to protect against overconsumption of certain nutrients, such as the fat-soluble vitamins. Vitamin A, for example, can be toxic to the body, mainly the liver, if taken in large amounts for a long period of time.

In this chapter, we will take a look at vitamins and minerals. After examining what vitamins and minerals are, we will discuss vitamin and mineral supplements—

the forms they come in, how much to take, and how to read the labels. We will then review the specific vitamins and minerals that are important for athletes.

WHAT ARE VITAMINS AND MINERALS?

Vitamins are organic substances that are essential for metabolism, growth, and development of the body. You need only small amounts of these "accessory food factors" for survival, but without them, you can become sick and may not be able to operate at your maximum physiological potential.

All vitamins must be obtained from food or supplement sources. However, some are often ingested in their precursor form—that is, the form that comes before the vitamin form—and are converted to the active substance within the body. For example, vitamin A can be made from beta-carotene, and vitamin D can be created from substances in our skin in a process that is initiated by sunshine.

Vitamins are organized into two groups—the fat-soluble vitamins, including vitamins A, D, E, and K; and the water-soluble vitamins, including the B vitamins and vitamin C. The fat-soluble vitamins are stored in the liver and fatty tissues of the body, whereas the water-soluble vitamins are excreted in the urine.

Unlike vitamins, minerals are inorganic components of the body's tissues and fluids. They work in combination with enzymes, hormones, and vitamins, and participate in nerve transmission, muscle contraction, blood formation, and energy production. Also unlike vitamins, minerals make up a large portion of the body—up to 5 percent. Two types of minerals are required for the body to function properly—major minerals, including calcium, phosphorus, and magnesium, which the body requires in relatively large amounts; and trace minerals, including chromium and copper, which it needs in minute amounts.

DAILY REQUIREMENTS OF THE VITAMINS AND MINERALS

To help you determine how much of each vitamin and mineral you need, the Recommended Dietary Allowances (RDAs) were created as a guideline to the daily requirements for these nutrients. First presented fifty years ago, the RDAs have reflected the changing findings of vitamin and mineral research. Today, the experts disagree on the exact amounts of the nutrients needed by the body, but they agree that the incomplete data make it impossible to set RDAs for all the vitamins and minerals.

To further confuse the issue, the RDA values that have been set are targeted at average body types of specific age and sex groups. For example, women twenty-five to fifty years old are assumed to be 5 feet 4 inches tall and weigh 138 pounds. Obviously, not every woman in that age group meets these requirements, making the dosages for them uncertain.

Sex, age, and size are not the only factors that must be considered when determining nutrient supplementation. Your diet, health, physical activity, biochemical individuality, and ability to absorb food elements all help dictate your vitamin and mineral needs, making dosages even more difficult to determine.

Increased energy needs and everyday stresses may necessitate taking nutritional supplements. Modern agricultural and food-preparation practices rob food of essential nutrients—crops are grown in nutritionally depleted soil; processing and refining strip vitamins and minerals from whole foods; and storage and cooking further diminish foods' nutritional values. Once you have eaten a food, the stress caused by the demands of modern living can rob you of whatever nutrients may have been remaining in the food. Although eating a well-balanced, healthful diet is the best way to obtain nourishment, supplements are sometimes needed to support the body so that it can function at its physiological optimum.

In addition to supplying nutrients for general health and well-being, supplements can also help prevent and cure illness. For example, vitamin C is used to treat the common cold, and calcium is often recommended to prevent age-related bone loss.

THE RIGHT BALANCE OF VITAMINS AND MINERALS

To help you determine whether you are getting the right balance of nutrients, the government has established the Reference Daily Intakes (RDIs) and Daily Reference Values (DRVs) as standards for nutrient intake. The RDIs include recommendations for twenty-seven vitamins and minerals, and the DRVs include recommendations for the macronutrients and two electrolytes. They are similar but not identical to the RDAs. The RDIs and DRVs are based on allowances set a number of years ago, so many of today's knowledgeable scientists know that a number of the values are out of date. The government has slowly been updating the recommendations. Recently, it updated the RDI for calcium.

The RDIs and DRVs are not requirements but rather estimates of the intake levels for the macronutrients, vitamins, and minerals that are safe and adequate for maintaining good health in most people. Each value was set to meet the requirements of the age and sex group with the highest need for the particular nutrient. For example, the RDI for iron is based on a woman's need and is overly generous for men. You should try to meet the RDIs and DRVs on a daily basis.

The Daily Values (DVs) compose a system created by the Food and Drug Administration (FDA) to help food and supplement manufacturers present their RDI and DRV information on their product labels. The DVs are the amounts of the nutrients in a product described as percentages, with 100 percent being equivalent to the total amount of a nutrient required by a "reference individual" consuming a 2,000-calorie-per-day diet. Note that the terms "Reference Daily Intakes," "Daily Reference Values," "RDI," and "DRV" never actually appear on nutrition labels.

As we will see throughout this book, scientific studies have shown that larger dosages of many vitamins and minerals are needed for our bodies to perform at their optimum. Therefore, the RDAs, RDIs, and DRVs have limited application for determining the optimum intake of the different vitamins for active individuals. Many nutritionists therefore prefer to use guidelines such as nutritionist Shari Lieberman's optimum daily intakes (ODIs)—the amounts needed for optimum health and performance. In this book, the intake recommendations for all the nutrients discussed are for the goal of optimum physiological performance.

To help athletes meet their special nutrition needs, a set of standards called the performance daily intakes (PDIs) was developed. The PDIs, the same as the RDIs and ODIs, are guidelines for the intake of nutrients based on the findings of scientific research studies. The PDI guidelines are for both men and women, and they compensate for the higher nutritional requirements that athletes have over nonathletes. They are dynamic, taking into consideration a wide range of needs, activity levels, and body sizes. They are for healthy adults who are currently in active training. In most cases, the lower limit of the PDI range is equal to the RDI value and can probably can be met with food sources. The upper limits are generally recognized as safe, but are intended for larger, more active individuals. The ranges will help you to keep your daily supplement intake within a safe range. If you use more than one supplement containing some of the same vitamins and minerals, add up your intakes of the affected vitamins and minerals from the different supplement sources to make sure that your total intakes are not too high. Always consult a healthcare practitioner before changing your diet or adding a new dietary supplement to your regimen to make sure that the change is appropriate for you.

VITAMIN AND MINERAL SUPPLEMENTS

Vitamin and mineral supplements come in many forms. Tablets and capsules are the most common, but powders and liquids are also available.

Be aware that many supplements contain additives. A filler such as salt or sugar may be used to fill up the space in a capsule. Cornstarch or molasses might be used as a binder to help keep a tablet intact. A disintegrator such as potato or cornstarch may be employed to promote tablet dissolution after ingestion, and artificial or natural colorings or flavorings are often added to make a supplement more appealing.

Many athletes wonder if there is a difference between natural and synthetic supplements. Although synthetic vitamins and minerals produce satisfactory results, the benefits from natural products surpass them on a variety of levels. The results of chemical analyses of both might appear the same, but there's more to natural vitamins because there's more to those substances in nature.

Synthetic vitamin C is just that—ascorbic acid and nothing more. Natural vitamin C from rose hips contains the bioflavonoids and the entire vitamin-C complex, which makes the vitamin C itself much more effective. On the other hand, people who are allergic to rose hips may experience an undesirable reaction to a natural vitamin C with pollen impurities. Natural vitamin E, which may include all the tocopherols, not just alpha, is more potent than its synthetic version. Nonetheless, as many who have tried both can attest, there is less gastrointestinal upset with the natural supplement than with the synthetic and far fewer toxic reactions when taken in higher than the recommended dosage. This is important, since many athletes take more than the recommended RDA for optimum health, performance, and recovery.

The Proper Dosage

Vitamin and mineral supplements offer a safe and effective way to improve your energy metabolism, health, and recovery. However, taking a larger dose than recommended is not always better. All substances, even water, can be harmful at high levels. Some vitamins and minerals, such as vitamins A and D, can cause acute poisoning when taken in massive amounts. Even slightly excessive levels taken over a period of time may lead to chronic toxicity. For example, vitamin K taken in megadoses can accumulate in the body and cause flushing and sweating.

When megadoses of vitamins and minerals are ingested, they can have a druglike effect. Therefore, you need to understand the dosages you plan to take before embarking on a megadosage-therapy program. Also, don't assume that you need to supplement with every vitamin and mineral. Iron, although found in many multivitamin-and-mineral formulas, should be taken only when indicated, such as in cases of iron-deficiency anemia. Excess iron can increase the risk of heart disease, cancer, and diabetes. For example, the buildup of iron in the tissues has been associated with a rare disease known as hemochromatosis, a hereditary disorder of iron metabolism that causes a bronze skin pigmentation, cirrhosis of the liver, diabetes, and heart disorders.

The Label

The list of ingredients on some vitamin and mineral supplement labels could tax the mind of even a PhD in nutrition! The challenge is to distinguish the truth from the marketing hype. Many companies select the ingredients or dosages for their products based on published research demonstrating a nutrient's effectiveness or the experience of skilled professionals. However, some companies select ingredients or dosages based on marketing strategies that take advantage of recent news reports on a specific nutrient.

The marketing strategies used by supplement companies are as varied as the manufacturers. For example, in order to make an ingredient list look longer and more beneficial, marketers may add nutrients that are present in useless amounts. Many vitamins and minerals may be included in the product, but the dosages may be incapable of improving health or performance. Therefore, you must learn the useful levels of the nutrients.

Some companies add items to their multi-vitamin-and-mineral formulas that sound good but have no real performance benefits. For example, vitamin E, to be effective as an antioxidant and at reducing muscle soreness, must be taken in dosages of at least 400 international units, not the RDA of 30 international units. So, if the label of an antioxidant formula says that it contains vitamin E, make sure that the vitamin is included in an adequate amount. Natural substances, such as the flavonoids and herbs, are often added to combination formulas in quantities that provide many benefits.

Some companies exaggerate the quality of their products by using just a little of a nutrient from a superior source and a lot of the nutrient from an inferior source, but not telling how much of each. For example, if a label lists "calcium (carbonate, citrate-malate)," you cannot tell how much of the calcium comes from carbonate and how much from citrate-malate. The product could contain as little as 1 percent of its calcium supply from citrate-malate, which is the much more expensive form. The label should state the amount of each source—for example, "calcium (carbonate), 400 milligrams, and calcium (citrate-malate), 100 milligrams"—or the ratio of the sources—for example, "calcium (four to one carbonate to citrate-malate)."

Most vitamins and minerals come in a variety of forms, such as inorganic salts, organic chelates, coenzyme forms, natural forms, and synthetic forms. Scientific studies show that some forms are better absorbed and utilized by the body than others. In general, natural vitamin E is better than synthetic vitamin E; vitamin-B coenzymes are better than regular B vitamins; and fully reacted chelates (such as aspartates, picolinates, citrate-malate, and glycinates) may be better absorbed and utilized than inorganic salts (such as carbonates, oxides, and sulfates). A supplement that includes multiple forms of a nutrient may be helpful if a person's ability to absorb one specific form is blocked or compromised. Look for brands that include well-studied and documented forms of specific nutrients.

The same as food labels, supplement labels must now also include nutrition facts. According to a recent ruling made by the FDA, the new "supplement facts" panel must include:

☐ An appropriate serving size.

☐ The amount of the product as a whole, with a list of the specific ingredients.

☐ The amounts of fourteen specific nutrients, including vitamins A and C, calcium, iron, and sodium, as well as of any other nutrients that are added or are part of the nutritional claim made on the label.

☐ The dietary ingredients for which RDAs have not been established.

☐ The plant parts used if the product is botanical.

This is just a quick course on reading supplement labels. For more information, check out the FDA's website at http://www.fda.gov. (For a brief run-down of the lingo normally used, see "Label Lingo" on page 76.) Discussing every label regulation and and highlight would necessitate a separate book. When in doubt about a supplement, form, or brand to buy, ask your local health-food-store staff for assistance.

When and How to Take Supplements

Your body operates on a twenty-four-hour cycle. Your cells do not go to sleep when you do, nor can they exist without continuous oxygen and nutrients. Therefore, for best results, take your vitamin and mineral supplements at evenly spaced intervals throughout the day.

The prime time for taking supplements is after meals. Vitamins are organic substances and should be taken with food or mineral supplements for the best absorption. In addition, our bodies tend to excrete in the urine the substances we ingested within the past four hours. This is particularly true of the water-soluble vitamins. When the stomach is empty, the B vitamins and vitamin C may be excreted as quickly as two hours after ingestion. (The fat-soluble vitamins, including vitamins A, D, E, and K, remain in the body for approximately twenty-four hours, though excess amounts can be stored in the liver and fat cells for much longer.) Taking your vitamins after breakfast, lunch, and dinner will help keep your body levels of the water-soluble vitamins as high as possible.

If taking supplements after each meal is not convenient, take half the amounts after breakfast and the other halves after dinner. If you must take your vitamins all at once, take them after your largest meal of the day. In other words, for the best results, take them after dinner, not after breakfast. And remember, minerals are essential for proper vitamin absorption, so be sure to take your minerals and vitamins together.

If vitamins are kept cool, away from light, and well-sealed, they should last for two to three years. To ensure freshness, though, your best bet is to buy brands that have an expiration date printed on the label. Once a bottle is opened, the product will be good for about twelve months.

THE ROLE OF VITAMINS AND MINERALS IN ENERGY PRODUCTION

Energy metabolism is the set of processes the body uses to break down the macronutrients into fragments and then use those fragments either to generate energy for muscle contractions or to build body compounds. Carbohydrates, lipids, and protein yield glucose, glycerol and fatty acids, and amino acids, respectively. Glucose can form chains of glycogen or break down into fuel fragments. Glycerol and fatty acids can form triglycerides or break down into fuel fragments. And amino acids can form protein chains or be stripped of their amine groups to yield fuel fragments similar to those derived from carbohydrates and lipids.

Within the metabolic pathway known as the Krebs cycle, the major energy pathway in the body, vitamins, minerals, and other nutritional components undergo a precisely orchestrated progression of reactions that ultimately yields energy. Releasing all of the energy contained in carbohydrates, lipids, and protein in one step would result in lost and wasted heat energy. Therefore, the energy is released in several steps. Several coenzymes assist in this multi-step process, with a number of vitamins lending helping hands.

In addition to assisting coenzymes, vitamins can also function as coenzymes in the body. A coenzyme is a heat-stable substance of low molecular weight that participates in a wide variety of biological processes, such as the Krebs cycle. Of the many compounds that can be considered coenzymes, clearly the most abundant and most active within the energy cycle consist of or originate from a common source—vitamins. When vitamins serve as coenzymes, they act principally as regulators of metabolic processes and play roles in energy transformations. For example, the primary function of the water-soluble vitamins (the vitamin-B complex and vitamin C) within the process of metabolism is acting as coenzymes. It is the coenzyme that combines with the inactive protein to create the active enzyme within the energy cycle. Coenzymes work together to help release energy from the three macronutrients. They stand alongside the metabolic machinery and help keep the disassembly lines moving.

Label Lingo

When choosing a supplement to meet your specific needs, do certain terms elude you? Do you find words such as "chelate," "elemental," or "enteric" confusing? If so, let's take a look at some of the more commonly used terms:

☐ *Bioavailability.* Bioavailability is the relative rate at which a vitamin or mineral reaches the general circulation. This rate is especially important when a supplement is taken orally. Factors that influence the bioavailability of a vitamin or mineral are its solubility in the stomach, the tablet size, the formula, and the other foods and drinks in the stomach.

☐ *Chelate.* A chelate is a compound formed by a mineral and its carrier. A carrier is a substance such as an amino acid that increases the absorbability of the mineral. A mineral, in its most basic form, cannot be carried through the body. It must link up with a transporter, which normally occurs during digestion. Once linked, the mineral is called a "chelated mineral." Unfortunately, the amount of a mineral generally absorbed can be quite low depending on such variables as the strength of the stomach acid, which tends to decrease with age. Purchasing chelated minerals ensures greater absorption and, hopefully, more health benefits.

☐ *Coenzyme.* A coenzyme is a recently discovered type of "active" vitamin sold either singularly or in combination formulas. Some vitamins are not active until they are absorbed through the intestinal wall and converted into a coenzymatic form. For example, vitamin B_6 is converted into its coenzyme form, pyridoxal-5-phosphate, once it is absorbed. Pyridoxal-5-phosphate is the compound that initiates metabolic activity in the body. Vitamins sold in coenzyme forms, such as vitamins B_2 and B_6, are purportedly better utilized by individuals who suffer from metabolic or digestive problems.

☐ *Elemental.* The term "elemental" refers to the amount of a mineral in a compound. For example, the "elemental amount of calcium" is the exact weight or potency of the calcium in a formula. If information is listed in parentheses immediately following the name, it is the form, chelating material, or source of the ingredient. If an ingredient's form, chelating material, or source is not in parentheses, the actual amount of the ingredient is less than the stated amount. For example, if the

---

Minerals are responsible for structural functions involving the skeleton and soft tissues, and for regulatory functions, including neuromuscular transmission, acid-base balance, water balance, blood clotting, oxygen transport, and enzymatic activity. They normally account for about 4 percent of a body's weight—for example, they compose about 6 pounds of the body weight of a 150-pound person—and are categorized according to their amount in the body. The minerals that make up more than 0.01 percent of the body weight are called major minerals, or macronutrient elements. Calcium and phosphorus are the most abundant major minerals, together accounting for 75 percent of the mineral content of the average adult. The minerals that make up less than 0.01 percent of the body weight are called trace minerals, or micronutrient elements.

ingredient were written as "magnesium aspartate" with no parentheses, you would actually be getting only about 20 percent of the listed amount of magnesium. This is because magnesium aspartate, by weight, is actually only about 20-percent magnesium; the remaining 80 percent is the carrier, aspartate. On the other hand, if the ingredient were written as "magnesium (aspartate)," you would be getting 100 percent of the listed amount of the magnesium.

☐ *Enteric.* An enteric coating is used on tablets to delay digestion of the tablet until it passes from the stomach into the intestines.

☐ *Krebs cycle complex.* The Krebs cycle is a process that produces energy within the cells. A Krebs cycle complex is the result of a method of chelation that utilizes substances that are part of the Krebs cycle, such as succinates, gluconates, and citrates. Commonly found in sports supplements, they enhance absorption and help increase the energy level.

☐ *Sublingual.* A sublingual tablet is a tablet that is placed under the tongue and allowed to dissolve through the buccal membrane. The nutrients bypass the digestive process and go directly into the bloodstream. Some people who have difficulty assimilating vitamins such as B$_{12}$ experience greater absorption with this form of supplement.

☐ *Unesterified.* An unesterified vitamin is a vitamin that is not in an ester form, which is a combination of an acid and an alcohol. The term is usually associated with natural vitamin E. Unesterified vitamin E is readily available to act as an antioxidant. Esterified forms of the vitamin, such as the succinate form, must undergo a digestive transformation before the vitamin is available for use.

There are also a number of terms that are popularly used on labels that are strictly regulated by the government. For example, manufacturers must follow certain rules if they use the terms "high potency" or "antioxidant." Products labeled "high potency" must supply 100 percent or more of the RDI or DRV of the nutrient. The term may be used on a multi-ingredient product if the formula supplies 100 percent or more of two-thirds of the ingredients. "Antioxidant" may be used if scientific research shows that the product will inactivate free radicals or prevent free-radical damage in the body.

Minerals can be a confusing subject, since not only do the functions of the different minerals vary, but the interactions of the different minerals do, too. In addition, some minerals affect the absorption, function, or excretion of other minerals, so pinpointing the exact characteristics and contributions of the minerals within complex biological systems becomes perplexing. However, one characteristic believed to be shared by all the minerals is the ability to directly or indirectly affect the body's energy level.

VITAMINS AND MINERALS AS ANTIOXIDANTS

A further function of certain vitamins and minerals is to serve as antioxidants. Antioxidants are the body's chief nutritional defenses against the detrimental effects of free radicals. Free radicals are reactive fragments of molecules that are produced during normal metabolism. However, they are produced in excess in reaction to external insults such as air pollution, ultraviolet light, stress, and the extra oxygen inhaled during exercise.

A stable compound has electrons in pairs. If an electron becomes unpaired, the compound becomes reactive and unstable. Such a compound will seek out another electron with which to unite in order to return to a stable state. The process, however, leads to the gradual degeneration of healthy tissue. A compound or element with an unpaired electron is called a free radical.

Among the havoc that free radicals wreak is attacking and altering cellular enzymes, the protein-derived catalysts that speed all metabolic processes. (For a complete discussion of enzymes, see Chapter Six.) A damaged enzyme is inactivated, which slows or halts all the processes dependent on that enzyme, including the liberation of energy. Additionally, free radicals activate dormant enzymes, which in turn can cause tissue damage or disease, such as emphysema, or can release neurotoxins affecting nerve or brain function or muscle soreness.

Little did you know that increased exercise can have a negative effect on your body. Yes, after all these years of telling us about the benefits of exercise—reduced body fat, increased cardiorespiratory fitness, increased strength, and reduced stress—scientists are now discovering a link between exercise and the formation of free radicals. Do free radicals sound like a group of terrorists in your body? They are. Oxygen is critical for life and for the production of the energy necessary to strength-train, run, cycle, and swim. But, ironically, some of the chemical reactions that oxygen triggers within your body can create free radicals. Free radicals attack the walls of your muscle cells, mitochondria, heart, and blood vessels. They cause problems for the body by damaging the structures of cells and by reducing the cells' abilities to function and regulate themselves.

If you exercise, you may even be at greater risk than "couch potatoes" because of the higher level of free-radical production in your body. Here's why: While exercising, you take in much more oxygen than you would if you were resting, leading to an increased number of muscle cells and an increased number of muscle-cell mitochondria (the structures involved in aerobic metabolism). The resulting increased mitochrondrial activity is thought to increase oxidation and free-radical production.

Exercise increases the release of the hormones epinephrine and norepinephrine to help charge up your nervous system, release fats from your fat stores, and increase the supply of glycogen to your muscles. The oxidation of these hormones has been shown to be related to free-radical formation.

Exercising in smoggy conditions can lead to increased intake of ozone and nitrogen oxide. With the increased rate and depth of breathing experienced during exercise, you are once again increasing the number of free radicals in your body. When the oxygen combines with the ozone or nitrogen oxide, an even greater number of free radicals is produced.

Free-radical damage has been linked not only to reduced exercise ability but also to problems specifically associated with aging, declining immune function, atherosclerosis, and Parkinson's disease. There may also be a direct link to cancer and heart disease, which together account for 80 percent of all the deaths in the United States.

Fortunately, our bodies are equipped to fight the ravages of free radicals with substances called antioxidants, which halt or inactivate these dangerous molecular byproducts and help repair the cellular damage. Antioxidants keep the damage from getting out of control in the body. Antioxidants are to the cells what traffic lights are to cars—they prevent destruction and mayhem. But the more oxygen cellular activity (traffic) there is, the more antioxidants (traffic lights) are needed.

The body creates its own antioxidants in the form of enzymes such as superoxide dismutase (SOD). But antioxidants are also found in vitamins C and E, as well as in beta-carotene, a precursor of vitamin A. The bioflavonoids, selenium, and zinc are other vitamins and minerals that have been found to be effective in the fight against free radicals. Additionally, there is good scientific news that shows specific herbs may be linked to combating free radicals in the body. Ginkgo, milk thistle, rosemary, Siberian ginseng, red Korean ginseng, grape seed extract, green tea, and turmeric are some of the more popular antioxidant herbs.

Free radicals are at least partially to blame for muscle damage, soreness, and reduced endurance. During intensive exercise, free radicals damage the muscle cells, which leads to inflammation and acute muscle soreness. Several studies have shown that optimum levels of antioxidants may reduce muscle injury and improve endurance.

Research coming out of the University of California showed that when athletes ran to exhaustion on a treadmill, two important enzymes normally found in muscle cells appeared in high concentrations in their blood. In a second trial, the runners were given daily doses of 1,000 milligrams of vitamin C, 10 milligrams of beta-carotene, and 800 international units of vitamin E for eight weeks. When the treadmill tests were repeated, the athletes had much lower concentrations of the two enzymes in their blood. This suggested that the athletes reduced their muscle-cell damage after taking the antioxidants. The athletes also had significantly higher blood levels of glutathione preoxidase, an antioxidant that helps prevent damage to muscle-cell membranes.

Vitamin C has many important functions, including enhancing iron absorption, producing collagen, assisting wound healing, and stimulating the immune system. As an important water-soluble antioxidant, vitamin C specializes in scavenging oxidants and free radicals in the water regions of the cells and the blood. The RDA for vitamin C is 60 milligrams, but many researchers recommend anywhere from 250 to 1,000 milligrams per day to prevent cell damage, serve as an antioxidant, prevent heart disease, and help prevent cancer. Remember also that vitamin C plays an important role in the uptake of iron in the body.

Beta-carotene and vitamin A are related. Beta-carotene serves both as a precursor to vitamin A and as an antioxidant by itself. Although vitamin A is not a very active antioxidant, it helps your body resist infection and neutralizes the effect of free radicals. It has also been shown to reduce the incidence of cancer. The RDA for vitamin A is 5,000 international units. Many people now believe, however, that you need about 10,000 to 20,000 international units of vitamin A per day to fight infections and battle free radicals.

Beta-carotene is not a vitamin, but a plant pigment that is converted to vitamin A once it is inside the body and the body has a need for it. When you eat a carrot or orange, part of the beta-carotene is converted to vitamin A. The remaining beta-carotene acts as an antioxidant, dousing free radicals and preventing oxidative damage. While no RDA has been established for beta-carotene, most scientists recommend a minimum intake of 5 to 10 milligrams per day.

Many in the medical community claim that vitamin E is the master antioxidant. Vitamin E has been shown to reverse some of the signs of aging and other changes that occur as a result of oxidative damage. Older individuals have greater levels of the markers of oxidative damage called lipid peroxides. However, when the elderly in one research study took a vitamin-E supplement in amounts twenty to forty times the RDA, the levels of these markers went down, suggesting a slowing of the aging of the cells.

The same results were found with a group of athletes. Athletes experience oxidative damage to muscle cells during exercise. A study on vitamin-E supplementation using as little as 400 international units per day showed decreased levels of malondialdehyde (MDA) after running. MDA is a marker for muscle-cell oxidation. Twenty-five female runners were measured for MDA before and after a thirty-minute treadmill run. The post-run levels of MDA increased over 30 percent in the group that did not take the vitamin-E supplements.

The RDA for vitamin E is 30 international units, but studies have used much higher levels, up to 800 international units daily, for three years without toxic effects. A minimum intake of 200 international units is recommended for those who exercise intensely or are routinely exposed to air pollutants during exercise.

Exercise may not only increase muscle and other cell damage, but may also have an effect on the immune system. Intensive training and racing suppress the immune system and increase susceptibility to colds, flu, and infection. There is most likely a link between intensive exercise, immunity, and antioxidants. After intensive exercise, the immune system needs a boost.

The stress your immune system experiences when fighting free radicals may make you susceptible to infections and colds when exercising vigorously and often. So, besides fighting free radicals, antioxidants are essential for optimum functioning of the immune system.

People who exercise intensively, are exposed to stress and poor air quality, eat too much processed food, and are exposed to radiation, whether from the sun or medical X-rays, may not be obtaining the key antioxidant nutrients. Even more problematic is the possibility that the RDAs of the antioxidants may be insufficient to provide a strong enough defense against free radicals and infections.

VITAMINS—YOUR BODY'S CATALYSTS

Vitamins are organic chemicals, substances that contain carbon, hydrogen, and oxygen. They occur naturally in all living things, plants as well as animals—flowers, trees, fruits, vegetables, chickens, fishes, and cows.

Vitamins regulate a variety of body functions. They are essential for building body tissues, such as bones, skin, glands, nerves, and blood. They assist in the metabolism of carbohydrates, proteins, and lipids so that you can get energy from food. They prevent nutritional-deficiency diseases, promote healing, and encourage good health.

Your body needs at least eleven specific vitamins—vitamins A, C, D, E, and K, and the members of the B-complex family including folate and vitamins B_1, B_2, B_3, B_6, and B_{12}. Two more B vitamins—vitamin B_5 and biotin—are now believed to be valuable for your well-being as well. You need only miniscule quantities of the vitamins for good health. In some cases, the RDAs may be as small as several micrograms.

The Fat-Soluble Vitamins

Vitamins are classified as either fat-soluble or water-soluble, meaning that they dissolve in either fat or water. If you take in a larger amount of a fat-soluble vitamin than your body needs, the excess will be stored in your body fat. Therefore, you must be very careful not to take more than the RDAs of these vitamins. The vitamins that are fat-soluble and require careful supplementation are vitamins A, D, E, and K.

Vitamin A and the Carotenoids

Vitamin A and its family members, including the carotenoids such as beta-carotene, lutein, and lycopene, all have a variety of important uses in healing and preventive medicine. If you use supplements, it's extremely important to know exactly what type of vitamin A–related substance you are dealing with, as well as the medical implications of using it.

Vitamin A (retinol) plays an important role in maintaining the quality and health of your eyesight, skin, teeth, bones, and mucous membranes (the mucous-producing cells that line such bodily surfaces as the nasal passages, respiratory tract, and intestines). Also, vitamin A assists in the growth and repair of body tissues and may bolster your resistance to infection. As an antioxidant, the vitamin-A precursor beta-carotene, in high blood levels, has been linked to a reduction in the risk of lung cancer.

But there is also a downside to vitamin A—the nutrient can be toxic if you allow too much to enter your body, especially through supplementation. When persons who are not healthy or in active training take doses in excess of 10,000 international units, the result may be vitamin overdose, with symptoms including blurred vision, hair loss, nausea, and dry skin. In the most severe cases, there may also be damage to the liver, birth defects, and enlargement of the spleen. But, except for birth defects, which may result when a woman takes more than 10,000 international units per day during pregnancy, serious vitamin-A problems may tend to occur only after a person has taken 50,000 international units a day for many years. Therefore, the PDI of vitamin A for men and women who are healthy and actively training is 5,000 to 25,000 international units.

Beta-carotene, a chemical precursor of vitamin A, presents a somewhat different picture. Beta-carotene, which is transformed into vitamin A after entering the body, is part of the carotenoid family of nutrients. The carotenoids' pigments are the sources of the yellow, orange, and green colors in certain vegetables and fruits, such as carrots, cantaloupes, sweet potatoes, spinach, collard greens, and kale. Higher blood-serum levels of beta-carotene have been linked to lowered risks of cataracts, heart disease, and cancer, including rectal cancer, melanoma, and bladder cancer. But the question is, how do you increase the amount of this nutrient in your blood?

The best way to take beta-carotene into your body is through foods high in the nutrient, such as carrots and sweet potatoes. Recent studies have cast doubt on the benefits of getting beta-carotene through supplements. Generally speaking, beta-carotene taken in supplement doses below 50,000 international units (30 milligrams) will have no effect. Until the findings are verified, the PDI of beta-carotene for men and women who are healthy and actively training will remain at 15,000 to 60,000 international units. For endurance athletes, the PDI of beta-carotene will remain at 20,000 to 80,000 international units.

Beta-carotene is usually sold in international units, but sometimes you will find a reference to it in milligram doses. For the purpose of conversion, 1 international unit of beta-carotene equals 0.6 microgram of the nutrient, or 0.0006 milligram. So, to convert international units of beta-carotene to milligrams, multiply the international unit by 0.0006. To convert milligrams of beta-carotene to international units, divide the milligrams by 0.0006. Suppose a bottle contains beta-carotene in 25,000 international units per capsule. You can convert the dosage to milligrams by multiplying the 25,000 by 0.0006, which would give you a result of 15 milligrams. If you read about a study in which the participants took daily supplements of 30 milligrams of beta-carotene, you can divide the 30 milligrams by 0.0006, which comes out to 50,000 international units.

Another member of the carotenoid family, lycopene, which gives tomatoes their red color, has been linked to lower rates of prostate cancer. A six-year study revealed that men of southern European ancestry, from countries such as Italy and Greece, were the most likely to eat tomato-based products and the least likely to develop prostate cancer. More specifically, researchers found that tomato sauce is the food most strongly linked to a lower prostate-cancer risk. The next best foods, in descending order of importance, are raw or cooked tomatoes, pizza, and tomato juice. Green leafy vegetables, fruits, and other common cancer-fighting foods also lower the risk of prostate cancer.

Lutein, found in all dark green leafy vegetables, is another excellent antioxidant. Lycopene and lutein are now added to some multivitamin supplements.

Vitamin D

Vitamin D is synthesized in the body through sunlight or is consumed with certain foods, such as vitamin-fortified cereals, margarine, milk, egg yolks, and liver. The vitamin helps make phosphorus and calcium available in the blood and contributes to the proper development and maintenance of the bones and teeth.

A deficiency of vitamin D in children may result in rickets, a disease characterized by bone deformities. In adults, vitamin-D deficiency may lead to bone problems such as osteomalacia, a disease marked by the softening of the bones through the loss of calcium and protein. In addition, any failure of the body to synthesize vitamin D allows calcium to leave the bones, which leads to the development of osteoporosis.

Vitamin D is essential to the absorption of calcium by the body and in this way helps prevent rickets in infants and bone deterioration in adults. In addition, the vitamin has been linked to reduced prostate cancer, improved parathyroid function, and lowered blood pressure. Vitamin D may also relieve the symptoms of Crohn's disease, an inflammatory disease of the lower intestine.

The average person's daily requirement for vitamin D is 400 to 800 international units, a dose that can be readily attained through the natural exposure of the hands, face, and arms to sunlight. About ten to fifteen minutes of exposure per day four to five days a week should be more than enough for light-skinned people. Dark-skinned people require longer exposure—thirty minutes four to five days a week. Foods fortified with vitamin D, such as certain cereals, milk, egg yolks, liver, butter, and fatty fish, can give you additional amounts of the vitamin. Individuals who are not frequently exposed to sunlight need more vitamin D from food sources or supplements than individuals who are frequently exposed. The PDI of vitamin D for men and women who are healthy and actively training is 400 to 1,000 international units.

Check the labels of the foods you consume to see if they are fortified and, if they are, how much vitamin D they contain. As little as 1 cup of most types of milk, for example, will provide 25 percent of your daily vitamin-D requirement, or about 100 international units.

Vitamin-D supplements are not needed unless you are unable to go outdoors or if recommended by your physician. The vitamin is quite powerful and, in excessive doses, can produce toxic effects, resulting in a variety of health problems. The initial symptoms may include headache, fatigue, loss of appetite, and excessive thirst. Chronic deficiency may lead to serious damage to the kidneys, lungs, and bones.

Vitamin E
Vitamin E is crucial to health and progress in the gym—it has been shown to reduce cramping and muscle fatigue, oxygenate the muscles, aid steroid production, and fight inflammation.

The most widely known use of vitamin E is as an antioxidant. Oxidized fats often accumulate in the body as free radicals, which have been shown to cause cancer. Antioxidants such as vitamin E work as free-radical scavengers. In its most complete form, vitamin E also contains several precursors for the production of the male and female hormones and the adrenal steroids needed to build muscle. In addition, it reduces muscle fatigue during exercise, reduces inflammation by supporting prostaglandin production, prevents muscle cramping by moving calcium and oxygen to the tissues, and increases injury resistance by mobilizing calcium reserves.

Muscle cramping is of special interest to athletes. It can be caused by several factors, including deficiency of calcium, magnesium, essential fatty acids, or vitamin E. Some athletes relieve their cramps with calcium or magnesium; others use vitamin E.

Unfortunately, it's next to impossible to get an adequate daily dose of vitamin E through diet alone. The richest food sources have relatively low amounts of the vitamin. Also, the best foods are oils and nuts, such as wheat-germ oil, soybean oil, almonds, and hazelnuts, which are high in calories and fat. For example, 1 tablespoon of wheat-germ oil has only about 30 to 35 international units of vitamin E but 120 calories; 1 cup of hazelnuts has only about 30 international units of vitamin E but more than 800 calories; and 1 cup of almonds has only about 20 international units of vitamin E but more than 800 calories. You can see that it would be very difficult to obtain 400 international units of vitamin E per day through diet alone without putting on many extra pounds. The most recent studies on vitamin E show that its most complete health and muscle-recovery benefits come from a daily intake of 400 to 1,200 international units. The PDI of vitamin E for men and women who are healthy and actively training is 200 to 1,000 international units. For athletes who compete at high altitudes, such as alpine skiers, the PDI is 600 to 1,200 international units. The only way to healthfully maintain this intake goal is to use a natural-vitamin-E supplement.

The word *natural* sometimes can, unfortunately, be misleading. In the case of vitamin E, a manufacturer can use a blend that is 10-percent natural vitamin E and 90-percent synthetic vitamin E, and still label the product "natural." Using synthetic vitamin E, which is much cheaper, a manufacturer can greatly reduce the quality of a product to reduce its manufacturing cost.

Make sure to read the label for the properly listed chemical name of the product in the contents description. The names of the natural forms of vitamin E begin with a "d," while the names of the synthetic forms begin with a "dl." For

ON THE CUTTING EDGE

Vitamin E Protects Muscles

The secret to avoiding muscle damage after intensive workouts may lie in a vitamin. According to an article in *Medicine and Science in Sports and Exercise* in 1998, Penn State researchers split twelve men into two groups. One group took a vitamin-E supplement every day for two weeks, while the other group took a placebo. At the end of the two weeks, both groups performed various weight-lifting exercises to exhaustion. Immediately after their workouts and up to two days later, the men who had taken the vitamin-E supplement had significantly less waste material circulating in their blood than did the men who had taken the placebo, indicating that their muscles had recovered better. The researchers concluded that the addition of 400 international units of vitamin E to the diet will help reduce muscle soreness and damage after weight-training exercises.

ON THE CUTTING EDGE

Vitamin E Decreases Free-Radical Damage of Weight Training

The majority of the research that has been done on free-radical damage and the protective effect of various vitamins has used different types of endurance exercise or training. The theory is that if you can prevent some of the free-radical damage caused by working out, you will recover quicker and make better gains in fitness. However, it was recently shown that the indicators of free-radical development increase after weight training and that vitamin E has a protective effect against free-radical damage. In a study reported in *Medicine and Science in Sports and Exercise* in 1998, recreationally weight trained males participated in weight-training sessions consisting of ten exercises. All the exercises were performed in three sets of ten repetitions at a ten-repetition maximum. One group was given 1,200 international units of vitamin E daily for two weeks prior to the weight-training session, while a second group was given a placebo. The markers of muscle damage and free-radical development were significantly increased after the workout in both groups, as would be expected. However, both markers were significantly lower in the vitamin-E group.

example, d–alpha tocopherol is a natural form of vitamin E, while dl–alpha tocopherol is a synthetic form.

Natural vitamin E is officially recognized as having 36–percent greater potency than its synthetic counterpart. However, recent studies using human subjects have indicated that natural vitamin E is probably twice as effective as synthetic vitamin E.

Vitamin E is usually sold in international units, but if you happen to buy a bottle that instead defines the product in milligrams, remember that 1 milligram of vitamin E is approximately equal to 1 international unit of the vitamin.

Vitamin K Vitamin K is a nutrient found in the small intestines, where it combines with protein to produce a substance necessary for blood clotting. Certain cases of vitamin-K deficiency have resulted in a failure of the clotting process and in hemorrhaging. In particular, there is a danger that hemorrhaging may occur in the brains of newborns, who lack sufficient vitamin K.

Vitamin K is so prevalent in the American food supply that anyone with a complete diet usually takes in more than enough for adequate blood clotting. The PDI of vitamin K for men and women who are healthy and actively training is 80 to 180 micrograms.

The food sources of vitamin K include green leafy vegetables, which are clearly the best dietary sources, supplying 50 to 800 micrograms of the vitamin in every 100 grams of food. You will get more than enough of the vitamin in one ample serving of a leafy green such as broccoli or cabbage. Roughly $1/2$ cup of broccoli, for example, provides 100 micrograms of vitamin K. Small but significant amounts of the vitamin are also present in milk and milk products, meats, eggs, cereals, and fruits. These foods supply 1 to 50 micrograms of the vitamin in every 100 grams of food. Vitamin K is also found in many multivitamin supplements.

The Water-Soluble Vitamins

Unlike the fat-soluble vitamins, the water-soluble vitamins are eliminated in the urine. While this generally prevents toxic buildup of these vitamins, it also means that they must be continually supplied to the body. The water-soluble vitamins include the B-complex vitamins and vitamin C.

Vitamin B_1 (Thiamine) When you look at the metabolism of carbohydrates, proteins, and lipids, you see that vitamin B_1, known as thiamine, plays a key role as a coenzyme. Without vitamin B_1, the cells have a difficult time taking energy from food. Vitamin B_1 is also important for a normally functioning nervous system.

Our bodies' vitamin-B_1 needs are related to the total amount of calories we consume. It is logical that, since vitamin B_1's primary role is in energy metabolism, increased calorie consumption means a greater demand for the vitamin. Luckily, when we eat more food, we usually take in more vitamin B_1 as well. However, a deficiency can occur when a large part of our daily calories come from "empty" sources, such as refined sugar and alcohol, which provide lots of calories but no essential nutrients.

Because of the extra calories and carbohydrates taken in during intensive training and competition, the need for vitamin B_1 is increased. The PDI of vitamin B_1 for men and women who are healthy and actively training is 30 to 300 milligrams. Additional vitamin B_1 can be obtained from a multivitamin supplement or through a sports rehydration drink. There are no known toxicity levels. Your body will excrete any excess of this water-soluble vitamin in the urine.

We get much of our vitamin B_1 from enriched grains and the products made from them, including bread, tortillas, pastries, and fortified cereals. Unlike many of the other vitamins, B_1 is not found naturally in substantial amounts in many foods other than pork.

Vitamin B_2 (Riboflavin) Vitamin B_2, popularly called riboflavin, derives its name from its chemical structure, a carbon-hydrogen-oxygen skeleton that includes ribitol (a sugar) attached to a flavonoid (a nitrogen compound). The same as vitamin B_1, vitamin B_2 is a coenzyme. Without it, your body could not digest or use proteins or carbohydrates. The same as vitamin A, it protects the health of the mucous membranes, the moist tissues lining the eyes, mouth, nose, throat, vagina, and rectum. The adult RDA for vitamin B_2 is 0.6 milligram for every 1,000 calories of food consumed, with a minimum of 1.2 milligrams required by anyone consuming less than 2,000 calories per day. The PDI of vita-

min B_2 for men and women who are healthy and actively training is 30 to 300 milligrams per day.

Milk is a major source of vitamin B_2 in the American diet. Although milk consumption has fallen off in recent years, it has been compensated for somewhat by an increased consumption of other dairy foods, such as cheese, yogurt, and ice cream. But when the dairy product is high in fat, as are cheese and ice cream, it contains less vitamin B_2. This is logical, since vitamin B_2 is a water-soluble, rather than a fat-soluble, vitamin. For example, 1 cup of 1-percent milk provides 105 calories and about one-third of the adult RDA for vitamin B_2. However, those 105 calories eaten instead as about $1/2$ cup of ice cream or 1 ounce of cheese provide less than one-tenth of the RDA of vitamin B_2. This is due to the increased amount of fat, which increases the total number of calories without a concurrent increase in the vitamin-B_2 content.

Vitamin B_2 is destroyed by ultraviolet light. This posed a problem in the days when milk was commonly bottled in clear glass and delivered to home doorsteps. When a milk bottle sat for too long on a doorstep, exposing the milk to daylight for too long, the vitamin-B_2 content fell. Direct sunlight can wipe out half of milk's vitamin B_2 in a couple of hours. Today, of course, most milk comes in waxed cartons or opaque plastic containers and is sold in grocery stores.

The livers, kidneys, and hearts of animals are very rich in vitamin B_2, but these organs are not commonly eaten. Other good sources of vitamin B_2 are meat, eggs, green leafy vegetables, and nuts such as almonds. The enrichment of bread and other grain products with vitamins has boosted the vitamin-B_2 intake in this country. Vitamin B_2 is also included in most multivitamin supplements.

Vitamin B_3 (Niacin)

Vitamin B_3, which is known as niacin, is really a pair of naturally occurring nutrients—nicotinic acid and nicotinamide. Vitamin B_3 is essential for proper growth and, the same as the other B vitamins, is intimately involved in enzyme reactions. In fact, it is an integral part of an enzyme that allows oxygen to flow into the body tissues. The same as vitamin B_1, it gives you a healthy appetite and participates in the metabolism of sugars and lipids.

Vitamin B_3 is available either as a preformed nutrient or through the conversion of the amino acid tryptophan. Preformed vitamin B_3 comes from meat. Tryptophan comes from milk and dairy foods. Some vitamin B_3 is present in grains, but it cannot be absorbed efficiently unless the grain was treated with lime (the mineral, not the fruit). Treating grains, such as the cornmeal used to make tortillas, with lime is a common practice in Central and South American countries. In the United States, breads and cereals are routinely fortified with vitamin B_3. The added vitamin B_3 is easily absorbed.

The RDA for vitamin B_3 is 6.6 milligrams for every 1,000 calories of food consumed, with a minimum of 13 milligrams of vitamin B_3 required by anyone consuming fewer than 2,000 calories a day. The term used to describe the vitamin-B_3 RDA is "niacin equivalent"—60 milligrams of tryptophan equal 1 milligram of vitamin B_3, which equals 1 niacin equivalent. The PDI of vitamin B_3 for men and women who are healthy and actively training is 20 to 100 milligrams.

A flush, called the niacin flush, occasionally occurs after vitamin-B_3 supplements are ingested. This flush, which is uncomfortable but usually harmless, consists of a red rash possibly accompanied by a tingling sensation. However, consuming more than 500 milligrams of vitamin B_3 daily for a prolonged period may cause liver damage.

Vitamin B_5 (Pantothenic Acid)

Vitamin B_5 is vital for the enzyme reactions that enable the body to use carbohydrates and that create steroid biochemicals such as hormones. Also called pantothenic acid, this B vitamin additionally helps stabilize the blood-sugar level, defends against infection, and protects the hemoglobin (the protein in red blood cells that carries oxygen through the body) as well as the nerve, brain, and muscle tissues.

Vitamin B_5 is obtained primarily from meat, fish, poultry, beans, whole-grain cereals, and fortified-grain products. No RDA has been established for vitamin B_5, but the Food and Nutrition Board of the National Academy of Sciences (NAS), which sets the RDAs and DRIs, has determined that an estimated safe and effective daily dietary intake range for adults and athletes is 4 to 7 milligrams. The PDI of vitamin B_5 for men and women who are healthy and actively training is 25 to 200 milligrams. The average individual eating a balanced diet is believed to get about 10 to 20 milligrams.

Vitamin B_6 (Pyridoxine)

Vitamin B_6, often called pyridoxine, is involved in more bodily functions than almost any other nutrient. It affects both physical and mental health, helps maintain sodium and potassium balance, and promotes red-blood-cell formation.

Vitamin B_6's involvement in amino-acid metabolism gives it a wide variety of jobs in the body. It is essential for the release of energy and nutrients from food. It is important in protein synthesis because B_6 coenzymes help make the nonessential amino acids by functioning in the transfer of the amino portion of one amino acid to the carbon skeleton of another.

The job of shuffling the amino portions of amino acids is also important when amino acids are used for fuel. The amino portions must be removed, a job that calls for B_6 coenzymes. Vitamin-B_6 coenzymes are also needed to convert the amino acid tryptophan to both vitamin B_3 and serotonin, a chemical messenger in the brain.

In light of the importance of vitamin B_6 in the metabolism of amino acids, it is not surprising to learn that the requirements for the vitamin are closely related to protein consumption. Since protein intake is high in the typical athlete's diet, the vitamin-B_6 requirement is correspondingly high. In addition, vitamin B_6 plays an important role in removing excess amounts of a substance called homocysteine from the blood. About 10 percent of the cases of heart disease in the United States have been linked to high blood levels of homocysteine.

The RDA for vitamin B_6 is 2.0 milligrams for men and 1.6 milligrams for women. The PDI of vitamin B_6 for men and women who are healthy and actively training is 20 to 100 milligrams.

The best food sources of vitamin B_6 are liver, chicken, fish, pork, lamb, milk, eggs, unmilled rice, whole grains, soybeans, potatoes, beans, nuts, seeds, and dark green vegetables such as turnip greens. In the United States, bread and other products made with refined grains are fortified with vitamin B_6. Vitamin B_6, the same as the other B vitamins, is found in most multivitamin supplements.

Vitamin B_{12} (Cobalamin)

Vitamin B_{12}, also known as cobalamin, makes healthy red blood cells. In addition, it protects the myelin, the fatty material that covers the nerves and facilitates the transmission of electrical impulses, or messages, between nerve cells. These messages make it possible for you to see, hear, think, move, and do all the things a healthy body does each day.

Vitamin B_{12} is unique. First, it is the only vitamin that contains a mineral, cobalt. Cyanocobalamin, a cobalt compound, is the form of vitamin B_{12} commonly used in supplements. Second, vitamin B_{12} is a vitamin that cannot be made by the higher plants (the plants that give us fruits and vegetables). The same as vitamin K, vitamin B_{12} is made by beneficial bacteria living in the small intestines.

The normal adult storage capacity of the vitamin is about 2,000 to 3,000 micrograms. The RDA, however, is only 2 micrograms, the smallest RDA of all the nutrients. So, for an average person, the B_{12} stores are not very quickly or easily exhausted. (An average person's stores hold about a two- to-four-year supply.) This means that an actual B_{12} deficiency may not occur for several years after the loss of intrinsic-factor-secreting cells. The symptoms usually appear gradually, rarely before the age of fifty.

However, many doctors still recommend taking daily supplements containing at least 500 micrograms. The PDI of vitamin B_{12} for men and women who are healthy and actively training is 12 to 200 micrograms. Taking extra B_{12} is a safe and inexpensive form of health insurance. If 500 micrograms seems excessive to you, take at least the PDI of the vitamin.

When we look at some of the biochemical roles of vitamin B_{12}, we can see why it is universally required by the cells. Among its functions, it is necessary for the formation of the nucleic acids, which hold the chemical blueprints of heredity and control our synthesis of proteins. Three of our body systems—the bone marrow (where the blood cells are made), the nervous system, and the digestive tract—make the primary demands for the vitamin. Failure of these processes—through an insufficient supply of the vitamin from food sources, insufficient absorption, or some combination of the two factors—suggests the origin of the leading deficiency symptoms. We can see why anemia, nervous-system defects, and diarrhea and other intestinal complaints are among the first signs of deficiency.

Meat, fish, poultry, milk products, and eggs are good sources of vitamin B_{12}. Grains are not natural sources of vitamin B_{12} but, in the United States, have it added along with the other B vitamins. For this reason, nutritionists strongly recommend that vegetarians take B_{12} supplements.

Biotin

Biotin is a B vitamin, a component of enzymes that ferries carbon and oxygen atoms between cells. Biotin helps metabolize lipids and carbohydrates, is essential for synthesizing fatty acids and amino acids needed for healthy growth, and seems to prevent the buildup of fat deposits that might interfere with the proper functioning of the liver and kidneys.

The best food sources of biotin are liver, egg yolks, yeast, nuts, and beans. If your diet doesn't give you all the biotin you need, bacteria in your gut will synthesize enough to make up the difference. No RDA has been set for biotin, but the Food and Nutrition Board has established an estimated safe and effective daily dietary intake range of 30 to 100 micrograms. The PDI of biotin for men and women who are healthy and actively training is 125 to 300 micrograms. The average diet is believed to provide about 100 to 300 micrograms daily. Athletes and individuals who exercise intensively should consider supplementing with 500 micrograms per day.

Folate
Folate, also called folic acid, is an essential nutrient for human beings and other vertebrates (animals with backbones). Folate takes part in the synthesis of DNA, the metabolism of proteins, and the subsequent synthesis of amino acids used to produce new body cells and tissues. This role makes folate vital for normal growth as well as wound healing, and for the creation of new fetal and maternal tissue during pregnancy.

The RDA for folate is 200 micrograms for men and 180 micrograms for women, or about four times what is believed necessary to prevent deficiency. The PDI of folate for men and women who are healthy and actively training is 400 to 1,200 micrograms. Lactation increases a woman's folate requirement, while pregnancy more than doubles it.

Beans, dark green leafy vegetables, liver, yeast, and various fruits are the best natural sources of folate. A good way to ensure an adequate folate intake is supplementation.

Vitamin C
Vitamin C, also called ascorbic acid, is essential for the development and maintenance of the connective tissue (the fat, muscle, and bone framework of the human body). Vitamin C speeds the production of new cells in wound healing and, the same as vitamin E, is an antioxidant that keeps free radicals from hooking up with other molecules to form damaging compounds that might attack the tissues. Vitamin C protects the immune system, helps fight off infection, reduces the severity of allergic reactions, and plays a role in the synthesis of hormones and other body chemicals.

Green peppers, broccoli, citrus fruits, tomatoes, strawberries, and other fresh fruits and vegetables are good sources of vitamin C.

Women twenty-two years old or older who are not heavy exercisers or overweight should consume up to 500 milligrams of vitamin C daily. Women twenty-two years old or older who weigh over 200 pounds should consume 1,000 to 2,000 milligrams daily. Men twenty-two to fifty years old who are not heavy exercisers or overweight should consume 1,000 to 2,000 milligrams daily, and men over the age of twenty-two who are overweight should consume up to 3,000 milligrams a day. Young men thirteen to twenty-one years of age should consume 500

ON THE CUTTING EDGE

Protect and Increase Muscle Strength With Vitamin C

The benefits of strength training may be compromised if significant free-radical damage occurs in the skeletal muscles. Ascorbic acid is a very effective antioxidant that protects against damage from free radicals. Ascorbic acid also plays a role in connective-tissue synthesis associated with strength gains. In a study reported in *Medicine and Science in Sports and Exercise* in 1998, the effect of long-term ascorbic-acid supplementation on the development of muscular strength in young adults during an eight-week isotonic strength-training program was examined. Sixty-three subjects were divided into four groups—two strength-training groups, one taking 1,000 milligrams of ascorbic acid daily and one taking a placebo, and two non-strength-training control groups, one taking 1,000 milligrams of ascorbic acid daily and one a placebo. The ascorbic acid and placebo were gel encapsulated and administered double-blind. The subjects' strength in four muscle groups, including the extensors and flexors of the knee and elbow, was measured before and after training. The relative changes in strength were then compared by group. The greatest relative change in all four muscle groups was experienced by the strength-trained group taking the ascorbic acid, but only in the knee extensors was the relative change significantly greater in the strength-trained ascorbic group than in the strength-trained placebo group. These results showed a clear advantage of taking ascorbic acid over a placebo in the development of strength.

Reduce Cortisol With Ascorbic Acid

A study of Junior National Team weight lifters showed that the daily ingestion of 1,000 milligrams of ascorbic acid had a significant impact on the cortisol level. According to a report in the *Journal of Strength and Conditioning Research* in 1998, the subjects were divided into two groups and given either ascorbic acid or a placebo every day for fourteen days. The subjects then participated in a competitive, high-volume, high-intensity weight-training program. Both groups lifted at the same intensity and had an equal lifting volume of training for the fourteen days. However, in the ascorbic group, the cortisol levels were lower at one hour after exercise and significantly lower statistically at twenty-four hours after exercise than in the placebo group. Lower cortisol levels are important since excessive cortisol has been shown to have a detrimental inflammatory effect on the muscle cells and to suppress the body's immune system.

milligrams daily. The PDI of vitamin C for men and women who are healthy and actively training is 800 to 3,000 milligrams.

To obtain up to 500 milligrams of vitamin C per day, food sources are adequate. However, to obtain more than 500 milligrams per day, supplements are necessary.

Vitamin C is usually sold in milligrams, but if you buy the vitamin in very large dosage amounts, you may also find references to grams. Remember that 1,000 milligrams equal 1 gram.

Vitaminlike Substances

There are some substances that are not vitamins but are generally grouped with those nutrients anyway. This is because these compounds do not fit the definition of vitamins—they're either synthesized in the body or needed in larger amounts than vitamins—but they do function in the body in some of the same ways. These vitaminlike substances include the bioflavonoids, carnitine, choline, conenzyme Q_{10}, lipoic acid, and para-aminobenzoic acid.

The Bioflavonoids The bioflavonoids are a family of related compounds, including rutin and the flavones, flavonols, and flavonones. The bioflavonoids are not vitamins or minerals, although at one time they were called vitamin P or substance P. They are found in the inner peel of citrus fruits, the white core of peppers, buckwheat, and leafy vegetables.

The bioflavonoids are essential for the proper absorption and use of vitamin C. They assist vitamin C in keeping collagen, the intercellular cement, in healthy condition. In addition, the bioflavonoids act as antioxidants, keeping vitamin C and adrenaline from being oxidized by copper-containing enzymes. Limited evidence shows the bioflavonoids might also prevent bruising and damage to the artery walls caused by free-radical attack.

No RDA has been established for the bioflavonoids. The PDI for men and women who are healthy and actively training is 200 to 2,000 milligrams. Besides a daily intake of good food sources of the bioflavonoids, you should take a supplement containing these nutrients every day to ensure proper vitamin-C uptake and to aid your antioxidant program.

Carnitine (Vitamin B-T) Carnitine, sometimes called vitamin B-T, plays a role in fat and energy metabolism in the body. Recently, carnitine received publicity as being useful for people with heart disease. However, more research is needed to establish its value, if any, for heart patients. Carnitine is found in greater amounts in foods of animal origin and in lesser amounts in foods of plant origin, so a vegetarian diet is apt to be low in carnitine. However, this is of little concern, since under normal circumstances, the substance is synthesized in the body. Some people may have an inherited inability to make sufficient amounts of carnitine. The symptoms of carnitine deficiency include muscle weakness, low blood sugar, and high blood-ammonia levels.

Several manufacturers recommend taking 2 to 4 grams of L-carnitine for two weeks, one hour before exercise, to help with fat burning. Taking this dosage to

ON THE CUTTING EDGE

If You Train in Air Pollution, Take Your Antioxidants

The adverse health effects of air pollution, specifically of ozone, are being increasingly recognized, according to an article published in *Occupational and Environmental Medicine* in 1998. A possible reason for the decreased lung function experienced after exposure to ozone is the pollutant's oxidant role, which induces injury to the lung tissues. Limited data suggest that vitamin C alone or in combination with vitamin E may protect against ozone-induced lung damage. In a recent study, lung function (forced respiratory volume, forced vital capacity, maximal mid-expiratory flow, and peak expiratory flow) with and without antioxidant supplementation was measured in twenty-six amateur cyclists during the summer, when the ozone concentration is normally high. The supplemented group received 15 milligrams of beta-carotene, 650 milligrams of vitamin C, and 75 milligrams of vitamin E every day for three months. In the supplemented group, the lung-function measurements were not affected in any way by the ozone. However, in the control group, all of the lung-function measurements after exercise except those for maximal mid-expiratory flow were negative, indicating decreased lung function at the higher ozone levels.

increase your fat-burning capacity or boost your weight loss is not dangerous, but it may also not produce results. Note that the DL-form of carnitine is not recommended for use, since it may be toxic.

Choline Choline is a substance found in most animal tissues. It can be found in combination with lecithin in nervous tissue, especially in the protective myelin sheaths surrounding the nerve fibers. Choline is also part of the structure of acetylcholine and phosphatidylcholine, and a deficiency in the body may have an effect on nerve transmission and exercise performance. It has been demonstrated that there is a significant reduction in the plasma-choline level following endurance training or extended exercise sessions. This reduction in the plasma-choline level associated with strenuous exercise may reduce the level of acetylcholine, and thus its release, and could thereby affect nerve impulses, which would impair endurance and performance. It has been hypothesized that the replacement of choline lost during exercise, or the prevention of this loss, could influence the neuronal release of acetylcholine and, subsequently, affect athletic performance and fatigue. The PDI of choline for men and women who are healthy and actively training is 600 to 1,200 milligrams.

In research conducted with runners, it was shown that taking 2,000 milligrams of free choline prior to exercise may prevent a fall in the blood-choline level during exercise, as well as raise the choline level above the baseline for up to two hours following exercise. Randomized placebo-controlled crossover studies found improvements in running and swimming times and suggested that performance in these activities is sensitive to changes in the choline level. In one study, long-distance runners improved their running times by an average of five minutes over a twenty-mile course when compared with runners taking a placebo. In a second study, a higher percentage of the swimmers who took choline prior to their swim experienced an improved performance on a timed swim test than did the swimmers who took a placebo.

Coenzyme Q_{10}

Coenzyme Q_{10}, also called ubiquinone, is chemically related to vitamin E, is synthesized by the body, and plays a role in energy metabolism. Coenzyme Q_{10} has attracted interest for its potential as an antioxidant. However, its primary job in the body is to help convert food into energy. Various studies have suggested that this coenzyme could play a role in protecting the body against tissue damage from heart attack, heart disease, retinal deterioration, breast cancer, and a number of other diseases.

The scientific literature indicates that a dosage of up to 300 milligrams a day of coenzyme Q_{10} should not produce any side effects. Extremely high dosages can cause diarrhea.

Lipoic Acid

Lipoic acid functions as a coenzyme along with vitamin B_1. Yeast and liver are good sources of lipoic acid, but it can also be synthesized by the body. Lipoic acid is now being used by some athletes as an "insulin mimicker" because it significantly increases the body's utilization of blood sugar, which helps the body build muscle glycogen.

Lipoic acid has also been shown to be a powerful antioxidant in dosages as low as 200 to 300 milligrams per day. Two studies have shown that lipoic acid helps protect the red blood cells and fatty acids from the type of oxidative damage caused by intensive training.

If you decide to try lipoic acid, start with a daily dosage of around 100 to 200 milligrams, taken with a meal. Eventually, work your way up to 400 to 500 milligrams, taken in three equal dosages with your three major meals of the day.

Para-Aminobenzoic Acid

Para-aminobenzoic acid (PABA) is part of the B vitamin folate and therefore isn't considered a separate vitamin. PABA is used in sunscreens, since when it is applied to the skin, it helps to protect against sunburn. Taken orally, however, PABA does not have the same effect.

If taken as a supplement, PABA should be limited to no more than 50 milligrams per day. Large doses taken over extended periods of time have been known to cause nausea and vomiting.

MINERALS—THE INORGANIC NUTRIENTS

Minerals are substances that occur naturally in nonliving things such as rocks and metal ores. Minerals are also present in plants and animals, but they are assimilated by them—that is, plants get their minerals from the soil in which they grow, and animals get their minerals from the plants they eat.

Minerals are elements, substances composed of only one kind of atom. In addition, they are inorganic; unlike vitamins, they usually do not contain the carbon, hydrogen, and oxygen atoms found in all organic compounds. Most minerals have names that reflect the places in which they're found or one of their characteristics, such as their color. For example, the word "calcium" comes from *calm,* the Greek word for lime (chalk), and "chlorine" comes from *choros,* the Greek word for the color green-yellow.

The Major Minerals

Nutritionists classify the minerals that are essential for human life as either major minerals or trace minerals. Nutritionally speaking, the difference between major and trace minerals is how much you have in your body and how much you need to ingest to maintain a steady supply.

The major minerals include calcium, chloride, magnesium, phosphorus, potassium, sodium, and sulfur. Although sulfur, a major mineral, is an essential nutrient for human beings, it is almost never included in nutritional books or charts. Why? Because it is an integral part of all proteins—any diet that provides an adequate supply of protein also provides an adequate supply of sulfur.

Calcium   Calcium plays an essential role in muscle contractions, in addition to its well-known role in the formation and maintenance of bones and teeth. Athletes who eliminate dairy products, rich in calcium, from their diets often experience muscle cramps. When these athletes reintroduce calcium into their diets, the muscle cramping often becomes significantly reduced. So, if you experience muscle cramping, make sure to include dairy products, salmon, dried figs, and dark green leafy vegetables in your diet to ensure an adequate calcium intake. It may also be wise to take a calcium supplement to make sure you meet your calcium requirement.

In 1997, the National Academy of Sciences published an entirely new set of nutritional numbers for calcium. The new numbers include 1,000 milligrams per day for adults thirty-one to fifty years old, and 1,200 milligrams per day for adults fifty-one years old or older. The recommendations for children include 500 milligrams per day for one- to three-year-olds, 800 milligrams per day for four- to eight-year-olds, and 1,300 milligrams per day for nine- to eighteen-year-olds. The recommendation for the last group—1,300 milligrams—is the amount of calcium found in $4\frac{1}{2}$ cups of milk or yogurt. The PDI of calcium for men and women who are healthy and actively training is 1,200 to 2,600 milligrams.

In addition, recent findings indicate that calcium citrate malate may be a superior form of the mineral for supplementation. It seems that dietary supplementation with an analog of calcium citrate (calcium citrate malate) and vitamin D may reduce bone loss and lower the incidence of nonvertebral fractures in men and women over the age of sixty-five. Using a dosage of only 500 milligrams of calcium, it was demonstrated that calcium citrate differs significantly from common calcium carbonate and oyster shell in reducing bone loss because it has a higher degree of calcium activity and greater bioavailability. Remember, bioavailability is the amount of usable nutrient a supplement delivers. Recent trials conducted at the Mayo Clinic and the University of Connecticut Health Science Center have also shown an enhanced bone response to calcium citrate. Researchers at these institutions have reported that 1,000 milligrams of calcium citrate produced more than twice the level of calcium in blood serum as did 1,000 milligrams of elemental calcium from calcium carbonate. Other unique benefits of calcium citrate malate are a reduced risk of kidney stones, elimination of the bowel-gas discomfort sometimes caused by calcium metabolism, and enhancement of iron absorption, which other calcium supplements inhibit. However, new research conducted by Dr. R.P. Heaney showed that the calcium from calcium carbonate, when the supplement is taken with food, is fully as absorbable as the calcium from calcium citrate.

Calcium is one of the minerals particularly important for women, especially women athletes. For a special report on women athletes' nutritional needs, see page 97.

Chloride
Chloride is the ionic form of the element chlorine, and its estimated minimum requirement is 750 milligrams per day. The PDI of chloride for men and women who are healthy and actively training is 1,500 to 4,500 milligrams. Chloride is found in the fluids within the cells, where it accompanies potassium, and between the cells, where it accompanies sodium. In fact, chloride accompanies sodium as part of the molecule sodium chloride, which is common table salt. Chloride is therefore found in any food that contains salt.

Chloride functions in fluid and electrolyte balance, and it is also needed to form the hydrochloric acid that functions in digestion in the stomach. There is some concern that chloride, rather than sodium, is the cause of hypertension (high blood pressure) among people who chronically overconsume salt. This connection, however, has yet to be confirmed.

Magnesium
Although the body contains less than 2 ounces of magnesium, this mineral is vital to its health and function. Magnesium plays a role in protein synthesis, muscle relaxation, and energy release, and also acts as a catalyst in important metabolic reactions, such as calcium metabolism. Magnesium is part of the mineral composition of the bones and teeth. Actually, the bones act as a reservoir for magnesium so that it is available when needed. Magnesium is also required for the normal circulating function of the parathyroid hormone, which regulates the level of calcium in the blood.

Magnesium is found in most foods, especially green leafy vegetables. This is because magnesium is part of chlorophyll, the pigment that makes plants green and facilitates the process of photosynthesis. Other good sources of magnesium are dairy products, breads and cereals, nuts, chocolate, and dried peas and beans. Hard water is also a reliable source of the mineral, and it is found as an additive in some rehydration drinks and sports nutrition bars.

SPECIAL REPORT
The Female Athlete

Women have a greater need for calcium, iron, and magnesium than do men. Athletic or active women need these nutrients even more. Following is a brief review of these three minerals that should be helpful to women engaged in intensive cardiovascular training or resistance training to increase muscle tone.

CALCIUM

Calcium is vital for athletic women because it is a major component of bone. The need for calcium starts when you're young, and if you get enough calcium early in life, you can build a "calcium bank" that can keep your bones strong. Unfortunately, women are at a disadvantage early in life because they begin with less bone mass than do men.

When your diet is deficient in calcium, this vital mineral is taken from your calcium bank and used for the other normal body functions that require it, such as nerve transmission and muscle function. This depletion can weaken your bones and increase your likelihood of developing osteoporosis in your later years.

Calcium also performs other vital functions, such as facilitating the production of hormones and the stimulation of enzymes. In addition, it has been linked to combating stress.

Calcium, along with a number of other important minerals, is lost in perspiration. It has been speculated that muscle cramping may be associated with calcium deficiency, as well as deficiencies of magnesium, potassium, sodium, and fluid. Make sure you consume adequate amounts of all these nutrients. For competition and training in hot weather, a rehydration drink that includes the electrolytes may be beneficial. Such a drink may also help if you find yourself cramping frequently during exercise. Many women, especially athletes who lose calcium while working out, have a particularly diffi-cult time the week before menstruation. Their calcium levels may drop sharply at this time, resulting in premenstrual syndrome (PMS). Doubling your calcium intake, as well as your magnesium intake, may prevent this problem.

By performing weight-bearing exercise, such as running, in-line skating, skiing, cycling, dancing, weight training, or walking, you're already increasing your chances of avoiding osteoporosis. Studies have shown that such activities increase bone mass and help women avoid osteoporosis, something to consider if you're a master's athlete (in most sports, an athlete who is over thirty or thirty-five years old).

The DRI for calcium is 1,000 milligrams for adult females up to the age of fifty and 1,200 milligrams for females who are older. The PDI for men and women who are healthy and actively training is 30 to 300 milligrams. The correct ratio of calcium to magnesium is two to one. Therefore, if you supplement with 1,200 milligrams of calcium, you should take 600 milligrams of magnesium.

Good sources of calcium are low-fat dairy products, almonds, broccoli, kale, salmon, sardines, spinach, and dried peas and beans. The best-absorbed sources are low-fat dairy products, such as low-fat yogurt and skim milk. If you are dieting or not eating properly, a calcium supplement can be good insurance that you obtain enough calcium in your diet.

IRON

Iron deficiency may cause certain types of anemia, which can hinder athletic performance. Iron is thus essential to an active woman's diet. Sports anemia, a condition that is common among endurance athletes with strenuous training regimens and poor diets, is one type of anemia that may result. Therefore, nutritionists recommend that women be tested for iron deficiency before beginning a new exercise program. The RDA for iron is 18 milligrams for women but should be increased to 30 milligrams or more during pregnancy. The PDI of iron for men and women who are healthy and actively training is 25 to 60 milligrams.

Iron is an essential trace mineral necessary for the formation of such oxygen-carrying compounds as hemoglobin and myoglobin, as well as for metabolically important enzymes. Hemoglobin, found in the red blood cells, carries oxygen from the lungs to the tissues by means of the bloodstream. Myoglobin ferries oxygen within the muscle cells. Obviously, a decreased level of hemoglobin or myoglobin will impair oxygen transport and limit a woman's ability to perform aerobic exercise. Insufficient iron consumption can result in iron-deficiency anemia, which can, among other things, lead to fatigue.

Do not be too quick to assume that the fatigue you feel during and after training is due to iron deficiency, however. Fatigue is caused by a multitude of factors. In fact, true iron-deficiency anemia is not common among athletes in general, especially male athletes. Female athletes are at a slightly greater risk, primarily as a result of iron loss from menstruation. Iron loss among athletes can also occur as a result of foot strike hemolysis (destruction of red blood cells as a result of the mechanical trauma of running), small blood losses due to bleeding from the intestines or kidneys during long runs, and poor dietary habits.

Although low hemoglobin values are one clinical sign of iron deficiency, hemoglobin levels in athletes must be interpreted with caution because plasma-volume expansion often occurs with training. This artificially lowers the hemoglobin level. The increase in plasma volume is actually beneficial to athletes because it reduces blood viscosity, increases cardiac output, and enhances thermoregulatory capabilities. The increased blood volume, and its resultant dilution of the hemoglobin level (often referred to as "pseudoanemia"), does not impair the blood's oxygen-carrying capabilities.

The occurrence of true iron deficiency is the same in athletes as in the general population, although reports of low blood-iron levels in both male and female middle- and long-distance runners give the perception that it is more prevalent in athletic groups. When the iron level is low, performance can be impaired and supplementation can be helpful. However, if a female athlete's iron status is normal, there is no scientific evidence that an iron supplement will have any beneficial effects on physical performance.

Regardless of the prevalence of iron-deficiency anemia among female athletes, analyses of athletes' diets have shown that iron intake is often below the RDA. Female athletes on self-imposed calorie-restricted diets for weight-control purposes are likely to have less-than-adequate intakes of iron. Also, female athletes and active women who obtain a high percentage of their calories from junk food may be at risk for iron deficiency.

Iron supplements, available at all pharmacies and health-food stores, generally contain ferric or ferrous citrate, ferric phosphate, ferric pyrophosphate, ferric or ferrous sulfate, ferrous ascorbate, ferrous fumarate, ferrous gluconate, or ferrous lactate, all of which have been approved by the government as nutritional additives. Compounds containing ferrous iron are generally more efficiently absorbed into the bloodstream than compounds containing iron in the ferric form.

Recent news stories have indicated that new research has linked high iron intake with heart disease. These news reports should not stop people from consuming adequate levels of iron, however. As is the case with most nutrients, iron can be the proverbial "double-edged sword"—too much iron may be harmful, but not enough iron can also be unhealthy and can limit athletic performance.

Good dietary sources of iron are meat, poultry, fish, eggs, vegetables, and fortified cereals. Meat sources of iron contain heme iron, which is absorbed more readily than nonheme iron, found in vegetable products.

People differ in their ability to absorb iron and this may be why some vegetarians become iron deficient. In addition, iron availability is enhanced by consuming foods high in vitamin C and by reducing your intake of coffee and most types of tea. There are substances in tea that may bind iron, making it unavailable for intestinal absorption.

Keep a list of the foods you eat to see if you are getting enough iron in your diet. If you think you may need a supplement, contact your health-care practitioner. If your physician tests you for iron, ask him or her to also check your ferritan level. Ferritan is the storage form of iron, and your blood-level reading will tell you if your iron stores are adequate, which is much more important to know than your blood level of the nutrient. Treat iron supplements as you would any medicinal drug. A relatively small amount may be necessary and helpful. Too much, however, may cause more harm than good.

MAGNESIUM

Magnesium plays an integral part in the normal functioning of an active woman's body. Magnesium helps convert glycogen to energy, aids in the development and functioning of the muscles, and regulates the heart rate and blood pressure.

Research has shown that strenuous activities, such as marathon running and cross-country skiing, tend to lower the level of magnesium in female athletes. In addition, this effect can linger for an extended period, causing potentially serious depletion of magnesium in the muscle tissue.

The National Research Council has set the RDA for magnesium at 280 to 350 milligrams for adult women. The PDI of magnesium for men and women who are healthy and actively training is 400 to 800 milligrams.

The best natural sources of magnesium are whole-grain breads and cereals, nuts, legumes, soybeans, and seafood. The mineral is also available in supplement form, which should always be taken if a calcium supplement is used. The correct ratio of calcium to magnesium, as mentioned above, is two to one. As a bonus, magnesium will help prevent the often constipating effects of calcium.

The RDA for magnesium is 350 milligrams for men and 280 milligrams for women. Athletes should consider taking 500 to 1,000 milligrams per day for optimum protein metabolism and muscle contraction.

Magnesium deficiency can lead to loss of muscle control by causing muscles to remain contracted. Nervousness, irritability, and tremors are other deficiency symptoms.

Magnesium, the same as calcium, is particularly important for women, especially women athletes. For a discussion of this, see "The Female Athlete" on page 97.

Phosphorus The same as calcium, phosphorus is essential for strong bones and teeth. It is also necessary for transmitting the genetic code (the genes and chromosomes that carry all the information about a person's special characteristics) from one cell to another when cells divide and reproduce. In addition, phosphorus helps maintain the pH balance of blood (keeps the blood from becoming too acid or alkaline) and is vital for metabolizing carbohydrates, synthesizing proteins, and ferrying fats and fatty acids among the tissues and organs. Phosphorus is also part of myelin, the fatty sheath that surrounds and protects the nerve cells.

ON THE CUTTING EDGE

Weight Training
Increases the Need for Calcium

High blood acidity is known to escalate calcium excretion. This explains why high-protein diets are often linked to increased calcium losses. But while weight training is good for bone health, it is also anaerobic, meaning that acidic metabolic waste products, such as lactic acid, are produced in the course of exercising. And wouldn't this increased acid lead to calcium loss? It certainly does, according to a study in the *Journal of Applied Physiology* in 1998. The study examined the effects of weight training on calcium loss in ten men. After exercising, the men underwent urine testing, which showed significant calcium losses. The losses were attributed to severe metabolic acidosis, which suggested that the mechanism behind the increased calcium excretion in the men during the weight training was an acid-induced loss of the reabsorption of calcium by the kidneys. The researchers concluded, therefore, that while women need to be especially conscious of calcium intake, men in training should also follow the new Dietary Reference Intakes (DRIs) of 1,000 milligrams of calcium per day from either food or supplement sources.

The RDA for phosphorus is 800 milligrams for adults over the age of twenty-five. For pregnant and nursing women, the RDA is increased to 1,200 milligrams. The PDI of phosphorus for men and women who are healthy and actively training is 800 to 1,600 milligrams. For most age groups, the RDA for phosphorus is the same as for calcium because keeping these two minerals in balance is important. A ratio of calcium to phosphorus of one to one is considered ideal. This makes milk a good source of phosphorus, since it contains phosphorus and calcium in approximately this ratio. In cheese, there is more phosphorus than calcium.

Some nutrition experts believe that an excessive phosphorus intake, especially when coupled with a low calcium intake, may be a factor in the development of osteoporosis. These experts believe that high levels of phosphorus can interfere with calcium absorption. The diets of some Americans consist mainly of high-protein foods such as meat, fish, and poultry; carbonated beverages or rehydration drinks; and ready-to-eat convenience foods, which contain phosphate additives, all of which can excessively increase the body's supply of phosphorus. The experts recommend that phosphorus-rich foods and drinks be consumed in moderation or at least in the proper one-to-one ratio with calcium.

Potassium   The element potassium, the principal electrolyte found within the cells, is third in abundance within the cells. Electrolytes are elements that can conduct an electric current when dissolved in water. In the human body, they control water balance, acid-base balance, and nerve-impulse transmission. Potassium functions in all of these phenomena, and it is also necessary for protein synthesis, muscle contraction, and maintenance of the regularity of the heart.

The estimated minimum daily requirement for potassium for adults is 2,000 milligrams. If the mineral is not present in adequate amounts, the symptoms may include mental confusion, muscular weakness, and paralysis. In extreme cases, death may result. Endurance athletes, such as marathon runners, may experience muscle cramping. The PDI of potassium for men and women who are healthy and actively training is 2,500 to 4,000 milligrams. Potassium is abundant in all whole foods, particularly meats, fruits, vegetables, and milk. Deficiency of the mineral usually results from dehydration due to large fluid losses, but it is also possible to flush potassium from the body by drinking too much water, perhaps a gallon or more a day.

Sodium
Sodium may be the only mineral that doesn't need to be obtained from food sources. Rather, it is routinely added to food in the form of table salt, or sodium chloride. In the body, sodium is found principally in the fluids between the cells, where it is important in maintaining the fluid balance and electrolyte balance. It is also important in nerve-impulse transmission.

The minimum daily requirement for sodium is 500 milligrams, an amount easily supplied by most diets. In fact, the abundance of salt in prepared foods has led the National Research Council to recommend a maximum daily sodium intake of 2,400 milligrams, an amount provided by about 1 teaspoon of table salt, which is regularly exceeded by many Americans. The PDI of sodium for men and women who are healthy and actively training is 1,500 to 4,500 milligrams. The kidneys remove excess sodium from the blood and excrete it in the urine. Sodi-

ON THE CUTTING EDGE

Salt Is Okay for Exercisers

It's okay to use salt. That's the word from the American Medical Association in an article published in its respected *Journal of the American Medical Association* in 1998. Compiling data from more than fifty studies published since 1966, researchers found that the general public doesn't have to pass on salt, although some patients with hypertension do benefit from sodium reduction. This is good news to remember on hot and humid summer days, when sweat loss is great. Unless you consume a decent amount of sodium, you'll simply urinate more regardless of how much water you drink during or after your long runs. For every pound you lose during intensive exercise, you lose approximately 16 fluid ounces of water. So, to win the battle against dehydration this summer, you can grab that salt shaker and add about 50 to 100 milligrams of sodium for every 9-ounce liquid serving, which is approximately the amount found in most rehydration drinks.

um is also lost with perspiration. After the age of forty or so, the kidneys become less efficient at removing and excreting sodium. As sodium accumulates in the blood, it tends to hold water, elevating the blood volume and blood pressure. Thus, excess sodium consumption has been linked to hypertension, a chronic condition.

Excess salt and water are removed together from the body by the kidneys. Hypertension develops from a lifetime of salt overconsumption. It is possible, although unlikely, to consume too little sodium. Faced with a deficiency, the kidneys will attempt to conserve the sodium that is present in the body with a sudden release of fluid through urination or perspiration. Usually, the lost sodium can be replaced through a normal intake of food and the use of rehydration drinks. The symptoms of sodium deficiency are loss of appetite, mental apathy, and muscle cramping.

Sulfur
Sulfur is the fourth most abundant mineral in the human body, but it cannot be classified as an essential nutrient. Because it is a component of the amino acids cystine and methionine, it is a part of virtually all the protein we eat. In addition, it is a constituent of vitamin B_1 and biotin.

It is probably more accurate to list the recommended intakes of the nutrients that contain sulfur than to provide a recommendation for sulfur itself. Cheese, eggs, fish, poultry, grains, nuts, and dried peas and beans are excellent sources of sulfur. Since no RDA has been established for sulfur, it is difficult to provide an intake recommendation. Furthermore, sulfur deficiencies are unknown.

The Trace Minerals

The trace minerals include chromium, cobalt, copper, fluoride, iodine, iron, manganese, molybdenum, selenium, vanadium, and zinc. They are classified as trace minerals because their recommended dosages are in the microgram to milligram range. Since some authorities classify a mineral as major or trace depending on its level in the body rather than recommended intake level, and some authorities even divide the minerals into more than two categories, other books may classify the minerals in this chapter differently. Trace minerals are also known as trace elements.

Chromium
Chromium is part of glucose tolerance factor (GTF), which regulates the metabolism of glucose in the body. GTF increases the action of insulin, a hormone involved in glucose metabolism. Insulin doesn't function properly when a chromium deficiency exists. Chromium supplements can improve the body's ability to handle glucose, but only if chromium was deficient in the first place.

Chromium's key function in the body is to act as a coenzyme in insulin action—that is, it helps insulin do its job. Science has shown that chromium deficiency indeed plays a role in the development of both insulin-resistant diabetes and hypoglycemia. These disorders can, in turn, lead to less-than-optimum muscle and fat metabolism. Many nutritionists suggest that supplementing the diet of non-insulin-dependent diabetics and hypoglycemics with at least 200 micrograms of chromium per day can significantly decrease their fasting glucose levels,

ON THE CUTTING EDGE

Combine Carbohydrate With Chromium for an Extra Boost in Exercise Capacity

In an article published in *Medicine and Science in Sports and Exercise* in 1998, the results of a project studying the effects of a chromium-carbohydrate supplement on exercise-performance capacity were described. According to the article, eleven male cyclists performed two separate trials at 75-percent of their maximum exercise capacity for sixty minutes, followed by forty-five-second sprint bicycle tests. The subjects drank either a chromium-carbohydrate beverage or a chromium-free carbohydrate beverage in four doses during the submaximum exercise. The beverages were administered using a double-blind counter-balanced protocol. The subjects consumed an average of 60.8 grams of carbohydrate during both trials, as well as 200 micrograms of chromium during the chromium trial. The subjects' blood-glucose and blood-lactate levels were measured during the submaximum exercise, immediately following the sprint tests, and five minutes after exercising. The total work performed was significantly greater following the chromium trial. In addition, the subjects' mean blood-glucose levels were lower and mean blood-lactate levels were higher during the chromium-carbohydrate trials at fifty and sixty minutes, respectively, suggesting a greater anaerobic-energy output. The authors concluded that chromium-carbohydrate ingestion improves maximum exercise performance after prolonged exercise.

Cut Fat, Maintain Muscle— Supplement With Chromium

Chromium supplementation can improve the body's insulin use. Improved insulin use in turn leads to decreased fat deposition as well as an increased amount of amino acids and glucose entering the muscle cells. The result is a change in body composition that favors the loss of fat and the maintenance of lean muscle mass. These observations were once again confirmed in a double-blind, placebo-controlled study reported in *Current Therapy Research* in 1998. In the study, one group of subjects was given up to 400 micrograms of chromium picolinate per day and a second group was given a placebo. After adjusting for the differences in caloric intake and energy expenditure among the subjects, the researchers found that the group taking the chromium picolinate lost significantly more weight and fat mass than the placebo group. The supplemented group also had a greater reduction in the percent of body fat without a loss of lean muscle mass.

improve their glucose tolerance, lower their overall insulin levels, and alleviate any symptoms of hypoglycemia. It appears that most of the population with an intake of less than 100 micrograms of chromium per day probably is marginally deficient. By supplementing the diet with chromium, the deficiency, along with its symptoms, can be eradicated.

As far as athletes are concerned, it is important to avoid a chromium deficiency because insulin resistance can lead to increases in body fat and can impair proper muscle metabolism. There have been some studies, reported by Michael Colgan in his book *Optimum Sports Nutrition,* showing that chromium supplementation may indeed help people lose excess body fat and gain muscle. In one study, the test subjects who consumed 200 micrograms of chromium per day for a ten-week period lost 3.3 pounds of fat and gained 1.5 pounds of lean muscle mass, while the placebo group lost only 0.4 pound of fat and did not gain any lean muscle mass. Keep in mind that these studies used subjects who were not highly conditioned athletes and probably had some type of insulin resistance and chromium deficiency to begin with.

Chromium is found in whole grains, meats, cheeses, eggs, and yeast. The more refined foods contain less chromium. No RDA has been established for chromium, but the PDI for men and women who are healthy and actively training is 200 to 600 micrograms. There are several forms of chromium, including chromium picolinate, chromium citrate, chromium chloride, and chromium polynicotinate. The picolinate and polynicotinate forms are the most popular. Chromium is included in many sports supplements.

Some athletes experience lightheadedness or a slight skin rash when taking chromium. If you feel lightheaded, stop taking the supplement. If you experience a rash, try switching brands, then discontinue its use.

Cobalt
As part of vitamin B_{12}, cobalt plays a major role in the body's metabolic processes. However, no RDA has been established for cobalt, since the amount needed is acquired as part of vitamin B_{12} and found in foods high in that vitamin.

Copper
Copper helps the body absorb and use iron. It's part of several enzymes that help form hemoglobin and collagen, and about 75 to 100 milligrams of the mineral exist in the body.

The sources of copper include shellfish, liver, dried peas and beans, nuts, cocoa, fruits, and vegetables. No RDA has been established for copper, but the suggested safe and adequate range of intake is 1.5 to 3.0 milligrams per day. The PDI of copper for men and women who are healthy and actively training is 3 to 6 milligrams. If you take a mineral supplement or use a sports nutritional powder, you're probably getting more than this amount. It's estimated that the average American diet provides about 2.0 milligrams, which qualifies as adequate. Copper deficiency is very rare.

Fluoride
Fluoride is the form of fluorine (an element) that is found in drinking water. In the body, fluoride is stored in the bones and teeth. While

researchers still have some question about whether fluoride is an essential nutrient, they know that it hardens the dental enamel, reducing the risk of cavities. In addition, some nutrition researchers suspect (but cannot prove) that certain forms of fluoride strengthen the bones.

No RDA has been established for fluoride, but there is a suggested safe and adequate range of intake of 1.5 to 4.0 milligrams daily.

Small amounts of fluoride are present in all soil, water, plants, and animal tissues. Fluoride is also supplied by fluoridated drinking water.

Iodine   Iodine is a component of the thyroid hormones thyroxin and tri-iodothyronine, which help regulate cell activities. These hormones are also essential for protein synthesis, reproduction, and tissue growth, including the formation of healthy nerves and bones.

The best natural sources of iodine are seafood and plants grown near the ocean, but athletes are most likely to get the iodine they need from iodized salt (plain table salt with added iodine). Iodates are also used as dough conditioners (additives that make dough more pliable), so you will find some iodine in most of the bread that is sold in stores.

The RDA for iodine is 150 micrograms. A teaspoon of iodized salt contains about 260 micrograms of iodine, nearly twice the RDA. The amount of iodine found in food depends on the amount of iodine that was present in the soil in which the food was grown and on how heavily the food is seasoned with table salt.

ON THE CUTTING EDGE

Female Athletes Should Monitor Their Iron Levels

Because iron plays an important role in oxygen transportation and energy metabolism, female athletes should closely monitor their hemoglobin levels to ensure continued health and maximum performance. Though full-blown iron-deficiency anemia is relatively rare among athletes, women who are on calorie-restricted diets frequently fail to meet their requirement of 15 milligrams of iron per day, according to an article published in *Training and Conditioning* in 1998. Since men have higher caloric needs and a lower iron requirement (10 milligrams per day), it is easier for them to avoid iron deficiency. Red meat, a food avoided by many athletes, who tend to strive for a low fat consumption, is one of the richest sources of iron. The average American diet supplies about 6 milligrams of iron with every 1,000 calories. Iron supplementation should be used cautiously, however, as iron is associated with increased free-radical production, in addition to toxicity, when taken in doses of over 75 milligrams per day.

Iron Iron is best known for its role in hemoglobin, the oxygen-carrying molecule found in red blood cells. Iron is also found in the compound myoglobin, which transports oxygen from the blood into the voluntary muscles. In addition, iron is part of some of the enzymes important in releasing energy from food, and it functions in other biochemical reactions within the cells.

The RDA for iron is 15 milligrams for women of child-bearing age and 10 milligrams for women after menopause. The reason for the higher RDA for younger women is that the mineral must be replaced every month after it is depleted during menstruation. The RDA for men is 10 milligrams.

Iron deficiency is probably the most common nutritional deficiency in the world, possibly because of the comparatively small amounts of animal protein that many people, particularly in the poorer nations, have available to them. Red meat, liver, fish, and poultry are excellent sources of iron. Eggs and shellfish are also good, as are legumes, dried fruits, and some dark green vegetables. Foods can become enriched with iron if they are prepared in iron cookware.

Because the absorption of iron is a complex process, simply eating iron-rich foods may not be enough to ward off iron deficiency. Much of the iron in animal protein is bound to either the hemoglobin or myoglobin of the animal protein and is referred to as "heme iron." The iron in animal foods that is not bound to hemoglobin or myoglobin and the iron in plant materials is called "nonheme iron." Of the two, heme iron is much more readily absorbed. Furthermore, vitamin C enhances iron absorption. Consequently, to avoid iron deficiency, it is necessary both to eat at least some animal foods and to have an adequate vitamin-C intake. Some foods contain materials that interfere with iron absorption. These foods include milk, coffee, tea, and whole grains. In summary, the amount of iron absorbed depends upon the form in which it is eaten and the interaction of the absorption promoters and inhibitors eaten with it.

Consuming too little dietary iron results in iron deficiency. The symptoms of deficiency include lethargy, irritability, and reduced athletic performance. If the iron deficiency becomes severe, it can affect the red blood cells and hemoglobin, reducing the blood's oxygen-transporting capacity. This condition is known as iron-deficiency anemia, and its symptoms include apathy, fatigue, and chill. Iron-deficiency anemia inevitably results in energy deficiency because, once the blood becomes affected, oxygen cannot be transported to the tissues in sufficient amounts for energy to be liberated from food. In general, women are at far more risk for iron deficiency and iron-deficiency anemia than are men because of their monthly menstrual blood loss. (For a discussion of iron and the female athlete, see page 105.) In addition, most women eat less than men. For these two reasons, many women rely on supplements to augment their iron intake, but there are disadvantages to this, too. First, not all supplements offer iron in an absorbable form. Second, some forms of supplemental iron are not well tolerated by the digestive system and can cause constipation.

Iron taken in amounts of more than 30 milligrams per day for an extended period of time can be toxic. Taken in amounts that are excessive but less than 30 milligrams per day, it may be toxic, but the risk is small. The intestines usually do not absorb much of the iron that passes through them unless there is an iron deficiency or an increased need, as in the case of pregnancy. Iron toxicity, called iron overload, usually results from an inherited trait that makes the intestines absorb too much iron, but alcoholism can aggravate the risk. Men are more vulnerable to iron overload than are women, and the outcome can include liver damage and heart attack.

Manganese About 20 milligrams of manganese are present in the average body. Manganese is involved in bone formation and the growth of connective tissue, and is an activator of many of the enzymes that function in metabolism. It may also play a role as an antioxidant as part of one form of the enzyme SOD.

Good sources of manganese are nuts, whole grains, and dried peas and beans. No RDA has been established for the mineral, but the suggested safe and adequate range of intake is 2 to 5 milligrams a day. Deficiencies of manganese have not been reported, suggesting that this level is readily attainable.

Some athletes take extra manganese when they suffer a muscle strain or sprain, since manganese has an important role in the function of glutamine synthetase, the enzyme that speeds up the production of glutamine, which plays a vital role in tissue healing. You may want to experiment with taking between 50 and 100 milligrams of manganese a day when you first experience a muscle or joint injury. Take this dosage for about one week, then reduce it to the PDI, which is 15 to 45 milligrams for men and women who are healthy and actively training.

Molybdenum Only about 9 milligrams of molybdenum are present in the average body. This mineral functions as part of the enzyme systems involved in carbohydrate, protein, and fat metabolism. Good sources of molybdenum are liver, wheat germ, whole grains, and dried peas. The molybdenum content of foods varies according to the level that was present in the soil in which the food was grown.

No RDA has been established for molybdenum, but a safe and adequate range of intake is 75 to 250 micrograms daily, an amount that is easily acquired through the diet. The PDI of molybdenum for men and women who are healthy and actively training is 100 to 300 micrograms.

Reports indicate that goutlike symptoms and other toxic side effects may be associated with excessive intake of molybdenum. Supplements of this mineral should not be taken unless directed by a doctor.

Selenium Selenium is a potent antioxidant that works synergistically with other antioxidant nutrients, such as glutathione peroxidase, vitamins C and E, and zinc, to combat cellular damage caused by free radicals. The RDA for selenium is 50 milligrams, but studies conducted at Colgan Institute, a leading center dedicated to sports-nutrition research, and other exercise-research institutes show that 200 to 400 milligrams of selenium per day may help in the fight against free-rad-

ON THE CUTTING EDGE

Vanadyl Sulfate Is a Safe Supplement

Vanadyl sulfate has been used by bodybuilders as an anabolic agent to boost strength and lean body mass. However, vanadyl compounds can be toxic in high doses, and concern has existed that they might increase blood pressure and blood viscosity, and damage red blood cells in some individuals. The effects of oral vanadyl-sulfate supplements were therefore evaluated in a study involving thirty-one bodybuilders, who consumed 0.5 milligram of vanadyl sulfate per day for every 1 kilogram (2.2 pounds) of body weight. At this dosage, vanadyl sulfate was found to have no effect on the blood system. In addition, it had no effect on the elastic properties of the red blood cells. The number of red blood cells was increased by the weight training but, according to the report published in *Medicine and Science in Sports and Exercise in 1998,* this was not associated with the vanadyl.

ical damage of heart-muscle tissue and decrease the incidence of cancer. Dr. Colgan also recommends the use of the seleno-L-methionine form of selenium for better absorption. Seleno-L-methionine is one of the most potent and nutritionally safe forms of selenium. The PDI of selenium for men and women who are healthy and actively training is 30 to 300 milligrams. Make sure to keep your daily intake of selenium to under 800 milligrams per day, since selenium can become very toxic when taken in excessive dosages, resulting in kidney and liver problems.

It is a well-known fact that many areas of the United States have too little selenium in the soil. Since plants don't need selenium, their growth will still be adequate. However, they will not supply enough selenium to the people who consume them.

Vanadium   Vanadium, or the form of the mineral called vanadyl sulfate, is popular with strength athletes. Some scientists believe that vanadyl sulfate is similar to chromium in that it "up-regulates" insulin. However, it may do this in some people, but not all. Remember that insulin is important for the transport of both glucose and amino acids into the muscles, possibly helping increase their endurance and cell size. It has also been reported that vanadyl sulfate may even help increase creatine uptake by the muscles. Up to 30 to 50 milligrams of supplemental vanadium or vanadyl sulfate can be taken per day to benefit athletic performance.

Zinc   Zinc stimulates SOD, the primary antioxidant enzyme manufactured by the body. SOD is crucial to the life of the cells. Most of the clinical research on SOD has been centered on the inflammation resulting from excess free radicals, such as in arthritis, bursitis, and gout. SOD supplements do not work because they are often missing cofactors or are almost completely destroyed in the digestive tract. Eating a balanced diet and taking zinc and other supplements will ensure production of SOD.

The RDA for zinc is 15 milligrams for men and 12 milligrams for women. The PDI of zinc for men and women who are healthy and actively training is 30 to 300 milligrams.

Meat, oysters, poultry, eggs, and liver are all high in zinc. Whole grains contain a fair amount of zinc, but they also contain phytates, which combine with zinc and prevent its absorption. Yeast counteracts the action of phytates, so eating whole-grain bread is a wise choice. Vegetarians, especially those who do not consume animal products of any kind, are likely to have a zinc deficiency. Vegetarians should eat whole-grain breads that are made with yeast, plus take zinc supplements.

Other Trace Minerals
While enough is not yet known about some of the trace minerals to establish requirements for them, evidence is accumulating that it may be essential for humans to acquire them in the diet. When the presence of a mineral in the diet promotes growth or improvement in a metabolic process, that mineral may be an essential nutrient. Another piece of evidence is a drop in the blood level of the mineral when it is not included in the diet.

The arguments for arsenic, boron, nickel, and silicon being essential for humans are growing. Nickel is present in all the tissues of the body. It is found firmly attached to DNA, and there is even a protein that binds to it in the blood. Silicon stimulates the growth of bones in animals. Boron's involvement in the bone growth of humans was reported in 1982. While it has no RDA, the PDI of boron for men and women who are healthy and actively training is 6 to 12 milligrams. Surprisingly, arsenic might be important for the metabolism of the amino acid methionine.

Colloidal Minerals

In recent years, many colloidal-mineral solutions have appeared on the market, sold as mineral and trace-mineral supplements. Colloidal-mineral manufacturers aggressively market their products to athletes, stressing the importance of minerals and trace minerals in improving health and athletic performance. While minerals and trace minerals are important for health, many of the claims concerning colloidal solutions have been exaggerated and unfounded, lacking scientific support and experimental evidence. An extensive search of over 2,000 medical and scientific journals revealed no references to colloidal-mineral intake by humans prior to 1996.

Basically, colloidal minerals are mixtures of clay and water. When water, the dispersing agent, is mixed with clay, the dispersed colloid, a colloidal mineral is created. The minerals contained in colloidal products evolved geologically in a lengthy process that included settling within clay during the Ice Age. In essence, clay is a glacial byproduct found throughout North America and northern Europe and Asia. The minerals in clay come from secondary minerals that were recrystallized by geothermal forces from minerals in granite rocks.

Clay minerals are essentially hydrous aluminum silicates. In some, magnesium or iron substitute in part for the aluminum, and alkalies or alkaline earths may be present as essential constituents. Herein lies the concern. Some colloidal-mineral products are claimed to contain between 1,800 and 4,400 parts per million of aluminum. By composition, foodstuffs contain no more than 10 parts per million as bound complexes, which are often hard to absorb. Because of the lack of any long-term research on the effect on humans of the consumption of colloidal minerals, it is unknown whether these minerals are contributing to the increased incidence of neurodegenerative diseases, such as Alzheimer's disease. Aluminum has been implicated as the possible cause of Alzheimer's, since aluminum deposits are found in microscopic clusters in the neurofibrillary tangles and granulovacuolar degeneration of the neurons that mark the disease. More research is needed to determine the exact role of the mineral, however.

Fortunately, there are many other products that offer athletes safe and reasonable levels of minerals. Until research has been completed on the benefits and safety of colloidal minerals, colloid products should be avoided. Long-term studies of the safety of colloidal minerals is certainly needed in light of the claims being made for these products.

The ever evolving and growing body of research in nutrition has led to a shift in beliefs regarding the need for supplemental vitamins and minerals. Many athletes have changed their thinking about who needs supplements and how much. These athletes no longer believe that we can rely solely on diet to meet our vitamin and mineral requirements. In some cases, the optimum amount of a vitamin cannot be obtained from dietary sources alone. Even for the vitamins that can be obtained strictly through diet, government surveys show that most people simply don't. In this hectic era, when so many of us eat our meals on the run, people don't have time to prepare and eat the well-balanced, varied diet necessary to meet the RDAs of all of the vitamins and minerals.

Most of all, however, evidence is mounting that antioxidants, vitamins, and minerals can help improve athletic performance and aid in the recovery from intensive training. Hopefully, this book will inspire you to look more carefully at your nutritional practices and to make the necesary changes to optimize your intake of the vitamins and minerals. When you do that, you will be taking a step on the path to optimum sports performance and health.

ENZYMES
THE KEYS TO HEALTH

6

No plant, animal, or human could exist without enzymes. During every moment of our lives, enzymes keep us going. At this very instant, millions of tiny enzymes are working throughout your body causing reactions to take place. You couldn't breathe, hold or turn the pages of this book, read its words, eat a meal, taste the food, or hear a telephone ring without enzymes. You'd be dead, pushing up daisies and fertilizing some living plant, if not for enzymes.

So far, researchers have identified more than 3,000 kinds of enzymes in the human body. There are millions of these energizers that renew, maintain, and protect us. Every second of our lives, these enzymes are constantly changing and renewing, sometimes at an unbelievable rate.

WHAT ARE ENZYMES?

Enzymes are protein-based substances found in every cell of every living plant and animal, including the human body. Without enzymes, the grass or trees would not grow, seeds would not sprout nor would flowers bloom, and beer and wine could not ferment. Even the autumn leaves would not burst forth in glorious colors without the help of enzymes. Mother Nature has blessed us with her wondrous magic in providing enzymes to ripen bananas from green to yellow-gold, or tomatoes from green to robust, juicy red.

Enzymes are the powerhouses of each and every cell. They either start chemical reactions, or they make them run faster. Enzymes remain unchanged even after a reaction is completed. Enzymes appear throughout nature, even in the food we eat. When the thinly sliced cabbage that your grandmother placed in a Crock-Pot fermented into sauerkraut, or your grandfather's elderberries slowly turned into wine, enzymes were at work.

The use of enzymes in food preparation probably began long before anyone knew what these little dynamos were or what they could do. Like a travelogue of enlightened civilizations, the history of enzymes takes us from ancient Egypt to Greece, Germany, Denmark, and Japan . . . around the world. All of these civilizations, knowingly or unknowingly, used enzymes in their food preparations. From the first bag of wine, round of cheese, keg of beer, vat of vinegar, or loaf of bread—in fact, any food that required fermentation (the word enzyme comes from the Greek word *enzymos,* which means leavened or fermented)—the action of enzymes helped our ancestors prepare and preserve the food they needed.

The ancients felt that the secret of life (and the difference between living and nonliving structures) was a certain "vitality." This is why the changes that occurred in foods as they fermented were considered to be almost magic—they possessed that special vitality. The ancients knew that milk could be magically changed into cheese, and grapes into wine. Couldn't this elusive vitality, this "magic," be harnessed and used to transform iron into gold? Such was the attempt of the early alchemists.

Though they probably didn't understand the process, our earliest ancestors knew that fermentation would change their food. Even cave dwellers discovered that aged meat had a more pleasing flavor and was more tender than the freshly killed variety. Your grandmother may have used *rennin,* an enzyme from calf's stomach, to clot milk—the first step in making cheese. Grapes left to ferment turned into wine, while grains, with a little coaxing (and the addition of malt, which is rich in an enzyme called *amylase*), produced beer.

Today, we know that fermentation is not magic but a chemical change caused by bacteria, microscopic yeasts, and molds. In some instances, fermentation is used to alter or change a material in a way that would be very costly or difficult if other methods were used. For example, modern medicine uses fermentation under controlled conditions to produce a number of antibiotics.

Although fermentation has been used for centuries in the processing of food, our knowledge of the science behind the way it works is relatively new. We now know that it is the action of enzymes in yeast (and not the yeast itself) that causes alcoholic fermentation. Eduard Buchner received the Nobel Prize in 1907 for this discovery. Enzymes act as natural catalysts that cause a chemical change without themselves being affected.

Now that scientists know how enzymes can affect our foods and our food-processing techniques, they have drawn on this knowledge to concoct better, faster, and cheaper ways to manufacture what we eat. And we see the results practically every day in almost every food or drink that we consume. For example, many beer drinkers, trying to cut down on calories, are opting for light beer, a product impossible to make without enzymes. Enzymes are also used in the production of cheese, wine, baked goods, soy sauce, fruit and vegetable juices, and food ingredients such as fructose, aspartame, modified oils and fats, and emulsifiers.

THE ENZYMES IN YOUR LIFE

All things living have enzymatic activity, whether it be the grass in front of your house, your dog Fido, or your food (if the enzymes have not been killed yet). Whatever is alive has enzymes in it. That includes *you.* In fact, enzymes make your body work.

All life processes, such as digestion, breathing, even thinking, consist at least in part of a complex series of chemical reactions called *metabolism.* But that explanation is a little too simple. Actually metabolism is composed of two parts: *anabolism* and *catabolism*. Anabolism is any process in which simpler substances are combined to form more complex substances. It is the process of building up (such as new tissue growth). Catabolism is the flip side. It is any process in which living cells break down substances into simpler substances (such as that which occurs in digestion). The sum of these two processes is metabolism. Enzymes are the catalysts (the jump-starters) that make these chemical reactions possible. In fact, many of the body's chemical reactions would never take place without enzyme catalysts.

In addition to their roles in metabolism, enzymes are also food potentiators. All foods have potential nutrients. Enzymes have the ability to turn these potential nutrients into available nutrients. For example, carrots contain beta-carotene. But we can't get the beta-carotene out if we can't unlock it from the carrot's cells. Therefore, we won't benefit from the carrot's nutrients. It's like Fort Knox—you've got to unlock the door in order to get the treasure out.

As long as our bodies can make enzymes, we live. But our bodies' production of enzymes can be decreased by illness, injury, stress, or aging. If the body can't produce them fast enough or with enough activity level, then enzymes must be acquired from an outside source. This is similar to a factory that uses a certain part faster than it can be made. Production can come to a standstill until the missing part is provided. Further, as the years go by, the machinery making the part begins to wear out and produces fewer parts. Therefore, more and more parts must be obtained from outside the factory in order to maintain the same production level. Your body works much the same way. When enzyme production falters or ceases, you're in trouble and enzyme supplements may be necessary. How long can your bodily functions remain active when breathing, circulation, or other systems are at a standstill?

Our bodies are magnificent machines containing over 3,000 kinds of enzymes, with each enzyme performing a different job. And without them, there would be no breathing, no digestion, no growth, no blood coagulation, and no reproduction. There are millions and millions of enzymes found in the lungs, liver, digestive system, and brain—in fact, in every system of our bodies. Some of these enzymes are secreted in an active form, while others (for instance, some enzymes involved in digestion) are secreted in an inactive form. They are activated when needed, sometimes by other enzymes, and are then ready to do their jobs.

From the top of your head to the tips of your toes, these enzymes are everywhere in your body. They help keep us alive and functioning. They keep us physically and mentally healthy, and they slow down that inevitable process of aging. Enzymes are so important that when their quantities drop and activity levels fall, illness is just around the corner.

SIX CLASSES OF ENZYMES

Because enzymes have so many applications, scientists have found it helpful to classify them based on what they do, what substances they act upon (substrates), and the reaction they start or accelerate. There are six main groups of enzymes, each having fundamentally different activities. *Hydrolases* break down proteins, carbohydrates, and fats such as during the process of digestion. They do this by adding a water molecule, thus the name *hydrolases. Isomerases* catalyze the rearrangement of chemical groups within the same molecule. The *ligases* catalyze the formation of a bond between two substrate molecules through the use of an energy source. *Lyases* catalyze the formation of double bonds between atoms by adding or subtracting chemical groups. *Oxidoreductases* make oxidation–reduction (the process by which an atom loses an electron to another atom) possible. *Transferases* transfer chemical groups from one molecule to another.

Your body contains many enzymes from each group.

HOW ENZYMES WORK

Most enzymes work by helping take something apart. For instance, your digestive enzymes are the forces that help break down that hamburger you ate last night into its smallest components, that is amino acids, mono- and disaccharides, esters, etc. Your teeth only do part of the work. The enzymes in your digestive tract actually snip apart the bonds that hold the various components of that hamburger together. Most enzymes work by taking bonds apart. Only about 3 to 5 percent of enzymes synthesize instead of breaking apart. These are the anabolic enzymes, not the cleaving catabolic enzymes.

In order to digest that hamburger, certain enzymes in your gastrointestinal tract break apart (lyse) the protein in the meat, while others work on the bread in the bun, and still others attack the onion, lettuce, pickles, ketchup, and mustard. Why so many enzymes? Because, with very few exceptions, each enzyme works on only one kind of substrate and in a specific way. Enzymes are very specialized. They are "substrate specific."

How does this work? There are at least two theories: the *lock and key theory* and the *induced fit theory.* The first theory—lock and key—likens the substrate to a key that must fit into a specific shape on the enzyme in order to activate that enzyme (much the same way a key fits into a lock to unlock a door). The induced fit theory states that the shape of the enzyme actually changes to allow the substrate to bind, similar to a glove conforming to the shape of a hand. The shape of the hand makes the glove's shape alter a little. Whatever the mechanism, the enzyme and the substrate come together and the enzyme is able to begin its work. The site of the connection between the enzyme and the substrate is called the *active site.* In order for the enzyme to do its work, the substrate (the molecule that is to be altered) must come into contact with the enzyme's active site. This recognition process ensures that only a specific molecule is recognized by an enzyme as being the proper substrate.

How Quickly Do Enzymes Work?

Each enzyme works under unique conditions and at its own speed—and they're fast. We can get some idea of the speed of enzymes by considering the slowest known enzyme, lysozyme. Lysozyme helps destroy bacteria and can process about thirty substrate molecules per minute. That is one substrate every two seconds! And as fast as that seems, it's nothing compared with the enzyme carboanhydrase, which processes an astonishing 36 million substrate molecules in one minute!

The speed of an enzyme is influenced by its work environment. It's like the work conditions in a factory. If a worker has pleasant conditions, he or she will be happier and work harder. If it's too cold or too hot, the workers will suffer and so will production. So it is with enzymes. They must have optimal working conditions.

Every enzyme also works best when in a specific range of pH—a measure of acidity and alkalinity. Some enzymes work better in an acid environment (like that of your stomach), while others need a more alkaline environment to do their jobs efficiently.

Coenzymes and Cofactors

Although enzymes stimulate a variety of chemical reactions, they can do so only in association with small molecules called coenzymes and cofactors. *Cofactors* are substances that must be present for an enzyme to function. Minerals, such as zinc, magnesium, copper, and calcium, are some cofactors. *Coenzymes* are organic substances that combine with an inactive enzyme (an apoenzyme) to form an active enzyme (a holoenzyme). A coenzyme may be a cofactor. Some coenzymes include the B vitamins and vitamin C.

Enzyme Inhibitors

Though some substances help enzymes work better, there are others that actually inhibit the activity of an enzyme. Sometimes these enzyme inhibitors are *competitive*. That is, they actually compete with the substrate, preventing it from getting to the active site where it bonds to the enzyme. Other inhibitors are *noncompetitive* and work by retarding the conversion of the substrate by an enzyme. Either way, enzyme inhibitors can terminate or retard enzyme activity.

We encounter a number of substances every day that can inhibit our bodies' enzymes. This includes most medicines (even aspirin). An example of other inhibitors would be organic solvents, the most frequently produced chemicals in the United States. Primarily obtained from petroleum or natural gas, these chemicals are used extensively in the chemical industry and in many manufacturing processes and are known to inhibit a wide variety of enzymes. Examples of organic solvents include methanol, ethanol, propenol, formic acid, ethylene glycol, hexane, benzene, and butanol. These and other organic solvents are used in the manufacture of, or are found in, a variety of products you encounter every day, including paints and numerous household cleaners.

How Long Do Enzymes Last?

Just like any other protein, enzymes do not live forever. They age and die. When an enzyme begins to show signs of wear and tear, another enzyme comes along and makes short work of it. The worn-out enzyme is broken down, dissolved, and transported away.

Some enzymes have a life of only about twenty minutes. After this, the enzyme is replaced by a newly produced enzyme of the same type. Other enzymes remain active for several weeks before they are replaced.

One of the most fascinating properties of all enzymes is their ability to work with each other to form cooperatives when necessary and to continually exchange information with other enzyme cooperatives. The equilibrium of all systems that they maintain and the mutual effort toward a common goal are all positive properties of enzymes.

ARE YOU ENZYME-DEFICIENT?

Our bodies' ability to function, repair when injured, and ward off disease is directly related to the strength and numbers of our enzymes. That's why an enzyme deficiency can be so devastating.

Disease, diets consisting of foods with dead enzymes, chemotherapy, stress, physical injuries, illness, aging, or digestive problems can all affect our enzyme levels. But sometimes eating right and living a healthy lifestyle are not enough. Certain individuals have genetic or inborn problems affecting their enzyme production or activity.

You've probably seen the label on diet soda warning that the soda contains phenylalanine. Most diet sodas use aspartame as a sweetener. But aspartame is made from two amino acids: phenylalanine and aspartic acid. Those individuals who are *phenylketonurics* lack the enzyme phenylalanine hydroxylase, which is necessary to break down phenylalanine. And if it can't be broken down, it will build up in the bloodstream leading to neurological symptoms and mental retardation. The only recognized treatment for this condition is to avoid taking phenylalanine—hence, the warning labels.

Those who suffer from *lactose intolerance* don't produce enough of the enzyme lactase, which digests lactose, so drinking milk, which contains lactose, can lead to diarrhea and pain. *Gaucher's disease* is a rare familial disorder of fat metabolism. This disease, which usually begins in childhood, is due to lack of the enzyme glucocerebrosidase.

Some of these enzyme deficiency diseases can be corrected with supplemental enzymes, some cannot. But an enzyme deficiency might not have blatant symptoms or be life-threatening. Many of us are suffering from suboptimal health *only* because we're enzyme-deficient.

SIGNS OF ENZYME DEFICIENCY

The first sign that you're not getting enough enzymes will probably be disturbed digestion. You know—indigestion, stomach upset . . . gas. Many people notice a bloated feeling after eating particular foods, such as beans or cauliflower. This could be a sign that they don't have the enzymes necessary to adequately digest that food. Many foods, including beans, contain complex sugars. If these sugars cannot be broken down, they will sit in the large intestine and putrefy, leading to a bloated feeling and gas. This is easily corrected by taking such enzyme supplements as BeSure; Beano; Beans, Beans . . . and More Beans Rx; or other digestive enzyme supplements.

Another sign of an enzyme shortage that's not so easy to see is free-radical formation. In a telephone interview, Hans Kugler, Ph.D., international authority on aging and former president of the National Health Federation, stated that we should be living to the age of 120 or better. But the average American lives to be about 72 years old. Why does this happen? Pollutants and free radicals in our environment—as well as free radicals produced within the body—cause our bodies to "rust" and age. Wrinkling is an external sign of free-radical damage. Certain enzymes are antioxidants, that is free-radical scavengers (some of the best known are superoxide dismutase, catalase, and glutathione peroxidase). These enzymes fight the free radicals that destroy our bodies.

Illness is probably the most obvious sign that you're not getting enough enzymes or that your body enzyme levels are depleted. As mentioned previously, enzymes make your body work. Any illness or disease process, such as cardiovascular disease, degenerative diseases, cancer, or even a slow recovery rate after an injury are all indications that your body's enzymes are not working optimally.

ENZYME SOURCES

Supplemental enzymes can be obtained from a variety of sources, including animals (usually hog or calf pancreas), plants (such as pineapple and papaya), and microbial fermentations (from bacteria or fungi—these are often called "plant-derived"), in combinations of the above, and in concentrated food or plant extracts, called "functional" foods.

Animal Enzymes

The human body produces and secretes a number of enzymes, many of which are also made by other animals. For instance, the enzyme trypsin, found in pancreatic juice, is also found in the pancreas of many vertebrates, as well as in insects, crayfish, and microorganisms such as *Streptomyces griseus*. Each form of trypsin (regardless of the source) is a hydrolase and catalyzes the same reaction. Enzymes taken from animal sources are commonly extracted from the pancreas, liver, or stomach of beef, oxen, and pigs. These enzymes include proteases, amylases, and lipases. Some of the best known are trypsin, chymotrypsin, pepsin, rennin, and pancreatin (which is not a single enzyme, but rather a combination of primarily amylase, lipase, and protease enzymes).

Protomorphogens (or glandulars) are organ- and glandular-based food supplements that contain a mixture of enzymes that naturally occur in the particular organ or gland from which the extract was obtained. They are taken from animal organs and glands, such as the pancreas, thyroid, ovaries, testicles, brains, and so on. The enzyme composition of protomorphogens varies depending on the animal and organ or gland used as a source, and the treatment the organ or gland received during processing into an extract.

Plant Enzymes

In addition to enzymes taken from animal sources, many enzyme supplements are derived from plants. Although every plant has enzymatic activity, some plants are particularly rich enzyme sources. The enzymes used in supplements are primarily those from pineapple (bromelain), papaya (papain), fig (ficin), and barley (malt diastase). Although available in purified form, most enzymes from plants are also found in plant or food extracts. In this book, concentrated food extracts are discussed and classified as "functional foods." These food concentrates often contain the amylase, lipase, and protease enzymes that naturally occur in the fruit or vegetable used in the product, as well as phytochemicals (beneficial plant chemicals), vitamins, and minerals. For example, pineapple extract contains the enzyme bromelain as well as vitamins A, B, C, D, E, and K; calcium; iron; phosphorus; potassium; sodium; and magnesium. Pineapple is one of the most nutrient-rich, enzymatically active fruits in the world and is considered an excellent source of natural antioxidants. In addition to pineapple, many other fruits, especially papaya, kiwi, figs, guava, and ginger root are known to have a high protease content.

Microbial Enzymes

Microbial (sometimes called "plant-derived") enzymes are of bacterial or fungal origin and are produced through fermentation using these microorganisms. In recent years, microorganisms have increasingly been used as a source of enzymes for supplements because they are relatively inexpensive and provide an abundant supply. In fact, microbial enzymes now represent about 90 percent of all enzymes produced commercially for any purpose, according to Tony Godfrey and Stuart West in their book *Industrial Enzymology,* 2nd Edition (New York: Macmillan Press, Ltd., 1996).

But before you back away in horror, be aware that fermentation is a source of many modern medicines. For instance, *Bacillus subtilis* is a common bacterium found in soil and water and is used to produce the antibiotic bacitracin. Even penicillin is derived from *Penicillium* and other soil-inhabiting fungi. Industrial microbiology is also used to produce vitamins (such as B_{12}, thiamin, and riboflavin), amino acids (such as lysine, arginine, and glutamic acid), and antibiotics (such as streptomycin, tetracycline, and cloramphenicol).

The best known sources of the many microbial enzymes used in supplements are *Aspergillus oryzae* (a fungus), *Aspergillus niger* (a fungus), *Rhizopus niveus* (a fungus), *Bacillus licheniformis* (a bacterium), *Bacillus subtilis* (a bacterium), and several *Saccharomyces* species (yeast).

Enzyme Combinations

Sometimes, manufacturers combine different types of enzymes from a number of animal, plant, and/or microbial sources. Because of their variety of origins and substrates, wide ranges of optimal temperatures and pH levels, synergism, increased percentage of absorption, and increased level of effectiveness, enzyme mixtures have a wider range of therapeutic advantages than do individual enzymes, according to Dr. Peter Streichhan, a world-renowned enzyme researcher from Geretsried, Germany.

Plant and microbial enzymes are still highly active at higher temperatures and in acidic environments, whereas most animal enzymes function best at body temperature and at a neutral to alkaline pH range. Very few animal enzymes demonstrate maximum activity at higher temperatures and in acidic environments (such as during fever or inflammation). This is why combining animal enzymes with plant or microbial enzymes is of value. The enzyme mixtures support one another in their range of activities. By combining enzymes from many sources, you can get wider pH, temperature, and substrate ranges. Because of this, you will have a broader range of activity and application. I like to think of these enzyme combinations as "cocktails."

There are a number of enzyme combinations on the market. In fact, most products sold in health-food stores are enzyme combinations, rather than individual enzymes.

Functional Foods

For centuries, humans have used foods such as fruits, vegetables, herbs, grains, and animal products to keep well, fight disease, and extend life. Our forefathers believed that these foods contained mysterious ingredients capable of keeping us healthy or curing us when sick. Today, extensive research is identifying the components responsible for the natural, health-giving properties of these foods. Scientists can now concentrate and standardize extracts from these fresh foods. Called by a number of different terms, including functional foods, pharmafoods, nutraceuticals, and designer foods, these extracts are excellent sources of enzymes, vitamins, minerals, chlorophyll, protein, phytochemicals, hormones, and other nutrients. These functional food products are available as tablets, capsules, powders, granules, liquids, elixirs, lozenges, and extracts.

The universe has a natural order. When we deviate from, or interfere with, this order (as our modern lifestyles cause us to do), illness results. Foods contain components that will keep our bodies in balance and help rectify these disorders whenever they occur. Therefore, functional foods, which contain these health-giving components, are effective in fighting diseases such as cardiovascular disease, diabetes, hypertension, cancer, and arthritis, improving wellness, and extending life.

Functional foods are helpful to our enzymes in many ways. They often serve as a direct source of enzymes. They provide coenzymes and cofactors (vitamins and minerals) needed for the proper function of your body's enzymes. Functional foods contain nutrients known to "kick-start" your body's enzyme production or function. For instance, among other nutrients, plant functional foods contain phytochemicals, and animal-derived functional foods contain hormones necessary for your body's enzyme function.

ENZYME THERAPY

Research has shown that a number of conditions, including acne, aging, allergies, autoimmune conditions, cancer, circulatory diseases, health conditions requiring detoxification, infections, inflammation, injuries, rheumatic diseases, skin problems, sports and other injuries, and viruses can all be treated with enzymes, according to Drs. D.A. Lopez, R.M. Williams, and M. Miehlke, authors of *Enzymes: The Foundation of Life* (Charleston, SC: Neville Press, Inc., 1994).

Although there is variation among individuals, our bodies' enzymatic activity generally begins to decline somewhere between the ages of sixteen and twenty, as our growth peaks. At this time, the rate of tissue reproduction tends to decrease, and what we refer to as aging begins. Since every activity in the body requires enzymes, replenishing the enzyme supply lost with aging can restore your body's natural enzyme balance. This, in turn, can help fight disease and improve your health status. This is why systemic enzyme therapy is effective against such a wide variety of conditions.

The type of enzyme you take, the dosage level, individual variables (such as height, weight, general health, lifestyle, and dietary patterns), and the condition being treated can all influence how rapidly you respond to enzyme therapy. For instance, if you are taking enzymes to improve digestion, you should notice an improvement within a couple of hours. If not, perhaps you need to increase the dose. If improvement still is not seen, analyze your diet and make sure you're taking the proper type of enzyme to digest what you eat, or that you don't have some other illness (for instance, a heart condition) that is mimicking a digestive problem.

Generally speaking, when enzymes are taken to treat an inflammatory condition or one involving pain, some improvement will be noted within three to seven days. Chronic conditions such as rheumatoid arthritis may require one to three months (or more) before you notice a change in your symptoms. In addition, some conditions have periods of waxing and waning (such as rheumatoid arthritis or multiple sclerosis)—times when the symptoms may be markedly worse or, perhaps, a little better. When the condition is worse (or when you notice an exacerbation of symptoms), it's important to increase the dose.

(For a discussion of the use of proteolytic enzymes to improve injury healing, see page 121.)

CHOOSING AN ENZYME SUPPLEMENT

Enzymes are specialized, and because the human body contains over 3,000 types of these catalysts (many of which act synergistically) it is impossible to say which particular enzyme is most important. However, a shortage of just one enzyme can mean poor health.

The enzyme supplement you choose will depend on your goal. If taking enzymes as digestive aids, you should choose enzymes based on your diet. For instance, those who have trouble digesting the protein in beef should take a proteolytic enzyme, such as pancreatin, trypsin, chymotrypsin, papain, or a microbial protease. Lipases assist in digesting fats, and a number of enzymes work on carbohydrates and sugars (including lactase, amylase, cellulase, alpha-galactosidase, and similar products).

If taking enzymes to fight free radicals, take an antioxidant enzyme (such as superoxide dismutase, glutathione peroxidase, and catalase). These enzymes are often enterically coated to improve absorption. Enterically coated enzymes are generally used for systemic purposes, although some (such as pancreatin) are also effective at improving digestion. Each enzyme has certain advantages, depending on what you want to achieve.

Enzyme supplements are available in many different forms—as tablets (uncoated, enterically coated, or microencapsulated), coated granules, powder, capsules, liquid, chewing gum, injections, creams and ointments, and retention

Proteolytic Enzymes Improve Injury Healing

Athletic injuries cause setbacks in training and downtime during the season. Because of this, in the 1960s, a number of scientists looked for natural products that can help improve the rate of injury healing. In animal studies, the use of proteolytic enzymes was shown to reduce the inflammation associated with injuries and to shorten healing time. Subsequent studies conducted in hospitals and using injured people, surgery patients, and women who had given birth also demonstrated that proteolytic enzymes can help quicken the healing process.

In 1967, P. S. Boyne and H. Medhurst applied these clinically verified benefits to athletes on the playing field. In a landmark study, they gave a proteolytic-enzyme concentrate (containing trypsin and chymotrypsin) to football (soccer) players from twenty-eight professional teams. The tablets were enterically coated, enabling them to pass through the stomach and not be digested until entering the intestines, since it had been learned in animal studies that the acidic stomach environment decreases the amount of proteolytic enzymes absorbed into the body by altering the enzymes chemically. During the study periods, any athlete who sustained a significant injury was immediately given two proteolytic-enzyme tablets, followed by two tablets at bedtime. The injured athlete then continued to take four tablets daily, in divided dosages, a half hour before meals, until he recovered from his injury and was able to return to training. At the end of the football (soccer) season, Drs. Boyne and Mehurst determined that less playing time had been lost per player when the injured players were given the proteolytic-enzyme product as compared to the previous season, when the proteolytic-enzyme product had not been given. In other words, the proteolytic-enzyme product reduced the amount of time it took to recover from injury and return to training.

Other researchers reported similar results when using proteolytic-enzyme preparations to help quicken injury-recovery time. The benefits to the healing process include improved blood flow to the injured area, reduced inflammation, reduced edema, and improved flexibility and motility. Along with the proteolytic enzymes (trypsin and chymotrypsin), the enzymes papain and bromelain have also been shown to be effective at improving the rate of recovery from injuries. Note that in the aforementioned studies, proper medical attention was also administered, along with drug therapy when indicated, as well as physical therapy, rest, and the application of ice. The oral proteolytic-enzyme products were well tolerated by the subjects, and side effects were rarely reported.

So, the next time you experience a sports-related injury—or any injury, for that matter—include a short course of proteolytic enzymes in your treatment. Try using a bromelain, papain, or trypsin-chymotrypsin product, or one that contains all four of these efficacious enzymes, in enteric-coated tablets or capsules. The effective daily dosages range from 300 to 500 milligrams three to four times a day. These enzymes are best taken on an empty stomach, with juice or water. (*Do not* take these enzymes if you are sensitive to papaya or pineapple.) Take them until the injury is healed, usually several days; take them longer only under a doctor's supervision. In addition to taking the enzymes, make sure you maintain a healthy diet and take your regular supplements, as well as other supplements known to improve healing—bioflavonoids, 1,000 to 2,000 milligrams a day; curcumin, 1,000 to 2,000 milligrams a day; glucosamine, 1,500 to 2,500 milligrams a day; and chondroitin sulfate, 1,500 to 2,500 milligrams a day. And don't forget to seek medical attention for the injury!

enemas. They may be formulated individually or in combinations of enzymes. You can choose your supplement based on your likes and needs.

Although many supplemental enzymes are taken orally, some can be taken sublingually (under the tongue), or rectally with an enema. Enzymes can also be applied topically in ointments, creams, salves, and lotions.

There are also some enzymes administered primarily by injection, which is done in a doctor's office or hospital. When administered in this way, absorption is not of critical importance, since they are injected directly into the bloodstream or into tissue. Those enzymes administered by injection include brinase, chymopapain, collagenase, hyaluronidase, lysozyme, plasmin, streptokinase, streptodornase, and urokinase. However, collagenase and hyaluronidase can also be administered topically. Other enzymes that can be taken by injection include carbohydrase, chymotrypsin, superoxide dismutase (SOD), and trypsin. It should be noted, however, that injectable enzymes should be used with caution. They can cause very serious side effects, such as anaphylactic shock, and are only used by physicians in severe life-threatening situations.

Enzymes are also of value in face and body creams. Papain and bromelain are probably the best known topical enzymes. Zia Wesley-Hosford, author of *Face Value* (San Francisco, Zia Cosmetics, Inc., 1990) believes that green papaya enzymes assist the healing of uneven pigmentation, fine lines, and brown spots by fighting free-radical damage and boosting cell production and are considered the "natural alternative to Retin-A." In fact, enzymes, especially papain, are being used in a number of facial products. Many of the larger cosmetic companies, such as Estée Lauder, are now beginning to add enzymes to their facial products.

Sometimes skin creams, salves, or exfoliants made with enzymes are purchased in powdered form and must be mixed with oil or other fluid to activate before application (follow the instructions on the bottle or box).

Food extracts contain many of the enzymes naturally occurring in the plants used in each particular formula. In addition, formulas containing enzymes combined with herbs, vitamins, minerals, and other nutrients are effective at improving the absorption and bioavailability of the nutrients, maximizing enzyme activity, and reducing the drain on the body's own digestive enzymes.

The price of enzyme supplements can vary widely depending on the activity level, the amount of enzyme in the tablet, and bottle size. The price of a bottle of enzymes can range from two or three dollars for a bottle of papain to $80 or more for certain enzyme combinations. Although the price is not always a guarantee of quality or potency, it can be one indication. Just like any other commodity, the bulk price for enzymes is fairly uniform. For this reason, you would expect to pay more for a bottle of one hundred 100 mg bromelain tablets than you would for a bottle of one hundred 50 mg bromelain tablets, regardless of the manufacturer, assuming that the enzymes in question had the same activity level. Comparing price gets a little trickier if the activity levels are different. Generally speaking, compare brands and choose the tablets or pills with the highest activity level regardless of price.

Keep in mind that when choosing an enzyme supplement, almost any choice is a good choice because the enzymes will help your body to function in a more effective fashion. Further, they will help you overcome the plight of enzyme-dead food, environmental problems (such as today's pollution and toxins), lifestyle changes, stress, premature aging, and the development of chronic disorders.

COMMON ENZYME SUPPLEMENTS

The following enzymes are those most frequently used by athletes. They can be purchased in health-food stores and drug stores, through mail order, or from multi-level marketing companies. Included are the sources from which they are taken, their actions and benefits, the best way to take them, and any additional comments.

Alpha-Galactosidase (or Melibiase)   Alpha-galactosidase, which is commonly sold as Beano, breaks down carbohydrates, such as raffinose, stachyose, and verbascose. Is is used as a digestive aid. It prevents the gas and other gastrointestinal symptoms that occur after eating a high-fiber diet of beans, grains, and other vegetables.

The microbial sources of alpha-galactosidase include *Aspergillus niger* and *Aspergillus oryzae*.

The food sources of alpha-galactosidase include cucumbers and legumes, such as soybeans and cowpeas (black-eyed peas).

Alpha-galactosidase is best taken orally.

Amylase (or Carbohydrase, Glycogenase)   Amylase breaks down carbohydrates, such as starch, glycogen, and related polysaccharides and oligosaccharides. It is used to aid digestion (usually in combination with other enzymes). It is used in pancreatic enzyme replacement therapy.

The animal sources of amylase include bovine and porcine pancreas. The plant sources include barley (*Hordeum vulgare*). The microbial sources include *Aspergillus aureus, Aspergillus niger, Aspergillus oryzae, Bacillus licheniformis, Bacillus stearothermophilus, Bacillus subtilis, Rhizopus niveus,* and *Rhizopus oryzae.*

Amylase is the most frequently found enzyme in plants and occurs most abundantly in raw sweet potato; corn, barley, wheat, oats, rice, and other grains; red lingzhi (or reishi) mushrooms; beet roots, leaves, and stems; banana; cabbage; egg; kidney bean; maple sap; milk; mushrooms; raw honey; and sugar cane.

Amylase is best taken orally.

Beta-Glucosidase (or Emulsin)   Beta-glucosidase breaks down carbohydrates, such as sugars and starches. It is used as a digestive aid (often in conjunction with amylase, as it facilitates its activity).

The plant sources of beta-glucosidase include sweet almonds. The microbial sources include *E. coli, Aspergillus niger,* and *Trichoderma longibrachiatum.*

The food sources of beta-glucosidase include almonds and green plants.

Beta-glucosidase is best taken orally.

Bromelain
Bromelain breaks down protein. It aids in the overall digestion and absorption of nutrients, particularly of protein. Bromelain is used in pancreatic enzyme replacement therapy. Because of its wide pH range, it can be used as a substitute for pepsin and trypsin in cases of digestive deficiency. Bromelain fights inflammation; reduces swelling; inhibits fibrin synthesis; degrades fibrin and fibrinogen; is used to treat conditions such as cellulitis, epididymitis, hypostatic and diabetic ulcers, numerous inflammatory conditions, furniculosis (boils), and epinephrine-caused pulmonary swelling. It speeds recovery from such injuries resulting from trauma, childbirth, sports, or surgery as sprains, strains, contusions, abrasions, hematomas, ecchymoses (small hemorrhagic spots), lacerated and/or perforated wounds, and fractures; and also reduces the swelling and hematomas that often follow surgery. Bromelain improves respiratory conditions including throat infections, pharyngitis, sinusitis, bronchitis, and pneumonia. It improves conditions associated with arthritis and other degenerative bone and joint disease. It is used to topically treat skin conditions, including infections and burns (it accelerates the elimination of burn debris and promotes healing), and is used in many cosmetics and personal care products (such as facial cleansers, bath preparations, and exfoliants). Bromelain fights cardiovascular problems, such as blood platelet aggregation, phlebitis (inflammation of a vein), varicose ulcers, peripheral venous disease, thromboses (in a variety of sites, including the central retinal vein), and heart attacks. It bolsters the immune system, uncovers the membranes of antigens (such as viruses and bacteria) and assists your body in better identifying and attacking these antigens, helps break up antigen-antibody complexes (immune complexes), and improves antibiotic absorption. It helps fight cancer and activates tumor necrosis factor (a tumor-fighting substance produced by the body). Bromelain helps prevent dysmenorrhea, allergies, and oral infections. It can be used for thyroid therapy. It can inhibit appetite. It prevents intestinal bacterial infections, which often cause diarrhea. Bromelain can help extend life.

The plant sources of bromelain include the stem or fruit of the pineapple (*Ananas comosus* or *Ananas sativus*).

The food sources of bromelain include fresh, raw pineapple.

Bromelain is best taken orally and topically.

Carboxypeptidase
Carboxypeptidase breaks down proteins. It is used as a digestive aid. Carboxypeptidase is used in pancreatic replacement therapy. It is one of four proteolytic enzymes found in pancreatin along with trypsin, chymotrypsin, and elastase.

The animal sources of carboxypeptidase include bovine and porcine pancreas. The plant sources include wheat. The microbial sources include *Pseudomonas* sp., *Penicillium janthinellum,* and yeast.

Carboxypeptidase is best taken orally.

Catalase
Catalase breaks hydrogen peroxide down into water and oxygen.

It reportedly lowers serum cholesterol. It is one of the most potent antioxidant enzymes.

The animal sources of catalase include bovine liver. The microbial sources include *Aspergillus niger* and *Micrococcus lysodeikticus.*

The food sources of catalase include peas, maize, soybeans, grape, mango, milk, mushroom, raw honey, and sugar cane. Catalase is found in almost all plant tissues.

Catalase is best taken orally.

Cellulase (or Endogluconase, Exogluconase) Cellulase breaks down cellulose (an indigestible fiber found in many fruits and vegetables). It is used as a digestive aid. Cellulase is used in pancreatic enzyme replacement. It is used in treating gastric bezoars (hard masses composed of hair and/or fruit and vegetable fibers that can form in the alimentary canal).

The microbial sources of cellulase include *Aspergillus oryzae, Aspergillus niger, Rhizopus* sp., and *Trichoderma longibrachiatum* (formerly *reesei*).

The food sources of cellulase include avocado, peas, oat sprouts, and red lingzhi (reishi) mushrooms.

Cellulase is best taken orally.

Chymotrypsin Chymotrypsin breaks down proteins. It is used as a digestive aid. Chymotrypsin fights inflammation and reduces swelling. It fights arthritis (osteo- and traumatic). It treats soft tissue injuries, acute traumatic injuries, sprains, contusions, hematomas, ecchymosis, infection, edema (of the eyelids and genitalia), charley horse, and sports injuries. Chymotrypsin aids in surgical recovery. It can be used in debridement, treatment of ulcerations and abscesses, and the liquefaction of mucous secretions. It can be used against enterozoic worms. Chymotrypsin can be used to treat cancer. It is one of at least four proteolytic enzymes found in pancreatin.

The animal sources of chymotrypsin include bovine and porcine pancreas.

Chymotrypsin is best taken orally, topically, or by injection. *Caution: Injectable enzymes should be used with care. They may cause severe, life-threatening side effects.*

Diastase (or Malt Diastase) Diastase breaks down carbohydrates. It is used as a digestive aid.

The plant sources of diastase include barley malt.

The food sources of diastase include barley.

Diastase is best taken orally.

Elastase Elastase breaks down proteins, including elastin, fibrin, hemoglobin, albumin, soybean proteins, and casein. It is used as a digestive aid. Elastase is often used in conjunction with other enzymes, such as trypsin, chymotrypsin, and collagenase. It is one of at least four proteolytic enzymes found in pancreatin.

The animal sources of elastase include bovine and porcine pancreas.

Elastase is best taken orally.

Enterokinase   Enterokinase breaks down proteins. It is used as a digestive aid. It is used in pancreatic enzyme replacement therapy.

The animal sources of enterokinase include porcine and bovine intestine (duodenum).

Enterokinase is best taken orally.

Esterase   Esterase breaks down ester bonds. It is used as a digestive aid.

The animal sources of esterase include bovine and porcine. The microbial sources include *Aspergillus niger.*

Esterase is found in many plant foods.

Esterase is best taken orally.

Ficin (or Ficain)   Ficin is similar in action to papain. It breaks down proteins. It is used as a digestive aid. Ficin fights inflammatory activity. It reduces swelling (edema). It fights intestinal worms in veterinary care.

The plant sources of ficin include the latex of the fig tree (*Ficus* sp.).

The food sources of ficin include figs.

Ficin is best taken orally.

Glucoamylase   Glucoamylase breaks down carbohydrates, specifically polysaccharides. It is used as a digestive aid.

The microbial sources of glucoamylase include *Aspergillus niger, Aspergillus oryzae, Rhizopus oryzae,* and *Rhizopus niveus.*

Glucoamylase is best taken orally.

Hemi-Cellulase   Hemi-cellulase breaks down carbohydrates, especially polysaccharides, such as hemi-celluloses, which are found in plant foods. It is used as a digestive aid. Hemi-cellulase is used in pancreatic enzyme replacement therapy.

The microbial sources of hemi-cellulase include *Aspergillus niger* and *Trichoderma longibrachiatum.*

The food sources of hemi-cellulase include green plants and plant seeds.

Hemi-cellulase is best taken orally.

Invertase (or Beta-Fructofuranosidase, Saccharase)   Invertase breaks down carbohydrates, especially sucrose. It is used as a digestive aid.

The microbial sources of invertase include *Aspergillus oryzae* and *Saccharomyces* sp. (Kluyveromyces).

The food sources of invertase include cucumbers, green plants, potato, and sugar cane.

Invertase is best taken orally.

Kallikrein (or Kininogenin)   Kallikrein is similar in action to trypsin. It breaks down protein. It is used as a digestive aid. Kallikrein is used as a vasodilator to lower blood pressure. It improves capillary permeability. It improves blood flow

in all cases of coronary artery and peripheral vascular diseases, migraine headaches, fractures, and delayed wound healing. It is used in the treatment of idiopathic infertility in men.

The animal sources of kallikrein include porcine pancreas.

Kallikrein is best taken orally.

Lactase (or Beta-Galactosidase)

Lactase, which is contained in Lactaid, breaks down lactose (milk sugar). It is used as a digestive aid. It is used to treat lactase insufficiency.

The animal sources of lactase include bovine liver. The microbial sources include *Aspergillus niger, Aspergillus oryzae, Saccharomyces lactis, Candida pseudotropicalis, Kluyveromyces lactis,* and *E. coli.*

The food sources of lactase include tomatoes, persimmons, apples, peaches, almonds, and milk.

Lactase is best taken orally.

Lipase

Lipase breaks down lipids and improves fat utilization in the body, and thus improves poor fat digestion in cases of lipid malabsorption due to liver or gall bladder insufficiency or surgical intervention. It is used as a digestive aid. It is used in pancreatic enzyme replacement therapy. Lipase decreases the fat level in stools. It synergistically intensifies the activity of lipase in the blood.

The animal sources of lipase include bovine and porcine pancreas and calf or lamb forestomachs. The microbial sources include *Rhizopus arrhizus, Rhizopus japonicus, Aspergillus oryzae, Aspergillus niger, Candida rugosa* (formerly *cylindracea*), *Staphylococcus aureus, Welchia perfringens, Candida paralipolytica, Mycotorula lipolytica, Geotrichum candidum, Pseudomonas, Rhizomucor (mucor) miehei,* and *Chromobacter viscosum.*

The food sources of lipase include avocado, wheat germ, rice, maize, green plants, soybeans, coconuts, flaxseeds, rape seeds, corn, and other germinating plants containing relatively large amounts of fats.

Lipase is best taken orally.

Maltase (or Alpha-Glucosidase)

Maltase breaks down the carbohydrates maltose and starch. It is used as a digestive aid.

The plant sources of maltase include barley (*Hordeum vulgare*). The microbial sources include *Aspergillus niger, Saccharomyces* sp., and various yeast species.

Maltase is usually found in plant tissues that contain amylase, such as brewer's yeast, rice, barley and other grains, beet leaves, green plants, sugar cane, banana, and mushrooms.

Maltase is best taken orally.

Nuclease

Nuclease breaks down nucleic acids. It is used as a digestive aid. It requires zinc to function.

The microbial sources of nuclease include *Aspergillus oryzae.*

The food sources of nuclease include mung beans.

Nuclease is best taken orally.

Pancreatin
Pancreatin breaks down proteins, carbohydrates, and fats because it contains many enzymes, principally trypsin, chymotrypsin, amylase, and lipase. There are at least four proteolytic enzymes (with different substrates) found in it. Pancreatin is used as a digestive aid. It is used to treat pancreatic insufficiency or after pancreas removal. Pancreatin is used to treat steatorrhea (excessive fat in the stools due to malabsorption). It is used after gastrectomy. Pancreatin is used in the treatment of cystic fibrosis. Calcium can increase its activity.

The animal sources of pancreatin include bovine and porcine pancreas.

Pancreatin is best taken orally.

Pancrelipase
Pancrelipase contains principally protease, amylase, and lipase enzymes, so it breaks down proteins, carbohydrates, and fats. It is similar to pancreatin, but with a higher ratio of lipase. Pancrelipase is used as a digestive aid. It is used to treat pancreatic insufficiency. It is used in the treatment of chronic pancreatitis, pancreatectomy, cystic fibrosis, and steatorrhea.

The animal sources of pancrelipase include porcine pancreas.

Pancrelipase is best taken orally.

Papain
Papain is similar to chymotrypsin in its actions and uses. It breaks down proteins (although other components degrade fats and carbohydrates). It is used as a digestive aid (especially to digest protein-rich foods). Papain treats chronic diarrhea and celiac disease. It is used in pancreatic enzyme replacement therapy. It treats gastrointestinal discomfort due to intestinal parasites (nematodes). Papain is used as a sedative. It is used as a diuretic. It fights allergies, infections, and inflammation. Papain treats soft tissue injuries, including strains, sprains, hematomas, contusions and abrasions, acute athletic injuries, charley horse, and pulled muscles. It is used in skin-care products, such as face creams, cleansers, moisturizers, exfoliants, and face-lift formulations; and treats psoriasis, warts, corns, skin cancer, and various skin ailments. It is used in many types of surgery to decrease inflammation, pain, and swelling. Papain treats ureteral obstruction, peritoneal adhesions, and children's enteritis. It treats infected wounds, sores, ulcers, tumors, hay fever, and catarrh. It is used to treat the intoxication caused by the stings of insects and jellyfish. Papain is used in dentrifices. It is used in ophthalmology to prevent corneal scar malformation. It is used to accelerate wound healing.

The plant sources of papain include the latex of the unripe papaya (*Carica papaya*).

The food sources of papain include papaya.

Papain is best taken orally, topically, and as a retention enema.

Pectinase (or Polygalacturonase, Pectin Depolymerase)
Pectinase breaks down carbohydrates, such as pectin (found in many fruits, such as apples). It is used as a digestive aid.

The microbial sources of pectinase include *Aspergillus niger* and *Rhizopus oryzae*.

The food sources of pectinase include citrus fruit, cucumbers, and green plants.

Pectinase is best taken orally.

Pepsin
Pepsin breaks down protein. It is used as a digestive aid, especially when pepsin secretion is deficient (an acid solution may be used in pepsin's administration to increase the gastric juice's effectiveness). It is used in pancreatic enzyme replacement.

The animal sources of pepsin include porcine stomach.

Pepsin is best taken orally.

Peroxidase
Peroxidase is one of the most effective antioxidant enzymes. It is capable of causing low-density lipoprotein oxidation. It may help fight idiopathic Parkinsonism.

The plant sources of peroxidase include horseradish roots and soybeans.

The food sources of peroxidase include horseradish, peas, oats, apple, egg, grape, mango, milk, and sugar cane. Peroxidase is widely found in fruits and vegetables.

Peroxidase is best taken orally.

Phytase
Phytase breaks down carbohydrates, specifically phytates (phytic acid), present in the leaves of plants. It is used as a digestive aid because it improves protein digestion and digestive enzyme activities. Phytase can increase mineral absorption and the bioavailability of iron, zinc, calcium, and magnesium. It can contain other enzymes, such as cellulase, pectinase, and xylanase.

The microbial sources of phytase include *Aspergillus oryzae, Aspergillus niger,* and *Aspergillus ficuum.*

The food sources of phytase include wheat.

Phytase is best taken orally.

Proteases (or Peptidase)
Proteases breaks down proteins. It is used as a digestive aid. It is used in pancreatic enzyme replacement therapy. Proteases fights inflammation. It fights acute conditions, such as sports injuries, surgery, and wounds. It fights chronic conditions, such as cancer and arthritis.

The animal sources of proteases include bovine and porcine pancreas. There are various plant sources, including pineapple and papaya. The microbial sources include *Aspergillus oryzae, Aspergillus niger, Aspergillus melleus, Aspergillus saitoi, Rhizopus niger, Bacillus subtilis, Bacillus licheniformis, Streptomyces caespitosus, Bacillus polymyxa, Streptomyces griseus, Staphylococcus aureau, Aspergillus sojae,* and *Serratia species.*

The food sources of proteases include pineapple, papaya, figs, guava, kiwi, ginger root, green plants, mushrooms, soybean, wheat, and kidney bean.

Proteases is best taken orally.

Rennin (or Chymosin, Rennase)
Rennin breaks down proteins. It is used as a digestive aid. Rennin coagulates (curdles) milk and converts casein (the

principal protein in milk) into insoluble curds that can be further digested by pepsin. It releases the valuable mineral elements (potassium, phosphorus, calcium, and iron) in milk. By doing this, the body can use rennin to strengthen bones and teeth, to stabilize water balance, to build nutrient-rich red blood cells in the circulatory system, and to aid in thinking more clearly by strengthening your nervous system.

The animal sources of rennin include calf stomach.

Rennin is best taken orally.

Ribonuclease   Ribonuclease is used as a digestive aid (it liberates nucleic acid).

The animal sources of ribonuclease include bovine pancreas and calf thymus. The microbial sources include *Aspergillus oryzae* and *Bacillus subtilis.*

Ribonuclease is best taken orally.

Serratiopeptidase (or Serratia Protease)   Serratiopeptidase breaks down proteins. It has fibrinolytic and anti-edema activity. It fights inflammation. Serratiopeptidase stimulates immune activity. It reduces sputum viscosity. It is used in the treatment of arthritis, fibrocystic breast disease, carpal tunnel syndrome, atherosclerosis, sinusitis, bronchitis, tuberculosis, bronchial asthma, cystitis, epididymitis, allergies, psoriasis, uveitis, ulcerative colitis, multiple sclerosis, some forms of cancer, bronchopulmonary secretions, traumatic injury (i.e., sprains and torn ligaments), and vaginal hysterectomy. Serratiopeptidase facilitates the effects of antibiotics in the treatment of infections.

The microbial sources of serratiopeptidase include *Serratia* sp.

Serratiopeptidase is best taken orally.

Sucrase (or Sucrose Alpha-Glucosidase, Sucrase Isomaltase)
Sucrase breaks down carbohydrates, specifically sucrose and maltose. It is used as a digestive aid. A liquid form of sucrase has shown effectiveness in enzyme replacement therapy for those suffering from congenital sucrase-isomaltase deficiency.

The microbial sources of sucrase include *Saccharomyces* sp.

The food sources of sucrase include green plants, beet leaves and stems, and banana.

Sucrase is best taken orally.

Trypsin   Trypsin breaks down proteins. It is used as a digestive aid. It aids gastric retention due to a malfunctioning stomach, pancreatic insufficiency, and intestinal obstruction. Trypsin is used in the debridement of ulcerations, empyemas, fistulas, necrotizing wounds, abscesses, hematomas, and decubitus ulcers. It is used as an auxiliary agent in meningitis therapy. It fights inflammation as occurs in intercostal neuritis, urticaria (hives), postoperative parotitis, decubitus ulcers, pleural effusion, infected wounds, old scars, pancreatitis, trench mouth, and eczematoid dermatitis. Trypsin treats circulatory problems, such as thromboembolic diseases, peripheral arteriosclerosis, pulmonary infarcts, peripheral vascular

diseases, milk leg (phlegmasia alba dolens), and ischemic purulent leg ulcers. It assists in surgical repair and reduces postoperative swelling from many surgeries. It speeds healing (inflammation and swelling) from injuries, including strains, sprains, contusions, fractures, black eyes, bruises, hematomas, tendonitis, and bursitis. Trypsin treats arthritis, such as acute rheumatoid arthritis and acute gouty arthritis. It treats skin disorders, including atopic dermatitis, pustular eczema, and acute eczematoid dermatitis. It helps respiratory and throat conditions, including influenza, bronchitis, tuberculous adenitis, lung abscess, infected bronchopleural fistula, bronchial asthma, sinusitis, peritonsillar abscess, pulmonary diseases, pulmonary emphysema, unresolved pneumonia–atelectasis, pulmonary tuberculosis, traumatic hyperemia, and viral pneumonia. Trypsin treats urogenital conditions, including lymphogranuloma venereum, acute gonorrheal urethritis, and proteus vulgaris infection of the urinary tract. It is used in eye care, such as in glaucoma, acute iridocyclitis, and thrombosis of the central retinal vein. It is used in diabetes management to prevent such problems as cellulitis, infected leg ulcers, and carbuncle. It helps fight cancer and such associated problems as ascites due to cancer or cirrhosis and lymphosarcoma with infection. Trypsin is one of at least four proteolytic enzymes found in pancreatin.

The animal sources of trypsin include bovine and porcine pancreas.

Trypsin is best taken orally.

You are dealing with an extremely powerful genie in a bottle when using enzyme supplements. The healing benefits of enzymes have been documented for centuries. The Greeks, Romans, Egyptians, Chinese, Germans, and Japanese have all used enzymes to maintain health and fight disease.

Because of our enzyme-dead, processed foods, polluted air and water, and high-stress lifestyles, supplements may be the only way we can ensure a sufficient daily enzyme intake. So, who needs enzyme supplements? Everyone.

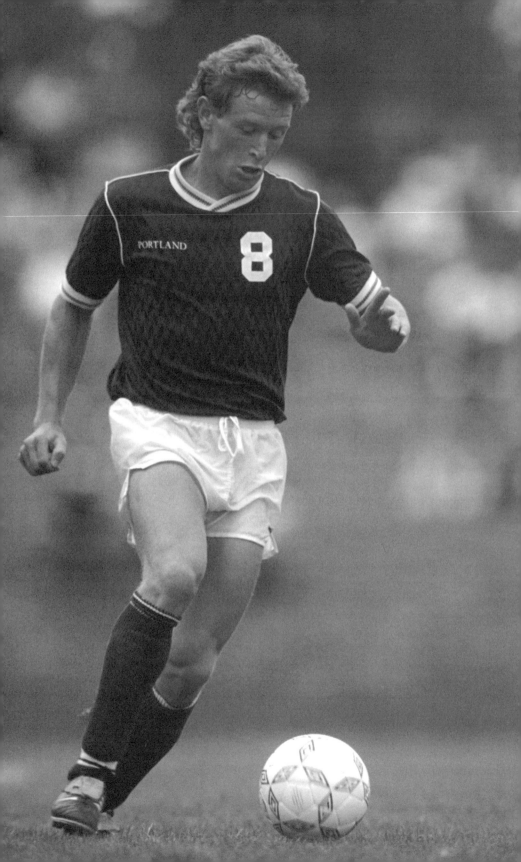

PART TWO

SPORTS-PERFORMANCE ENHANCERS

I t is often noted that we are living in the age of the information revolution. For more than a decade, this revolution has had an effect on how well we are able to keep up with what is new in sports nutrition and supplementation. Where once we could grasp the basic tenets of a discipline by reading a book that was under development for two or three years prior to its publication and often read for up to five years afterwards, today we are finding that those basic tenets are constantly being updated by new information and perspectives, which at times are even fundamentally challenging them.

Individuals interested in sports nutrition are frequently hard-pressed to keep abreast of the advances in the field. Often, their attempts to remain informed and aware are limited by the difficulties of keeping up with the scientific and consumer literature. As a result, they often miss out on the most valuable information that is available to them.

In Part Two of *Avery's Sports Nutrition Almanac,* we will discuss the cutting-edge, high-tech supplements that have only recently become widely available. Also included is new information on some familiar supplements that are now being sold in new and improved forms or have lately been the subject of ground-breaking news. In either case, Part Two not only describes the supplement, but also explains how to use it. Not every supplement is good for everyone; therefore, you will also be cautioned about the conditions in which a supplement is not appropriate.

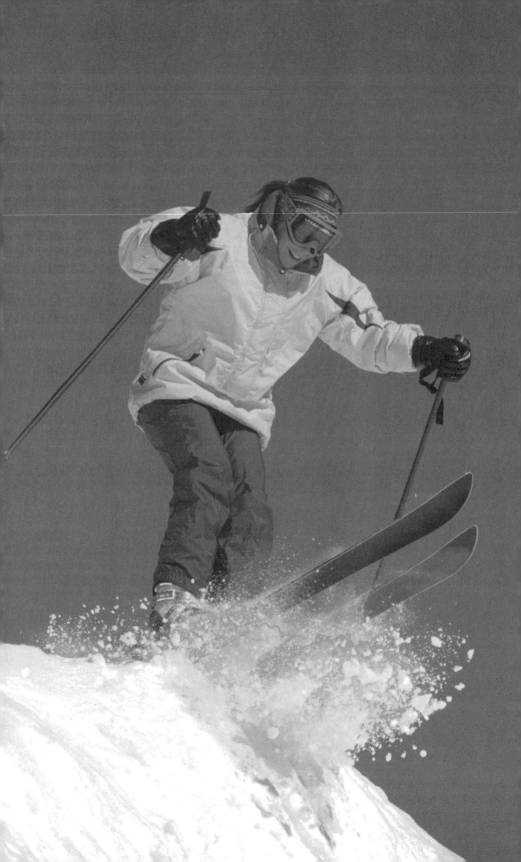

HERBS AND MUSHROOMS

7

NATURE'S OPTIMIZERS

Herbs and mushrooms have been utilized by humans for centuries. Some are used as seasonings in cooking, while others are used for very specific medicinal purposes. Some, such as the herb ginseng, act as adaptogens, substances that help the body adapt to stress. Because of their many health and performance benefits, herbs and mushrooms are becoming increasingly popular among athletes and nonathletes alike. In this chapter, we will discuss the herbs and mushrooms that are the most appropriate for the fitness-minded.

HERBS

The study of herbs and the practice of prescribing them for health and performance have become a real science. Many herbs have powerful components that can be of great benefit. In fact, the pharmaceutical industry got its start when druggists began isolating these components and making them available in their purer forms. Herbalists believe, however, that the other components in an herb are present to enhance the primary components' beneficial effects and to offset their undesirable actions. They feel that an herb should be used in its complete form to allow the body to benefit from the balanced package provided by nature. Many people believe that herbs are just as effective as medications and do not have the side effects.

Herbs do offer many health and performance benefits, but they must be used with care. Some herbs should be used for only short periods of time, to help heal the body of an illness or to treat a symptom. Some herbs should not be combined with certain medications or other herbs, since their primary components may interact negatively. Some herbs should be avoided by competitive athletes, since they contain a substance, such as caffeine, that may be banned by sports governing organizations. Furthermore, not all plants are beneficial to humans. Some herbs are toxic, even deadly, especially if used for prolonged periods of time. Before you use any herb for more than two to three months, seek the advice of a knowledgeable health-care practitioner or a competent herbalist. Including herbal preparations in your performance-nutrition program can prove advantageous if you use them correctly—or disastrous if you do not.

In general, the bitter-tasting herbs are medicinal and the pleasant-tasting herbs are less toxic. Plant roots and bark are naturally fungicidal and bactericidal, since if they were not, they would be destroyed in the ground. In addition, the active components in herbs tend to be most potent when the herbs are freshly picked. At the same time, roots, bark, and other herb parts can remain potent for years if they are properly dried and stored.

Herbalism tends to be geographic in practice, as herbalists have direct access only to the herbs growing in their local areas. Luckily, however, these different areas all seem to have herbs that serve the same purposes. There are two main herbal approaches that are popular today. In one approach, herbs are used for their specific active ingredients, such as the caffeine in guarana. In the other approach, which is Asian, herbs are used to balance the body's flow of energy. Both approaches have advantages, and a practitioner of either can help you improve your health and performance.

Standardizing Herbal Supplements for Consistency

It is often the concern of athletes that not all herbs or herbal products are created equal. The reason: Herbs are plants, and the chemical composition of plants varies greatly depending on where the plants were grown, the soil in which they were grown, the weather conditions during their growing season, and how they were harvested.

Our everyday experiences confirm this variation in plant quality. For instance, have you ever bitten into a big orange only to discover that the fruit had hardly any taste or flavor? Well, the poor growing conditions (for example, a winter freeze or too little rain) that affect oranges are similar to the factors that act upon herbs.

And, just as oranges can look delicious but be tasteless, herbs can appear healthy but lack the ingredients that normally convey their health benefits. Appearance is no guarantee of potency. That's why standardization was developed. Standardization guarantees that herbal ingredients are consistent from bottle to bottle.

Ever since humans first began ingesting herbs, variations in content have influenced the processing of the plants. Originally, the only way to ingest the active ingredients from medicinal plants was to consume the plants fresh and raw.

One of the first significant technological breakthroughs in connection with herbs occurred when it was learned that steeping liberates the active chemicals from plants while leaving behind, in the plant, the unwanted substances. To steep an herb—that is, to make tea—place the dry herb in hot or simmering water for several minutes. While heating a plant may break down and destroy some of its chemicals, steeping retains and even enhances the potency of many botanicals.

A second method that is effective at liberating the active chemicals from herbs is making an extract. Liquid extracts are made by soaking the whole herb in a liquid that will release and concentrate its active ingredients. Water is the most commonly used liquid for this process, but alcohol is also effective. When making an extract, the active ingredients are pulled from the herb and the nonactive parts are discarded. This has several advantages. First, our digestive tracts do not have to expend energy to break down the cellulose, lignin, and other plant structures in which the active constituents are held. Second, the active ingredients are concentrated and rendered soluble in our digestive juices, so they are quickly and efficiently absorbed. It is estimated that over 95 percent of many liquid and powdered extracts is absorbed, depending on the types of constituents involved. So, an extract is a plant preparation "containing a high concentration of active constituents and a low concentration of inactive ones," according to Christopher Hobbs in his book *Handbook of Herbal Healing*.

Extracts are commonly used in many parts of the world where herbal medicine is more evolved. In Europe, many extract forms are available and may even be more popular than bulk herbs. In China and throughout the Orient, thousands of patented extracts are available and are extremely popular. Liquid extracts, sometimes called tinctures, come in several forms. They are usually made with a solvent of grain alcohol and water. The proportion of alcohol to water varies according to the active constituents of the herb and whether they are more soluble in water or alcohol.

In more recent times, herb users discovered that when tea evaporates, it leaves a powdery residue that often possesses many of the characteristics of the original plant or tea. This residue frequently has a greater potency than the original plant or tea because the active ingredients are more concentrated. When the active "principals" of 10 ounces of an herb are concentrated into a single ounce of powder, the resulting substance is said to be a 10x, or ten-to-one, concentration.

Nowadays, most herbs come in pill and capsule forms, which are far more convenient and easy to use than the materials available to the early herbalists. When pills and capsules are made, the herbal ingredients are extracted in a process similar to steeping, but using cold alcohol. Cold alcohol avoids the damage caused by heating. After the alcohol has evaporated, the concentrated material that is left is dried, pulverized, and pressed into tablets or poured into capsules.

A mere list of ingredients on a label does not indicate the strengths or amounts of the active ingredients in a supplement. If a label claims that each capsule contains 100 milligrams of a certain herb, you still do not know if those 100 milligrams were extracted from a weak herb that suffered unhealthy growing conditions or a robust plant that was harvested in prime time.

At the same time, a label may claim that each capsule has 100 milligrams of the herb in 10x strength, which means that the product has ten times the concentration of the unprocessed herb. But, if the original whole herb was deficient in the active ingredients, the 10x concentrate is also weak. A tenfold increase of not very much remains not very much.

To cope with inconsistency, the herbal-supplement industry has adopted a system, called standardization, that records the minimum concentration of the active constituents (or of the components closely correlated to an activity) in a product. For example, citrus aurantium, an herb used for weight loss, is sold in both standardized and nonstandardized forms. (For a discussion of citrus aurantium, see page 141.) Packages of standardized citrus aurantium indicate the synephrine content on the label. And, although synephrine is not the only active component in citrus aurantium, extracts containing from 1.5- to 3.0-

ON THE CUTTING EDGE

Maximize Your Lactate Clearance With Herbs

In a double-blind, randomized, placebo-controlled study reviewed in *Medicina Dello Sport* in 1998, researchers evaluated the effect of a formulation of standardized herbal ingredients (sold under the brand names of Metaflex and 2nd Wind) on lactate clearance after exercise performed at maximum capacity. Lactate clearance is the amount of lactate metabolized by the body in a specific amount of time. The researchers randomly assigned thirty male subjects aged eighteen through twenty years to one of three groups. Group A received a placebo; group B, 600 milligrams a day of the herbal formula; and group C, 1,000 milligrams a day of the formula. The researchers took the subjects' blood-lactate measurements before exercising, at VO_2 max (the point at which oxygen is consumed at the maximum rate), and fifteen minutes after stopping the exercise. The tests were performed on all three groups at the beginning of the trial period and after two weeks. After four weeks, group C also performed a third treadmill test. Among the group-C participants, the blood-lactate metabolism improved significantly—that is, the lactate was quickly cleared from the blood after exercising. The researchers concluded that the higher dosage of the herbal formula caused faster utilization of the lactate as part of the energy production during recovery.

percent synephrine have been found to be the most active. Extracts with less than this concentration of synephrine have demonstrated less efficacy and may have been derived from plants that were harvested prematurely, processed incorrectly, or grown in poor conditions.

Herbs for Improved Sports Performance

We all seem to want more energy for improved training and competition. In this modern era of creatine and sports drinks, however, we sometimes forget that herbs, within limits, can help provide this energy, act as stimulants, and provide vitality. When used properly, herbs can bring our energy forces into balance to keep us healthy, improve our recovery, and keep us active. Following are the most popular herbs among today's athletes.

Ashwagandha
Ashwagandha (*Withania somnifera*) is also known as Indian ginseng. In Ayurveda, an Indian philosophy of medicine, it is considered an adaptogen that facilitates learning and memory. (For a discussion of these special substances, see "Adaptogens" on page 139.)

In a 1993 clinical study in India, fifty people complaining of lethargy and fatigue for two to six months were given an adaptogenic tonic made of eleven herbs, including 760 milligrams of ashwagandha, once a day. None of the participants had responded to a vitamin-and-mineral supplement, taken for at least two months, and they had no recognizable diseases. After one month of taking the ashwagandha mixture, the patients reported an average 45-percent improvement in mood. Their blood-plasma-protein levels and hemoglobin, two factors used to measure overall health, also increased significantly, providing a statistical measurement of the tonic's effect.

A 1994 study in India compared the adaptogenic and anabolic effects of Asian ginseng and ashwagandha in mice and rats. Three groups of six mice were fed either a ginseng extract, an ashwagandha extract, or saline for seven days. On the eighth day, the animals' endurance levels were tested with swimming. The average swimming times were 62.55 minutes for the group fed the ginseng, 82.14 minutes for the group fed the ashwagandha, and 35.34 minutes for the group fed the saline.

Ashwagandha is often blended with other adaptogenic herbs, such as Siberian ginseng. A typical dose is 1 to 2 teaspoons of extract two to three times a day or a 500-milligram capsule three times a day. Ashwagandha may cause gastrointestinal upset in some people.

Astragalus Widely used in Chinese medicine, astragulus (*Astragalus membranaceus*) has both antiviral and immune-enhancing properties. It is available alone and in a variety of combination formulas.

Astragalus increases the body's resistance to disease in general and also boosts

Adaptogens

The term "adaptogen" was first introduced into scientific circles by Soviet pharmacologists conducting scientific experiments with ginseng. These scientists coined the term to refer to natural plant substances that are safe to use in even relatively large quantities and produce no or minimal adverse side effects. Adaptogens have a toniclike effect on the body, helping it to adapt to many types of nonspecific stressors, such as heat, cold, fatigue, emotional stress, and time changes.

Adaptogens increase the efficiency of the healing system or help it neutralize the harmful effects of stress or overtraining. Herbs that function as adaptogens are often called tonics. The word "tonic" derives from the Greek word for "stretch"; adaptogens and tonics stretch and tone our systems the same way that physical exercise stretches and tones our muscles. Working our bodies—subjecting them to graduated tension followed by relaxation—increases our natural resilience, an essential quality of health, because it determines our responsiveness to environmental stress. The more resilient we are, the greater is our ability to bounce back from any kind of stress or injury.

Adaptogens are supplements for healthy, active athletes. They promote wellness, enhance resistance, speed recovery, and help the body adapt to stress. The most popular adaptogenic herbs used by athletes include ashwagandha, ginseng, gotu kola, and schisandra.

the functioning of other herbs that are known to increase energy, aid digestion, and stimulate the production and circulation of the blood. Pharmacological studies have confirmed that astragalus enhances the immune system. It increases the activity of several kinds of white blood cells, as well as the production of antibodies and interferon. These properties have to do with the root's content of polysaccharides, large molecules composed of chains of sugar subunits. Polysaccharides are structural components of many organisms. Until recently, they did not excite much interest among Western physicians because conventional wisdom held that they could not be absorbed even from the gastrointestinal tract. But polysaccharides are a common feature of many herbal medicines that enhance immunity and scientists are now beginning to realize their importance, even though they do not yet understand their properties. (For other herbs that enhance immunity, see "Herbal Antioxidants and Immune Enhancers," below.)

Astragalus is an excellent herb for athletes and active individuals who suffer from chronic infections such as bronchitis and sinusitis. It is also beneficial for individuals who lack energy or feel vulnerable to stress or overtraining. Astragalus is available at most health-food stores. The recommended dosage is 200 to 1,000 milligrams a day of Astragalus membranaceus root extract standardized to provide 0.4-percent isoflavone or 0.4-percent 4'-hydroxy-3'-methoxy isoflavone 7-sug. Higher dosages may be prescribed by herbalists who use whole powder in unstandardized form.

Cat's Claw
Cat's claw (*Uncaria tomentosa*), an herb that grows in South America, is known not just for its immune-enhancing qualities, but also for its ability to reduce inflammation. It was given its name because of its clawlike stems. While becoming popular in the United States only in recent years, it has been part of the health arsenal of the Peruvian Indians for centuries. It is used to treat a number of disorders related to the immune system, including rheumatoid arthritis, Crohn's disease, herpes, and cancer. (For other herbs that fight pain and inflammation, see page 141.)

Cat's claw, called *uño de gato,* is found most often in tincture and pill form.

Herbal Antioxidants and Immune Enhancers

Herbs are natural substances that protect the healing system and help it neutralize harmful influences. Athletes often use herbal products when debilitated, recovering from illness or injury, or coping with excessive stress. There are several herbs that are particularly good for athletes who are fatigued or feel slightly overtrained. They include astragalus, echinacea, garlic, ginger, ginkgo, green tea, milk thistle, and turmeric. Many of these herbs also function as antioxidants and protect the body against free-radical damage.

Even if you are not ill or lacking in energy, you may want to experiment with herbal antioxidants and immune enhancers to help strengthen your immune system and protect your body from the stresses of everyday life and intensive training.

Herbs That Fight Pain and Inflammation

Herbs that are known to reduce inflammation can also help stop pain. Another advantage of these herbs is that they do not have the long list of dangerous side effects that result from the long-term use of anti-inflammatory medications.

Most of the herbs suggested for sports injuries do little to fight the actual injuries, but they do reduce the pain. If you suffer from chronic pain, you know this is important. You must have patience—it can take several weeks to notice any improvement—but the results can be dramatic. Some herbs can help increase the mobility of arthritic joints. In many serious cases, herbs have even enabled people with chronic pain in their joints or muscles to reduce the amount of anti-inflammatory medication they were taking.

Among the herbs that help fight pain and inflammation are cat's claw, feverfew, and ginger. Other herbs are meadowsweet and willow bark.

High-quality cat's claw dietary supplements consist of cat's claw bark or wood-stem extracts standardized to provide 15-percent polypenols. Commonly recommended dosages of standardized cat's claw are 500 to 1,000 milligrams a day.

Citrus Aurantium
Citrus aurantium, the immature fruit of the green orange, is an important herb used in traditional Chinese medicine to improve digestion, circulation, and liver function. It has been used for approximately the past 1,000 years as an energizer, and its effects seem to be very similar to those of ephedrine.

Most athletes are certainly more familiar with the ephedrine-containing herb ephedra (ma huang) than with citrus aurantium. Citrus aurantium, which contains synephrine, has effects that are similar to ephedrine, as well as to other thermogenic substances, such as caffeine, guarana, and kola nut—but without the side effects. The reported side effects of many of these substances include high blood pressure, tremors, insomnia, and nervousness. (For a discussion of stimulant herbs, see page 142.)

Synephrine-containing citrus aurantium may be an excellent alternative to the ephedrine-containing herbs for many individuals. Animal research has found no serious side effects even when synephrine was given intravenously. Also, synephrine does not act on the nervous system the way ephedrine does. As a matter of fact, synephrine has not been shown to be habit-forming in any way.

Synephrine is a compound used in medicine for its stimulating abilities. Clinical research has shown that synephrine has antidepressant capabilities and can increase the heart's cardiac output. Most interesting is the ability of synephrine, the same as epinephrine, to increase the activity of adenosine 3,5-cyclic monophosphate (AMP). Such an increase can be directly tied to the boost in metabolism that increases fat burning.

The recommended dosage is 200 to 400 milligrams a day of citrus aurantium

Stimulant Herbs

The use of herbs as pharmacologically active stimulants is considered controversial. Many health-conscious athletes avoid even the relatively mild stimulant caffeine, which has been used along with tonic herbs for thousands of years.

It has often been pointed out in traditional Chinese medicine that using adaptogenic or tonic herbs is similar to "feeding a tired horse," and using stimulant herbs is similar to "beating a dead horse." Many athletes would rather use herbs such as ashwagandha, ginseng, and schisandra to increase attention and alertness than strong stimulants such as ephedra and guarana. Other stimulant herbs are kola nut, licorice, maté, and synephrine.

The use of stimulant herbs is one of personal choice. Some people use them sparingly to help energize themselves before intensive workouts or competitions. Moderation, rather than reliance, is the key to using central-nervous-system stimulants to their best advantage.

standardized to provide 1.5- to 3.0-percent synephrine. This will furnish 3 to 6 milligrams of synephrine a day. Citrus aurantium comes in capsule and tablet forms.

Ciwujia

Ciwujia, pronounced *su WAH ja,* is the whole root and rhizome of Siberian ginseng. (For a discussion of Siberian ginseng, see "Ginseng" on page 147.) Grown in the northeast section of China, it has been used continuously as part of traditional Chinese medicine for almost 1,700 years. It is employed by the Chinese to treat fatigue and bolster the immune system. It does this without the aid of caffeine, and it does not produce any stimulant or anabolic-steroid side effects.

Ciwujia first intrigued researchers because of published reports of mountain climbers enjoying improved work performance at high altitudes and low oxygen. Studies showed that laboratory animals administered ciwujia survived longer under low-oxygen conditions than animals not given the herb, and that the herb increased oxygenation of the heart-muscle tissues.

Extensive research done at the Academy of Preventative Medicine in Beijing, China, and the Department of Physiology of the University of North Texas Health Science Center has shown ciwujia to significantly improve workout performance through a carbohydrate-sparing action. During exercise, ciwujia shifts the body's energy source from carbohydrate to fat, thereby increasing fat metabolism by up to 43 percent. This carbohydrate shift also improves performance by delaying the lactic-acid buildup associated with muscle fatigue. In addition, in the research, ciwujia raised the lactate threshold by 12.4 percent and increased recovery following exercise as determined by measuring the heart rate.

Ciwujia has been shown to be remarkably safe. The usual human dosage is 9 to 27 grams of raw herb daily. However, in a number of studies, ciwujia has been successfully administered to laboratory animals at dosages ranging from sixty to two hundred times the recommended human dose. Ciwujia also comes in tablets and capsules, and the recommended dosage for these forms is 100 to 1,000 milligrams of the herb standardized to provide 0.5- to 0.8-percent Eleutherosides.

Echinacea

Echinacea (*Echinacea*), native to North America, has been used by the American Indians for more purposes than any other herb. And echinacea is still one of the most used herbs for fighting infections, colds, flu, and a host of other minor and major ailments.

Modern scientific research coming out of Europe shows that echinacea increases the number of immune-system cells in circulation as well as their activity, enhances the body's production of interferon and other immuno-active compounds, and has other immune-stimulating effects. Today, echinacea is still touted for its ability to strengthen the immune system, fight infections, and promote wound healing. An estimated 350 scientific studies have investigated its pharmacology and clinical uses.

Echinacea is often taken in capsule form alone or in combination with other immune-enhancing herbs. The recommended dosage is 200 to 400 milligrams two to three times a day. Of the nine species of echinacea that exist, only two—*Echinacea purpurea* and *Echinacea angustifolia*—have been studied extensively in the scientific literature, so look for these species on the label for maximum therapeutic effect.

Ephedra

Ephedra (*Ephedra sinica*), commonly referred to by its Chinese name, ma huang, has received so much publicity recently that it's hard to read a newspaper or magazine without coming across a reference to it. The ephedra products commonly sold in health-food stores consist of the green stems of several species of the herb native to central Asia.

Ma huang has been used in China for the treatment of bronchial asthma and related conditions for more than 5,000 years. The therapeutic value of the herb is due to several closely related alkaloids, of which ephedrine is both the most active and the one present in the largest amount. North American species of ephedra, one of which is referred to as Mormon tea, contain no active alkaloids. Ephedrine was researched in the United States during the 1920s and was a standard over-the-counter medication for many years.

Ephedra has both an upside and a downside. The alkaloids' vasoconstricting effects make the herb a useful nasal decongestant, but also cause it to raise the blood pressure and increase the heart rate. They also make it an effective bronchodilator, but additionally cause it to stimulate the central nervous system, with side effects ranging from nervousness to insomnia. This stimulation is greatly increased if caffeine or a caffeinated beverage such as coffee, tea, or cola is consumed along with the herb. (For a discussion of caffeine, see page 144.) Consequently, ephedrine has been replaced to a large extent in over-the-counter cold and cough products by related chemicals, such as pseudoephedrine or phenylpropanolamine. These chemicals have actions similar to those of ephedrine, but with reduced effects on the central nervous system.

In recent years, ephedra-and-caffeine combination products have been used as

Caffeine

Coffee beans are the seeds of *Coffee arabaica* and other coffee plants grown primarily in Africa and South America. Coffee is consumed on a daily basis by millions of individuals seeking an energy boost. The energy boost comes from the alkaloid caffeine, which acts on both the cardiovascular and central nervous systems to reduce fatigue, increase alertness, and improve endurance.

Although caffeine is a common ingredient in many beverages, foods, and over-the-counter medications, some experts have recently suggested that it cannot be called a food or a drug. Dr. Jeffrey Bland, of HealthComm, Inc., a company specializing in health and nutrition education, says that caffeine falls into a newly defined in-between category called nutraceuticals. A nutraceutical is a food-derived substance that can have pharmacological effects on the body. Caffeine fits this definition perfectly.

By definition as a nutraceutical, caffeine can have negative and positive effects on the body, depending on the dose consumed and the metabolism. There has been evidence published showing that excessive and chronic use of caffeine can lead to episodes of anxiety and high blood pressure. It has also been shown that subjects taking the substance in high doses performed worse than when they consumed a placebo. When taken in excess, caffeine can irritate the stomach lining, disrupt sleep, cause diarrhea, and accelerate dehydration—race-day problems that you certainly can do without. It can cause calcium depletion and may help to weaken the bones in menopausal women. Lastly, if you chronically drink high levels of coffee or caffeinated beverages and try to back off, you will most likely suffer withdrawal symptoms.

But, as many athletes know, caffeine in moderate doses can have a positive effect on athletic performance. During exercise, the muscles always use some combination of carbohydrate and fat for fuel. As you increase the intensity of your effort, the tendency of the muscles is to use a greater proportion of carbohydrate. However, after you consume caffeine in the form of cola, coffee, a sports bar, or tablets, your body switches to using free fatty acids as the preferred fuel, mobilizing fat from your body's fat deposits. This causes glycogen sparing, allowing your body to have more glycogen available for your final climb or sprint in the race.

The optimum dose of caffeine before long training sessions or races is 2 milligrams for every pound of body weight, taken about thirty to sixty minutes before exercising. A cup of drip coffee has approximately 125 milligrams of caffeine, a cup of instant coffee has approximately 100 milligrams, a cup of most soft drinks has from 30 to 60 milligrams, and a No-Doz tablet has 100 milligrams. Therefore, for a

appetite suppressants, metabolic stimulants for weight loss, and athletic-performance enhancers. There is considerable literature about the effects of the drug ephedrine on weight loss. Detailed studies of the herb's effect on athletic performance do not exist, however. Regardless, ephedra should be avoided and taken on a continuing basis only under the guidance of a qualified health-care practitioner. Many herbal products do not list the concentration of ephedrine present. Some manufacturers almost certainly "spike" their dosage forms with additional quantities of synthetic ephedrine.

170-pound athlete, about three and a half cups of coffee or a combination of caffeinated beverages and No-Doz tablets can provide a sports-enhancing effect.

At these levels of ingestion, caffeine, because it is a diuretic, causes increased loss of water through the urine thirty minutes to two hours following ingestion, which may dangerously compound your loss of water during long races. And, once again, caffeine-induced acid secretion in the stomach may lead to heartburn.

Caffeine may also have physiological benefits, however. For many years, cyclists have been drinking small viles of expresso with 10 kilometers to go in road races, and sprinters have been known to carry canisters of strong coffee with them during competitions on the track. Both of these athletes are hoping to take advantage of caffeine's effects on the central nervous system. Caffeine has been shown to help reduce the sense of physical effort that is experienced during intensive exercise and to stimulate the brain, increasing alertness. In addition, caffeine may be linked to the release of calcium in the muscles, which is linked to muscle contraction.

In a recent study on caffeine use and motor reactions, scientists tested three groups of subjects. The first group ingested 300 milligrams of caffeine, the second group ingested 600 milligrams, and the third group served as the control and ingested no caffeine. The 300-milligram group reported the fastest reaction times. A surprise to the research team was that the 600-milligram group reacted no faster than the control group. Thus, although some caffeine may boost performance, too much may prove ineffective.

Finally, people with coffee or soft-drink habits probably have built up a tolerance to caffeine, which causes a reduction in the side effects such as nervousness, increased heart rate, and increased urination—as well as in any improvement in performance. If you can wean yourself from caffeine for the few days before a race, however, caffeine may give you a lift on race day. One recent study examined the results of caffeine dosing in coffee-drinking athletes who abstained from caffeine for four days prior to a race. The research team found that the blood levels of free fatty acids were greater following the withdrawal from caffeine than they were when the athletes stuck to their regular caffeine habits. These results indicated that the benefits from caffeine may be greater for athletes who don't regularly drink beverages containing it or who abstain from it for a few days.

The bottom line of this story is that caffeine is a plant-derived nutraceutical that can have pharmacological effects on the body. Some of the effects are beneficial, while others may be harmful. As is true of all things related to nutrition, you should evaluate caffeine's specific effects on your body and consume it at levels that take advantage of its benefits but minimize the negatives.

In October 1995, the FDA convened a special advisory group on ephedra that made a number of recommendations regarding the sale of ephedra products. Among those recommendations were imposing strict dosage limitations, prohibiting sale to persons under the age of eighteen, placing warnings on the product labels to individuals with specific health risks, and advising against chronic use.

Some sports federations have determined that specific amounts of ephedrine in an athlete's system are grounds for disqualification, due to the use of the drug by certain individuals for its speedlike effect. Most sports organizations have

ON THE CUTTING EDGE

Caffeine-Ephedrine Combo
Extends Time to Exhaustion

A study published in the *European Journal of Applied Physiology* in 1998 examined the effects of the drugs ephedrine and caffeine—taken separately and together—on the time to exhaustion during high-intensity exercise. The researchers weren't interested in any fat-mobilizing effects, but instead wanted to see if using either substance alone or a combination of the two would allow more intensive training before fatigue set in. They tested eight men, who exercised at high-intensity levels on stationary cycles. Before exercising, the men took either 5 milligrams per kilogram (2.2 pounds) of body weight of caffeine, 1 milligram per kilogram of body weight of ephedrine, a combination of the two substances, or a placebo. Only the combination of ephedrine and caffeine increased (by 38 percent) the training time to exhaustion.

banned its use. It is a reasonable response by these authorities to try to stop the use of ephedra. Unfortunately, these sports officials have not been properly informed of the benefits provided by the herb. The use of ephedra is not a black-and-white issue, but a gray one requiring some understanding of the medical, botanical, and legal issues surrounding the herb.

Ephedra comes in powder form or combined with other herbs in capsule and tablet forms. A common dosage range is 50 to 150 milligrams of ephedra per day. Note that ephedra should not be taken for an extended period of time because it is addictive.

Feverfew   Feverfew (*Tanacetum parthenium*) is one of the "natural aspirins" that stops inflammation and the resulting pain. It does this by reducing the prostaglandin levels, according to several studies conducted in the United States— and it often works even better than aspirin. In addition, feverfew slows down platelet aggregation and the release of histamines. Because of these actions, it is also used to relieve migraines and allergies. A tonic and a stimulant, feverfew is also commonly used for cramps, digestive upsets, and parasites. It is best known as a prophylactic to reduce the frequency, duration, and severity of migraine headaches.

Feverfew is available in tincture and tablet forms, alone and in combination with other herbs. A recommended dosage range is 100 to 200 milligrams per day. To make feverfew tea, use 1 teaspoon of dried herb to 1 cup of water, and drink 1 cup a day.

Garlic   Garlic (*Allium sativum*) is a potent antibiotic, with antibacterial and antiviral effects as well. Garlic has many active constituents, including alliin, allicin, and sulfur compounds. These ingredients account for garlic's famous potency as an antibiotic and fungicide, and for its use in lowering the blood pressure and cholesterol level. In addition, alliin is an antibiotic agent, which means that it kills bacteria and many viruses, and sulfur compounds strengthen the immune system, lower high blood pressure, and fight infection. These two major properties of garlic make it an infection fighter easily comparable to penicillin. Take garlic in capsule or tablet form; a common dosage is 600 to 1,200 milligrams per day of garlic extract standardized to provide 1-percent allicin. For fresh garlic, eat two raw cloves every day.

Ginger
Ginger (*Zingiber officinale*) is known to most people as a spice rather than a medicinal plant. However, it has been used for hundreds of years in Indian and Chinese medicine for its tonifying and energizing properties. Today, ginger is better known for its ability to settle an upset stomach, stimulate digestion, and relieve aches and pains.

Ginger improves the digestion of protein, relieves nausea and motion sickness, protects against intestinal parasites, and strengthens the mucosal lining. It also mediates healing, strengthens the immune system, and reduces inflammation.

Ginger can be taken in the form of the fresh rhizome or as a honey-based syrup. It also comes as an encapsulated extract or loose dried herb. Ginger is often consumed as a tea or as a drink make by adding the honey syrup to hot water or another liquid. Since its chemistry changes when it is dried—its anti-inflammatory properties and analgesic effects are increased—the best forms to take for inflammation are the dried powder and capsules. A recommended daily dosage is 2 to 4 grams of the fresh rhizome or the equivalent in the other forms.

Ginkgo
Research abounds on the use of ginkgo (*Ginkgo biloba*) as an herbal antioxidant. One of the major effects of ginkgo is as a free-radical scavenger. Compounds within the plant can absorb reactive free radicals that would otherwise cause damage to the cells and DNA. Ginkgo has also been shown to improve circulation by making the blood vessels more flexible. Because of this vasodilating effect, ginkgo not only neutralizes existing free radicals but helps prevent the formation of new ones by improving blood flow. The increased blood flow in the body and brain also helps improve neurological performance. (For a discussion of this, see "Herbal and Nutritional Supplements for Improved Neurological Performance" on page 148.)

The recommended dosage of ginkgo is 60 to 240 milligrams per day of ginkgo leaf extract standardized to provide 24-percent ginkgo flavones; most herbalists do not recommend higher doses. In large doses, ginkgo may cause diarrhea, irritability, and restlessness. Ginkgo comes in tablet, capsule, softgel, and liquid forms.

Ginseng
Ginseng, one of the more popular herbs in the United States, is touted for its ability to increase vitality and combat stress. The root of this plant contains active compounds, called ginsenosides, that are known to reduce stress, enhance the immune system, relieve mental and physical fatigue, and normalize

Herbal and Nutritional Supplements for Improved Neurological Performance

The subject of feeding the brain using nutrition and dietary supplements has become very popular. It is widely understood that the typical adult lifestyle in this decade is one that perpetuates mental, emotional, and physical stress. Herbal products, as well as combination products also containing amino acids, vitamins, and minerals, are now being used by athletes to overcome fatigue, boost neurotransmitter levels for better training, and combat overtraining.

The brain runs on nutrients, and several herbal and nutritional products provide the brain with the ideal combination of nutrients to run smoothly and efficiently. Combination products containing such natural ingredients as St. John's wort, ginkgo, vitamins B_6 and B_{12}, folic acid, and vitamin C taken on a regular basis will enhance mental concentration, improve sleep, decrease mental fatigue, improve mood, and increase energy. St. John's wort, for example, has been shown to alleviate depression and elevate mood. According to a study published in the *British Medical Journal* in early 1997, St. John's wort is as effective as pharmaceutical antidepressants but has fewer side effects. It works by influencing the levels of the neurotransmitters in the brain thought to affect well-being, including dopamine and serotonin. Its active ingredient, hypericin, apparently slows down the breakdown of these neurotransmitters. This is important to athletes, since depression may be a trigger to overtraining.

Another example is ginkgo, which is often prescribed by doctors in Europe to increase the cerebral circulation, thus improving mental alertness and overall brain functioning. According to a number of studies, ginkgo works by increasing the blood flow throughout the body, including the brain. It elevates the production of adenosine triphosphate (ATP), the universal energy molecule, and also improves the brain's ability to metabolize glucose, prevents platelet aggregation inside the arteries by keeping the arterial walls flexible, improves the transmission of nerve signals, and acts as a powerful antioxidant. It has been shown to be helpful in short-term memory loss, depression, tinnitus, slow thinking, and slow reasoning.

These are very exciting times for the natural-therapy movement. We now have quite a number of herbs and vitamins that can provide therapeutic relief to millions of individuals by helping sustain a healthy emotional balance and positive outlook for effective training—naturally.

body systems. Many athletes claim that ginseng increases the overall vitality with no negative side effects. It has been used by Russian athletes for years to improve endurance and recovery.

Ginseng is an old-time restorative. It works by improving the general health, resistance, and energy. Traditional Western medicine puts all types of products that claim to have restorative powers in the snake-oil category. Eastern medicine is more holistic in its approach and also more interested in preventive medicine.

Soviet scientists initially used the word "adaptogen" to refer to Asian ginseng (*Panax ginseng*) and so-called Siberian ginseng (*Eleutherococcus senticosus*). American ginseng (*Panax quinquefolius*) is also considered adaptogenic.

In traditional Chinese medicine, American ginseng is used to cool and soothe, quench, and reduce fevers. Asian ginseng, which is said to possess warming properties, is used to revitalize, especially after long illnesses. In Germany, Asian ginseng products are approved for use as a tonic to take during times of fatigue, reduced concentration, and lowered work capacity.

Since the early 1960s, Siberian ginseng has been studied and used extensively for medicinal purposes. Its effects on mental alertness, work productivity, and work quality have been studied, and the results have been generally positive.

The ginsenosides contained in the ginsengs are believed to be the constituents responsible for most of the herbs' actions. The ginsenoside content can vary considerably in samples of the same species of ginseng and is always different between the species.

One double-blind, placebo-controlled study conducted in Europe involved 232 people aged twenty-five to sixty years old with nonspecific fatigue. Participants were given 80 milligrams daily of a standardized commercial extract of Asian ginseng that also contained small amounts of vitamins and minerals. All the participants were rated with "fatigue scores" before the study, then after twenty-one days, and finally after forty-two days. The patients given the ginseng generally reported improvements in their feelings of fatigue, nervousness, anxiety, and poor concentration after twenty-one days, but the improvements weren't statistically significant until after forty-two days. The amount of vitamins and minerals in each dose was very small, so the ginseng may have played the major role in counteracting the fatigue in this study. However, the researchers didn't rule out that the vitamins may have had an impact on the results.

A dose of 100 milligrams of standardized extract in capsule or liquid form two to four times daily is recommended. Long-term use has been linked to gastrointestinal upset and overstimulation in some people. Individuals with high blood pressure should avoid using ginseng, as should pregnant women.

Many Western scientists have a special dissatisfaction reserved for Eastern scientific discoveries. There is a general attitude that most Eastern scientific breakthroughs are unsubstantiated fluff that doesn't hold up under Western scientific scrutiny. Admittedly, enough "breakthroughs" have been shown to be fluff to make you want to proceed with caution, but let us not confuse ginseng (and other useful herbs) with other unproven sports-performance aids.

Gotu Kola

Gotu kola (*Centella asiatica*), a well-known tonic herb, is usually shelved in the "energy" section at health-food stores. However, do not confuse this herb with the caffeine-containing herb kola nut. Gotu kola, a staple of Ayurvedic medicine and traditional Chinese medicine, is a weedy-looking herb that contains active triterpenoid compounds. It is used as a tonic in the East and West to increase energy and endurance, improve memory and mental stamina, and alleviate depression and anxiety. Gotu kola is available in capsule and tablet form. A common dosage range is 50 to 150 milligrams per day of gotu kola leaf standardized to provide 10-percent asiaticosides.

Green Tea

For thousands of years, various regions in the Orient have

enjoyed the refreshing and health-promoting effects of a beverage brewed from the leaves of *Camellia sinensis*. In its unfermented form, *Camellia sinensis* imparts a soft, rich green tone to tea. Over the past six years, green tea has been the focus of hundreds of biomedical and epidemiological studies and scientific symposia. Groups such as the National Cancer Institute have intensively investigated green tea and its constituent polyphenol catechins as possibly having anticancer, anticarcinogen, and antioxidant effects in humans.

Green tea, the national beverage of Japan, is made from the unfermented leaves of the tea plant. In preparing the more familiar black tea, the leaves are piled up in heaps and "sweated," a natural fermentation process that darkens the leaves and changes their aroma and flavor. Recently, medical researchers have discovered a number of health benefits in the catechins, which are mostly destroyed in the fermentative conversion of the leaves to black tea. Oolong tea is somewhere in between, since it is only briefly sweated, resulting in a color, flavor, and catechin content intermediate between green and black tea.

If you are a heavy coffee, black tea, or cola drinker, you should consider switching to green tea. Green tea contains theophylline, a close relative to caffeine, but it additionally offers you immune-enhancing and general health-tonic benefits. For these benefits, drink six to ten cups of the tea a day, preferably with meals. Green tea is also available in capsule and tablet forms. A common dosage range is 50 to 300 milligrams per day of green tea leaf extract standardized to provide 50-percent to 80-percent polyphenols.

Guarana

Guarana (*Paullinia cupana*) is a climbing evergreen vine native to the Amazon region. In Brazil, a carbonated soft drink made from the seeds and produced commercially is considered the national beverage. Guarana has more caffeine than most other plants; the seeds contain as much as 7-percent caffeine and are used to naturally increase mental alertness and fight fatigue. Guarana is also used regularly to treat headaches, paralysis, urinary tract irritation, and diarrhea.

Guarana is often added to sports-nutrition products. It can also be purchased alone in capsule or tablet form, or in combination products including other herbs. A common dosage range is 50 to 250 milligrams per day in divided dosages.

Kola Nut

The kola tree (*Cola nitida*) is native to Africa, where it grows wild, and is commonly cultivated in South America and the West Indies. The seeds, large flat red or white nuts housed in a woody dull yellow pod, are used in soft drinks and herbal-stimulant products. This is because the seeds contain up to 3-percent caffeine, which is more caffeine than coffee beans contain. Kola nut is used as a stimulant to prevent fatigue. It also functions as a heart tonic and relieves headaches and the pain of neuralgia. Kola nut is available in powder, capsule, and tablet forms. A common dosage is 250 to 1,000 milligrams per day of kola nut seed extract standardized to provide 8-percent to 12-percent methylxanthines.

Licorice

Licorice (*Glycyrrhiza glabra*) is an herbal stimulant that doesn't contain alkaloids. Its stimulating action is provided by glycyrrhizin, known best for its sweetening character, and other biochemicals, including flavonoids. Licorice stimulates the adrenal cortex and prolongs the action of the adrenal hormones, which play a major role in regulating the metabolism.

When licorice is used to jump-start the adrenal system to help recovery from overtraining, it is relatively safe. However, it seems to lose its effect with long-term use and may cause side effects such as fluid retention, hypertension, and reduced stomach-acid secretion. Licorice used excessively, the same as any drug, can be quite toxic. People with heart disease, liver disease, or hypertension should avoid licorice, and it should not be used during pregnancy.

To regain energy, use 1 to 2 grams of a licorice-root product containing at least 4-percent glycyrrhizin three times daily for up to six weeks. Then, over the course of two weeks, taper the dose to nothing. Look for a standardized extract in the form of a liquid or capsules.

Maté
The same as guarana and kola nut, maté is a stimulant herb used for its caffeine content. Maté, more properly known as yerba maté (*Ilex paraguariensis*), is a small evergreen holly tree that grows in several countries in South America. The tea made from the dried leaves contains about 2-percent caffeine. In recent years, it's been implied that the caffeine in maté, kola nut, and guarana is more healthful than that found in coffee and tea. While each plant contains a variety of compounds that may subtly alter the effects of caffeine, each of these plants is primarily a source of caffeine with all of its positive and negative effects. Maté comes in capsule, tablet, and tea forms. An average dosage is 3 grams per day of unstandardized powder.

Meadowsweet and Willow Bark
The best-known commercial pain reliever is aspirin. But did you know that there are natural aspirins such as meadowsweet (*Filipendula ulmaria*) and willow bark (*Salix*)? The magic ingredient in these herbs is salicin, which converts in the stomach to salicylic acid, a compound you have probably heard about in aspirin commercials on television.

Salicylic acid was first synthesized by chemists in the mid-nineteenth century. It was hoped that this new purified form would not irritate the stomach the way natural aspirins did, but the new drug turned out to be even more irritating, and it tasted terribly bitter. Then the slightly less irritating acetylsalicylic acid was developed. Reflecting its herbal heritage, this new compound was commonly called "aspirin," from "spirea," the old name for meadowsweet (the herb, not the ornamental bush).

Herbalists use willow bark and meadowsweet to fight many of the same symptoms for which aspirin is used. The best dosage for both is 2 cups of tea or 1 to 2 dropperfuls of tincture. Ironically, it turns out that these natural aspirins are far less irritating to the stomach than the synthetic drug. This is especially true of meadowsweet, which herbalists even recommend for treating the pain of a stomach ulcer.

Both natural and synthetic aspirins decrease pain by reducing the levels of pain-producing prostaglandins, hormonelike chemicals that are manufactured in the body. Prostaglandins serve many important functions, but for various reasons, the body sometimes makes too much of them. Medical researchers believe that high levels of these chemicals are a typical cause of menstrual cramps and a contributor to migraine headaches and various types of arthritis.

Milk Thistle
Several hundred scientific research and clinical studies have found silymarian, an extract of milk thistle (*Silybum marianum*), to be ten to twenty times stronger than vitamin E, which many scientists find to be the strongest vitamin antioxidant. Besides its antioxidant properties, silymarian stimulates the body to produce superoxide dismutase and glutathione peroxidase, two primary antioxidants manufactured by the body. Milk thistle also enhances the metabolism of liver cells, then protects these cells from toxic injury, and is often used by individuals who take medications that are hard on the liver.

Milk thistle is available in all health-food stores. Select standardized extracts in tablet or capsule form. A common dosage range is 300 to 600 milligrams per day. Milk thistle can be used indefinitely.

Schisandra
Schisandra fruit is from a hardy perennial vine sometimes referred to as magnolia vine or Chinese magnolia vine. Schisandra is in the family of plants known as the *Schisandraceae,* although some botanists place it in the magnolia family, *Magnoliaceae.* The vine is native to the eastern portions of Siberia and the Sakhalin peninsula, as well as to northeastern China, Korea, and Japan.

There is growing scientific evidence concerning the general health benefits of schisandra. Some scientists classify schisandra as an adaptogen, a term that is usually reserved for the highest quality herbs, such as ginseng. Schisandra is also considered adaptogenic based on its traditional use. Interestingly, animal and human studies indicate that schisandra acts as a stimulant and tonic as well as an adaptogen. A stimulant generally increases metabolism and working capacity in one dose, while a tonic increases them during and after the administration of repeated doses.

In traditional Chinese medicine, the schisandra fruit was used primarily for nervous conditions, especially neurasthenia, a neurological disorder characterized by physical and mental fatigue and often including depression, headache, and gastrointestinal and circulatory problems. Schisandra was also used for insomnia, weakness, chronic coughing and wheezing, liver ailments, diarrhea, and perspiration. Modern scientists took an interest in the herb in the 1950s, when reports indicated that the extract of the dried fruit stimulates the central nervous system, resulting in increased mental and physical capacity.

Schisandra is available in tincture form. A typical recommended dose is 1 to 2 teaspoons two to three times a day. There are no known side effects associated with schisandra use.

Tribulus Terrestris
In Ayurvedic medicine, Tribulus terrestris has been prescribed for centuries as both a general tonic and a remedy for impotence.

Recently, a preparation of Tribulus terrestris was used to treat fifty subjects complaining of fatigue and lack of interest in performing their daily activities. The subjects showed a 45-percent improvement in their symptoms after taking the herb.

Of greater interest are studies in which Tribulus terrestris was found to have a stimulating effect on the libido. One study showed that when healthy men were given a daily dose of 750 milligrams of standardized Tribulus terrestris, they enjoyed a 30-percent increase in their testosterone level after just five days. For a complete discussion of this, see page 228.

In another study of men suffering from impotence and infertility, the administration of a standardized extract of Tribulus terrestris caused an increase in the testosterone levels and improvement in libido without any side effects.

Tribulus terrestris comes in capsule and tablet forms. A reasonable intake is 250 to 750 milligrams a day of the herb standardized to provide 40-percent furostanol saponins.

Turmeric
In addition to being a favorite culinary spice, turmeric (*Curcuma longa*), which originated in Asia, has been employed in the traditional health-care systems of many nations for centuries. Curcumin is the main pharmacological agent in turmeric. Curcumin has been shown in several studies to have protective properties similar to those possessed by the nutrient antioxidants vitamins C and E.

Turmeric is also used in the Indian and Chinese systems of medicine in the treatment of inflammation. This use seems to be substantiated by recent scientific research demonstrating that curcumin possesses significant anti-inflammatory action. An herb that combats inflammation is known as a nonsteroidal anti-inflammatory (NSAID).

The recommended dose of turmeric is 400 milligrams three times a day. This helps with inflammation, pain, and muscle soreness.

MUSHROOMS

Mushrooms contain unique compounds that are used in Eastern medicines to strengthen the immune system and allow the body to handle larger amounts of stress and training volumes. Athletes looking to support their training programs would benefit from the use of mushroom products. Mushrooms have been consumed for thousands of years, not only for their taste and nutrient contents but also for their medicinal properties.

A mushroom is the fruiting body and reproductive structure of a fungus. It also includes the mycelia, the fine hairlike strands that grow into the host body. A mushroom begins to grow when its mycelia begin to consume the host, which can be wood or a dead worm. As the mycelia grow, the mushroom blossoms. However, a mushroom is at its maxiumum potency, as far as the compounds important for immune function are concerned, just before it is completely mature. Mushrooms can also be cultivated in commercial vats in a medium of sugars and starches. When combined with the use of herbs and the consumption of a healthy diet, mushrooms will greatly improve training and health.

The medicinally useful compounds discovered so far in mushrooms include numerous polysaccharides, sterols, lipids, proteins, and triterpenes. The long-chain sugars known as polysaccharides have received the most scientific attention because of their ability to stimulate the immune system and inhibit tumor growth. Mushroom polysaccharides enhance a healthy cell's ability to fight off foreign substances such as viruses and cancer cells.

Several types of mushrooms have become particularly popular in sports nutrition for their ability to enhance health and performance. They include the cordyceps, maitake, reishi, and shiitake mushrooms.

Cordyceps
In 1993, the women of China's national track-and-field team broke the record for the 10,000-meter run by an unbelievable 40 seconds. They also improved on the previous world records for the 1,500- and 3,000-meter events, and went on to set further record times at the Asian Games in Japan in 1994. Since then, many articles have been written about a tonic mushroom that was attributed with having a large impact upon their performance. The mushroom, known as the caterpillar fungus, or cordyceps (*Cordyceps sinensis*), initially received a lot of unfavorable press, and many people called it an illegal "drug." Little did any Westerners know that cordyceps has been widely used by millions of Chinese for thousands of years and is a safe medicinal.

Cordyceps grows not on trees but on the living bodies of certain moth larvae. The mushroom organism, in the form of fine threads, penetrates the larva, eventually killing and mummifying it. The mushroom then sends up its fruiting body—a slender stalk with a swollen end that will release spores. The mushroom is cultivated because it is in great demand as a supertonic that builds physical stamina, mental energy, and sexual power. Chinese doctors say that it is simultaneously invigorating and calming, as well as life-prolonging. Chinese people usually buy it in its whole dried form, consisting of the mummified larva and attached fruiting body of the mushroom, which they add to a soup or stew made with duck or chicken. In addition, extract of cordyceps is included in many compound tonic formulas. Cordyceps is considered safe and gentle, indicated for both men and women of any age and state of health.

Caterpillar fungus takes its Chinese name, which means "winter worm, summer grass," from the fact that it grows on the larvae of caterpillars that inhabit the ground in winter. In early spring, high in the mountains of China and Tibet, the harvesters stoop to spot the little brown bladelike growths as they protrude above the melting snow. The individual growths are then graded, dried, and tied with bright threads to make small bundles to be sold to the wealthy. The flavor of the fungus is reminiscent of licorice. Today, thanks to modern technology, the far less expensive mycelia of caterpillar fungus is available. Tests have shown the mycelia to be just as active as the bladelike fruiting bodies.

In traditional Chinese medicine, caterpillar fungus is prized as a potent tonic having properties similar in action to ginseng, one of the very few medicinal plants with demonstrated performance-enhancing effects in animals and athletes. The oldest prescriptions called for 8.5 grams of the fungus to be cooked inside a duck; when eaten, the effects were equal to those of 28.35 grams of the best quality ginseng. Today, caterpillar fungus is also cooked with chicken.

Cordyceps is available in capsule form, alone or in combination with other nutrients, and as an extract, which can be used to make a tea to be drunk once a day. It is also available in whole dried form for use in soups and stews.

Maitake
The maitake mushroom (*Grifola fondosa*) has long been known for its ability to lower the cholesterol level and blood pressure. It has also been shown to reduce liver and blood fats, resulting in the loss of body fat. It additionally has anti-viral and immune-enhancing properties.

One of the more tasty mushrooms used in cooking, the maitake, pronounced *my TAH key,* grows wild in Japan and in some parts of the United States. Try eating fresh dried maitake two or three times a week. Fresh dried maitake is available at many specialty health-food stores. Maitake can also be taken in capsule or liquid form. In liquid form, take five drops of d-fraction extract three times a day.

Reishi
Reishi (*Ganderma lucidum*) is one of the most popular mushrooms in both the Orient and the West for strengthening a compromised immune system. The same as the cordyceps, maitake, and shiitake mushrooms, the reishi mushroom's immunologically active constituents are polysaccharides. The primary polysaccharide is beta-D-glucan, which has immune-stimulating qualities, as well as antioxidant and liver-protecting qualities. Because the liver is responsible for a multitude of metabolic reactions, which increase dramatically during intensive training, reishi, along with other mushrooms, is essential for the optimum health of the liver.

Herbalists in China recently began to examine the antifatigue effects of reishi. A large study involving 196 medal-winning athletes found that during competitions in cold conditions at high altitudes, taking an extract of 80-percent reishi and 20-percent ginseng caused an improvement in sleep, even though sleep is frequently compromised at higher altitudes. Compared to the control group, the athletes given the extract also were less fatigued.

Shiitake
Shiitake (*Lentinus edodes*) is among the better known mushrooms with healing applications. Shiitake, pronounced *she TAH key,* is a known source of the nontoxic drug lentinan, a polysaccharide, which is used in Japan to potentiate the immune system. Shiitake has also been used by individuals suffering from chronic fatigue syndrome. The same as maitake, shiitake has known liver-protecting compounds and is also effective at lowering the cholesterol level and blood pressure.

Most herbalists believe that a small amount of medicinal mushroom extract goes a long way toward increasing energy and improving recovery. A daily formulation that can be used during periods of intensive training or when you feel fatigued should include 40 to 50 milligrams of shitake, 50 to 60 milligrams of maitake, 50 to 60 milligrams of reishi, and 100 milligrams of cordyceps. When shopping for shiitake, make sure to select a standardized extract.

Traditionally, the Western medical establishment has lumped all herbs and mushrooms that claim to have restorative powers and improve performance into the snake-oil category. Eastern science does not suffer from this preconception. Eastern medicine has always been more holistically oriented and more interested in preventive medicine and natural products.

It is amusing to observe the contrasts between Western and Eastern thoughts when discussing this particular topic. To the Eastern mind, it is logical, even obvious, that medicinal herbs and mushrooms exist. The more holistic Eastern point of view sees all systems as interrelated and most natural products as having general, whole-body actions. To the Western mind, which is more accustomed to thinking in terms of disease and discrete physiological mechanisms, it is almost impossible to imagine a plant or fungus with such a general health-promoting action. As usual, each argument contains some truth.

There has been criticism of athletes for using natural products to help recovery and improve performance. Athletes' use of these products is a healthy sign, however, a step toward helping the body, rather than abusing it. Comparing the destructive state of mind that motivates athletes who use amphetamines or steroids with the constructive attitude that underlies the use of health-promoting and energizing herbs and mushrooms brings to mind an interesting lesson in contrasts.

Mt. Everest was first ascended by Sir Edmund Hillary and Sherpa guide Tenzing Norgay. When they were interviewed after their return, Hillary spoke repeatedly of conquering the mountain, but Norgay, his mind deep-seated in the East, said that he and the mountain together had achieved the summit. Both Hillary and Norgay made it to the summit. You decide who chose the superior way.

The scientific validation of many natural products places them among the most effective and safe performance-enhancing supplements available to modern athletes. Whether you're a weekend jogger or an Olympian, herbs and mushrooms will help you achieve your optimum performance—and like Tenzing Norgay, you can do it the better way.

SPORTS-SUPPLEMENT PRODUCTS

8 METABOLITES AND OTHER PERFORMANCE ENHANCERS

I n addition to the macronutrients, traditional micronutrients (vitamins and minerals), enzymes, herbs, and mushrooms, several other substances have been shown to benefit performance and health. These items fall into the remaining category of metabolites and other performance enhancers. Metabolites are substances that take part in metabolism. Some are produced in the body as part of the metabolic process, while others are derived from food sources. Some are now also available in supplemental form. Even though the body is able to make many of these substances, loading up on them allows athletes to prevent shortages during exercise and to have an immediately available supply on hand. Much of the pioneering research to determine which metabolites are important to athletes was conducted in clinical settings using both individuals with metabolic disorders and patients recovering from injuries or surgery. The researchers discovered that the subjects not only overcame their disorders but often went on to attain a state of health better than what they had started with. Studies conducted with athletes demonstrated that certain metabolites improve such athletic-performance factors as strength, agility, speed, and aerobic capacity.

Metabolite supplements are sold in health-food stores, pharmacies, and gyms and through mail-order catalogs and professional trainers. As their popularity continues to grow, some are even making their way onto supermarket shelves. Metabolites, the same as herbs, are available as single-ingredient formulations and as part of multi-vitamin-and-mineral formulations. They come in tablet, powder, and liquid forms. To have an ergogenic (sports-enhancing) effect, most must be ingested in large amounts for short periods of time or taken daily in smaller amounts for longer periods of time to build up stores in the body. Many of the supplements are expensive, and care should be taken to select products manufactured by reputable companies. If one product is much cheaper than similar products, it is probably of a lesser quality.

Use caution when taking any dietary supplement. To be extra safe, keep a record of your daily intake. For the dosage you should take, see the label on the supplement bottle, consult your health-care practitioner, or check a reference source such as *Dynamic Nutrition for Maximum Performance* by Daniel Gastelu and Dr. Fred Hatfield (Garden City Park, NY: Avery Publishing Group, 1997). Competitive athletes should also check with the organization that governs their sport to make sure that the supplement ingredients are acceptable.

Beta-Hydroxy Beta-Methylbutyrate
Beta-hydroxy beta–methylbutyrate (HMB) is one of the newer metabolite supplements to gain popularity. It is being touted as an aid to muscle gain when used in association with a weightlifting program.

Beta-hydroxy beta–methylbutyrate seems to be a breakdown product of the amino acid leucine and may play an important role in protein metabolism. Studies have indicated that when it is taken in supplemental amounts, it boosts nitrogen retention, thereby helping the body to hang onto more amino acids, which are necessary for muscle growth and repair. HMB therefore may be useful for individuals training to increase muscle mass. According to studies, supplemental amounts ranging from 1,500 to 4,000 milligrams yield positive results. However, if you choose to try HMB, use it as part of a rounded supplement program, not alone.

(For a special report on HMB, see page 159.)

Bicarbonate
Bicarbonate is a member of a group of metabolites that has been creating excitement in the sports world in recent years. Known as blood buffers, these metabolites are substances that help maintain the pH balance in the blood. When the blood becomes too acidic due to lactic-acid buildup, fatigue sets in and performance is impaired. Bicarbonate, in particular sodium bicarbonate, is the blood buffer that has gotten most of the attention.

ON THE CUTTING EDGE

Reduce Muscle Damage With HMB

A study presented at the Experimental Biology 1998 conference, held in San Francisco, revealed that beta-hydroxy beta-methylbutyrate, a supplement popular with strength athletes, may also offer significant benefits to endurance athletes. In the study, runners who added 3 grams of supplemental HMB to their daily nutrition program experienced 50 percent less muscle damage than athletes who used a placebo. The HMB-supplemented runners showed an average increase of only 145 units per liter of blood of a muscle-damage byproduct called creatine phosphokinase (CPK) twenty-four hours after a 20-kilometer race. The placebo group had an average increase of 230 units of CPK per liter. The greater elevation of CPK in the placebo group showed that an enhanced degree of muscle damage had occurred. The HMB-supplemented runners also maintained or improved their leg strength, whereas the placebo group lost leg strength. HMB may be important in reducing the amount of muscle damage associated with almost any type of strenuous physical activity that normally results in soreness and/or muscle damage.

SPECIAL REPORT

Building Muscle Strength With HMB

One of the best-selling anabolic supplements to come to market during the last few years is beta-hydroxy beta-methylbutyrate (HMB), a byproduct of leucine metabolism. The most common pathway of leucine metabolism involves the conversion of the amino acid to alpha-ketoisocaproate (KIC), which is then transported into the mitochondria, where it is converted to ketones. In an alternative pathway, the leucine is converted to KIC, and the KIC is oxidized to HMB by an enzyme called KIC-dioxygenase.

The HMB is then further metabolized in one of at least three ways. In one, it plays a role in cholesterol synthesis. In a second, it is lost in the urine. Studies have indicated that up to 40 percent of the HMB consumed is lost in the urine, which likely accounts for its relatively short half-life of about one hour. In the third way, it is used by the cell. In muscle cells, HMB seems to affect protein synthesis and may help maximize the anabolic effects of exercise. Studies have indicated that HMB is the bioactive component of leucine metabolism that plays a regulatory role in protein metabolism. HMB meets the criteria of a dietary supplement because it is found in some foods, such as catfish and citrus fruits, in small amounts; is found in breast milk; and is used and produced by body tissues.

HMB AND MUSCLE GROWTH

Early human-performance studies using HMB were conducted at Vanderbilt University and Iowa State University, where it was found that HMB increases strength and lean body mass in athletes. These two universities hold several patents on HMB and have licensed its production and distribution to several companies.

In the first part of a two-part study published by S. Nissen and associates, forty-one male volunteers aged nineteen through twenty-nine years and weighing an average of 180 pounds were given one of three dosages of supplemental HMB—none, 1.5 grams, or 3.0 grams—on a daily basis while consuming a normal-protein diet or high-protein diet. The subjects controlled their food intake by selecting meals from a list of prepared entrées. The same meals were used during the baseline-data-collecting week and during the study. The participants also lifted weights for an hour and a half a day, three days a week, for three weeks.

The results of this first study indicated that HMB improves strength and lean body mass. The subjects gained lean body mass in a dose-responsive manner—the group taking no HMB gained an average of 0.88 pound per subject; the group taking 1.5 grams of HMB gained an average of 1.76 pounds per subject; and the group taking 3.0 grams of HMB gained an average of 2.64 pounds per subject.

The researchers also found that the HMB-supplemented subjects were able to lift more weight than the unsupplemented subjects during all three weeks. The supplemented subjects additionally were able to perform more abdominal exercises, with the unsupplemented subjects increasing their performance by 14 percent and the supplemented subjects by 50 percent. Finally, total strength increased by 8 percent in the unsupplemented subjects, 13 percent in the 1.5-gram group, and 18.4 percent in the 3.0-gram group.

In the second part of Nissen's study, thirty-two male volunteers participated in an additional strength-training study. These men were divided into two groups, receiving either no HMB or 3.0 grams of HMB per day, with both groups lifting weights for two to three hours a day, six days a week, for seven weeks. The early measurements in the study indicated that the subjects taking the HMB developed significantly more fat-free mass than the subjects not taking HMB. The bench-press strength of the HMB group was almost three times greater than that of the non-HMB group, and the strength increases for the squat of the HMB group, although not statistically significant, were also greater. These increases occurred independent of the amount of protein consumed by the subjects. However, it is important to note that the group consuming the least amount of protein still ingested more than twice the RDA recommended for maintaining nitrogen balance. So, it could be that a protein intake considered normal by non-bodybuilding standards limits the benefits of HMB.

At the 1997 meeting of the Federation of Applied Science and Experimental Biologists, several studies were presented showing the continued benefits of combining HMB with resistance training. In one study, researchers looked at the effects of HMB on body composition and strength in both exercising and non-exercising women. They wanted the answers to two questions: Does HMB work as well in women as it does in men? And will HMB work even if the subjects don't exercise? The research presented mixed results.

In the exercising group, the women supplementing their diets with 3.0 grams of HMB a day during the four-week study period showed impressive results compared to the women taking a placebo. On average, their strength increased by 77 percent over the placebo group, they gained more than twice as much lean muscle mass, and they lost almost three times as much body fat. However, in the nonexercising group, the women taking 3.0 grams of HMB a day showed no significant changes in lean body mass or body fat compared to the women taking the placebo. This study showed that HMB may play a role in the muscle-building and fat-burning response to exercise.

Two studies were presented by Dr. Richard Kreider and associates from the University of Memphis in which the effects of combining HMB with creatine on both strength parameters and body composition in collegiate football players were investigated. The researchers had hypothesized

that combining these two supplements could have a synergistic effect, but the results of the two studies did not support this assumption. There were definite trends, which led Dr. Kreider to state, "Results revealed that adding creatine to HMB may enhance strength and/or anaerobic capacity," but the results were not statistically significant.

Although there were no significant differences, the average changes in the supplemented groups were positive and paralleled those found in previous HMB studies showing significant differences. Dr. Kreider pointed out that the length of the supplementation period was a variable that could lead to significant differences in strength gains.

An in vitro study investigating how HMB helps decrease body fat was also presented at the 1997 meeting. This study, performed by Dr. Cheng at the State University of New York at Stony Brook, revealed that when muscle cells in a test tube were exposed to HMB, they burned fat faster. In other words, HMB may help people more efficiently utilize their body-fat stores for fuel, thus both decreasing stored fat and sparing protein and carbohydrates for muscle building and energy production.

HMB MECHANISMS

The exact mechanism of the effect of HMB on muscle metabolism is not known, but at least two hypotheses can be put forth to explain the results. In one, HMB is thought to be an essential component of the cell membrane. Under stressful conditions, scientists propose, the body either does not make enough HMB to satisfy the increased needs for the substance, or the concentration of certain enzymes or biochemicals is altered, resulting in a decrease in HMB production. Either scenario would require dietary supplementation with HMB for the muscle tissue or immune system to function maximally.

In the second hypothesis, HMB is believed to regulate the enzymes responsible for muscle-tissue breakdown. This theory is supported by evidence found in several studies in which the biochemical indicators of muscle damage were decreased. Additionally, a recent study using isolated chick and rat muscle indicated that HMB can directly decrease muscle-protein breakdown.

Currently, research is underway ranging from basic studies designed to explain the biochemical action of HMB to more complex studies intended to assess the impact of HMB on wasting diseases and the maintenance of lean muscle mass in women who are losing weight. Several studies that have been completed and others that are still in progress all show that HMB is safe and effective for men and women. Human studies have been conducted in which up to 4.0 grams per day of HMB have been administered for up to four weeks. The authors report no toxicity at these levels.

All the research reported to date seems to point to HMB as a dietary supplement that offers benefits to athletes and individuals trying to gain lean body weight and muscular strength. HMB appears to be safe and seems to display a rather consistent degree of positive health gains in clinical trials with humans.

Many studies have reported that sodium bicarbonate produces ergogenic effects in individuals repeatedly exercising to capacity, for several seconds to several minutes. These ergogenic effects have all been confirmed in studies performed with sprinters and world-class rowers. Large amounts of sodium bicarbonate are needed, however—about 100 milligrams for every 1 pound of lean body mass. This means that if you had, for example, 150 pounds of lean body mass, you would need about 15,000 milligrams of sodium bicarbonate. The exact dosage would depend on whether you experienced any side effects, which include diarrhea, nausea, cramps, and flatulence. If you suffered no side effects, you could take your dosage on an empty stomach one hour before your activity. If you experienced gastrointestinal side effects, you would do better starting two hours before your activity and taking one-fourth of your dosage with water every fifteen minutes. Sodium-bicarbonate loading also packs the body with a few thousand milligrams of sodium, so be careful if you have blood-pressure problems or hypertension. Always follow the product directions, and consult your health-care practitioner if you notice any side effects.

Carnitine   *See* Carnitine (Vitamin B-T) *on page 92.*

Coenzyme Q$_{10}$ *See* Coenzyme Q$_{10}$ *on page 94.*

Colostrum   Colostrum is the special milk that is secreted by mammals after they give birth. It contains important growth factors, immune-system compounds, and other nutrients that help the new offspring get a jump-start on life. Colostrum production slows down forty-eight to seventy-two hours after birth.

Commercial colostrum, which is primarily bovine (cow) colostrum, has been on the market for a long time and, like cow's milk, is consumed by humans. While the benefits of colostrum for newborns are clearly understood, the benefits for human adults are of growing interest. Dr. Bernard Jensen, a pioneer in the field of nutrition, is one of the great proponents of colostrum, which he calls "white gold." Colostrum's clearly proven benefits are to the digestive system. Its immunoglobulins (Ig's) and growth factors—in particular, its insulin-like growth factors (IGFs)—help keep the lining of the digestive system healthy. They also assist with the maintenance of the intestine's "good bacteria," which help keep the "bad bacteria" in check. Studies with adults and children have shown that colostrum combats severe diarrhea. In athletes, colostrum helps normalize the gastrointestinal system and reduces diarrhea. This leads to better digestion and better absorption of other nutrients, which means better nitrogen balance and recovery. (For a discussion of nitrogen balance, see page 21.) Additionally, the Ig's in colostrum can benefit the immune system. Athletes' immune systems are constantly being stressed by exercise.

The second-level benefits that colostrum has to offer are less certain but are supported by indirect evidence and case studies. The IGFs found in colostrum are known to be critical in the promotion of growth and have been clinically shown to improve nitrogen balance and to increase muscle growth. This is why colostrum exists in mother's milk during the critical first few days of lactation (milk production). The voluminous research data on these powerful growth factors is compelling. Without exception, studies document how two of the most important growth factors found in colostrum, insulin-like growth factor I (IGF-I) and insulin-like growth factor II (IGF-II), enhance DNA and protein synthesis. IGF-I and IGF-II are the healing properties of colostrum. Their muscle-building and connective-tissue-repair characteristics are biochemically unsurpassed. They are essential ingredients in muscle growth, primarily through their roles in the repair and conversion of broken-down muscle fibers.

All told, colostrum has potential as a component in the athlete's diet. Please note, however, that if you choose to take a colostrum supplement, you should look for a standardized product, since the Ig content does tend to vary. Colostrum with an Ig content of 26 to 33 percent may be ideal. Colostrum is available as a supplement both alone and as part of a formulation.

Creatine
Creatine is manufactured in the body during protein metabolism. It is also present in food and available in supplemental form as creatine monohydrate. Creatine monohydrate is consumed to increase the body's stores of creatine and creatine phosphate (CP). CP is produced in the body by the combination of creatine and phosphate. In the body, CP is stored in muscle tissue along with ATP. Together, CP and ATP store the chemical energy of the body. The more energy they store, the better the muscles can perform in short-term maximum-strength events.

The body uses CP to quickly replenish ATP, a process that takes just seconds. Creatine loading can therefore bring about improved training intensity and recovery in anaerobic sports involving all-out effort for short periods of time (a few seconds). Dosages of creatine monohydrate that have reportedly been used for this purpose range from 1 to 24 grams per day. For long-term building-up of the creatine level, the recommended daily dosage is 8 milligrams for every 1 pound of lean body mass, or about 1 to 2 grams total. For short-term creatine loading, take

40 to 80 milligrams for every 1 pound of lean body mass, or about 5 to 10 grams total, every day for several days. Some people take as much as 80 to 160 milligrams for every 1 pound of lean body mass, or about 10 to 24 grams total. Use the product as directed on the label for up to two or three months at a time.

(For a special report on creatine, see page 164.)

ON THE CUTTING EDGE

Creatine Increases Gains in Muscle Mass

Does taking creatine while weight training increase muscle mass more than just weight training alone does? In a study of football players, this very important question of the effect of creatine supplementation on body composition and strength was investigated. According to an article in *Medicine and Science in Sports and Exercise* in 1998, every day for twenty-eight days, two groups of football players were given either a placebo or a creatine supplement containing 15 grams of creatine. During this time, the athletes participated in a comprehensive weight-training program. The creatine group showed a significantly greater increase in weight than did the placebo group (4.8 pounds versus 1.7 pounds). The creatine group also showed a significantly greater increase in muscle mass (5.3 pounds versus 3.9 pounds). In addition, the creatine group showed a greater increase in a strength test using a four- to eight-repetition maximum. The major findings were that the creatine supplementation resulted in greater gains in muscle mass and strength than did the weight training alone.

Creatine Use Is Safe

When three wrestlers died during weight-cutting episodes, a number of researchers began to look at the possible link to the athletes' creatine intake. A team of experts from the Centers for Disease Control (CDC) investigated the three cases in-depth and published their findings in 1998 in the *CDC Morbidity and Mortality Weekly Report*. Each case was described, and autopsy analyses of various substances were provided. The findings? The wrestlers, tragically, died because they lost too much weight too quickly and their bodies overheated from being unable to adequately cool off due to dehydration. The report cited the fact that all three of the wrestlers used rubber suits, exercised vigorously in hot environments, and had elevated sodium and urea in their postmortem fluids, indicating dehydration. Practices such as exercising in heat and wearing rubber can adversely affect cardiac function, electrical activity, thermal regulation, renal function, electrolyte balance, body composition, and muscular endurance and strength. But what about taking creatine? Well, remember the reports that the wrestlers were all taking creatine? As it turned out, only one had supplemented with creatine, and he had stopped taking it two weeks before his death because he thought it was preventing him from losing weight.

SPECIAL REPORT
Muscle Up to Creatine

Creatine supplementation is being touted as one of the most significant developments in sports-related nutrition since the discovery of carbohydrate loading three decades ago. Creatine is now the ergogenic supplement of choice of athletes looking for an edge in training and competition. Scientific research has verified that creatine is not just an energy source that powers the muscles but also an important supplement because it:

☐ Increases muscle strength and power.

☐ Promotes significant increases in lean body mass and muscle without increasing body fat.

☐ Improves performance during short-duration high-intensity exercise, as well as intermittent exercise.

☐ Hastens energy recovery between bouts of high-intensity exercise. For example, with creatine supplementation, a second sprint could be run at the same intensity and greater speed.

☐ May reduce fatigue by decreasing the lactic-acid buildup in high-intensity and sprint exercises.

☐ May increase the anaerobic threshold.

☐ Allows more intense training, further improving strength and muscle growth by delaying muscle fatigue.

Creatine is derived from the amino acids arginine, glycine, and methionine. It is normally found in meat and fish in quantities of approximately 5 grams of creatine for every 1 kilogram (2.2 pounds) of meat. Therefore, you would have to eat 4 kilograms, or about 9 pounds, of meat to ingest 20 grams of creatine. The initial loading dose often prescribed during the first phase of creatine supplementation is 20 to 25 grams.

Several studies have indicated that the total creatine content of muscle can be increased 20 to 30 percent following supplementation with creatine monohydrate. Furthermore, many studies have been conducted demonstrating that the performance of intermittent high-intensity (not endurance) exercise is improved following creatine supplementation. The improved performance is attributed to increased pre-exercise concentrations of creatine and phosphocreatine and/or to a greater resynthesis rate of phosphocreatine during the recovery period between exercise bouts. Recent evidence supports a greater role for the latter mechanism. A quicker resynthesis of phosphocreatine during recovery should increase the body's ability to sustain maximum force or power production during intermittent high-intensity exercise.

PERFORMANCE ENHANCEMENT

Because of creatine's important role in energy metabolism, as well as the fact that its supply is finite, loading the muscles with creatine seems a logical means of enhancing muscle performance during anaerobic exercise. The first question, however, is whether supplementation can expand the muscle stores of creatine.

So far, research has shown that, while there is significant individual variation, supplementation can allow muscle to increase its holdings of creatine. Overall, the degree of creatine uptake appears to be dose-related; it is dependent on the athlete's current stores, and the major portion of the uptake occurs during the initial days of supplementation. One study showed that doses of less than 1 gram produced a negligible effect, while doses of 5 grams resulted in a fifteen-fold increase in muscle creation.

The dosage protocol most frequently used in research studies is to "load" with 20 to 25 grams of creatine per day—specifically, 5 grams four or five times a day—for the first four to five days, resulting in an average

20-percent increase in muscle creatine, of which 20 percent is in the form of creatine phosphate. There is an upper limit to the creatine level that can be achieved and, once the muscles reach that saturation point, any extra creatine is excreted by the kidneys.

Individuals with the lowest levels of muscle creatine achieve the most pronounced effects from creatine supplementation, while those who begin with high levels accumulate a negligible amount of additional creatine. Women have slightly higher creatine levels than men. Vegetarians have lower creatine pools, suggesting that they may benefit the most from supplementation.

MUSCLE BUILDING

As any serious athlete or weight lifter knows, the best way to build up your muscles is to push them to their limits. It stands to reason that if creatine lets your muscles perform more work at a higher intensity, you're going to be able to stimulate even more muscle growth with creatine than you would without creatine.

Creatine's muscle-building powers seem to lie in its ability to enhance the body's capacity to create two key muscle proteins—myosin and actin. Muscle cells must have adequate amounts of these two proteins for continued contraction.

Athletes in sports such as powerlifting, bodybuilding, football, and baseball, and in events such as swimming and running sprints, the shotput, and javelin will greatly benefit from creatine supplementation. So will tennis, hockey, and soccer players, and wrestlers.

Athletes over the age of thirty may also benefit from creatine supplementation. Since creatine boosts protein synthesis and muscle-energy stores, it should help maintain muscle mass in older athletes as they age.

ADEQUATE DOSING

The most efficient method of increasing your creatine stores and then maintaining the increase is to creatine load for five days and then follow a maintenance program. During the loading phase, consume 20 to 25 grams of creatine per day in 5-gram doses every two to three hours. Since changes in the creatine stores are directly related to changes in exercise performance, it is particularly important to optimize the creatine uptake by your muscles during this phase. A factor that has been shown to increase creatine uptake into the muscles and to reduce urinary-creatine excretion is the ingestion of carbohydrates. Thus, during the loading phase, carbohydrates should be consumed along with the creatine. Once the creatine-loading phase is complete, the muscles should be fully saturated and further increases unlikely.

To maintain your elevated creatine stores, a much lower intake of creatine is required. Recent research suggests that as little as 2 grams of creatine per day will maintain elevated creatine stores in individuals not engaged in physical exercise. However, due to the increased breakdown of creatine associated with training, a more appropriate maintenance dose for athletes is 5 grams a day. Furthermore, a number of large (weighing more than 220 pounds) strength-trained athletes have been known to take up to 10 grams of creatine per day because of their increased muscle mass and their muscles' increased creatine needs. The form of creatine used in all studies showing an ergogenic effect is creatine monohydrate. Creatine is sold commercially by several nutritional-supplement companies under a variety of trade names, as either capsules or a tasteless white powder. A single 5-gram serving of creatine equals approximately 1 teaspoon of powder. This should be dissolved in some form of liquid immediately prior to consumption.

While some athletes may wait until an important event to creatine load, this might minimize many of the positive effects creatine supplementation could have on training. Thus, unlike carbohydrate loading, in which athletes typically begin their regimen of tapered training and increased carbohydrate consumption one week prior to their event, creatine loading should be undertaken during the preseason or long before an important event. Beginning creatine supplementation at this time may enhance the quality of the practice sessions by allowing the athlete to train at an increased intensity, possibly inducing greater physiological adaptations and improved exercise performance.

MEDICALLY SAFE

The science surrounding the efficacy of creatine supplementation for enhancing many types of athletic performance is virtually indisputable. However, the media is now trying to discredit the supplement by raising questions about its safety. Creatine's critics focus purely on anecdotal and unsubstantiated accounts of the substance's supposed implication in everything from muscle cramping to kidney stress to the deaths of three college wrestlers. The science behind creatine simply does not support the claims being made regarding any health hazards.

Although no adverse side effects have been reported in the literature from clinical trials, some of the concerns being raised involve suppression of endogenous creatine synthesis, enhanced kidney or liver stress, muscle cramping when exercising in heat, and muscle strains and pulls. Concerns have also been raised about certain possible long-term effects of supplementation. While all these concerns should be evaluated and addressed, it should be noted that there is no evidence from any well-controlled clinical trials to indicate these concerns have any validity. The only side effect that has thus far been reported is weight gain, and this has been in clinical studies investigating dosages of 1.5 to 25.0 grams taken daily for three days to one year by preoperative and postoperative patients, untrained subjects, and elite athletes.

Creatine is a very hot topic due to its ability to enhance performance. Currently, creatine supplementation appears to be a safe practice when performed as recommended. Individuals who supplement with this powerful substance can expect to see an increase in their body weight along with a decrease in their body fat when combining their supplementation with physical training.

Dehydroepiandrosterone Dehydroepiandrosterone (DHEA) entered the dietary-supplement market during the last few years as, among other things, a longevity substance. However, take note that DHEA is not for everyone; most health authorities do not recommend it for individuals under the age of forty. The DHEA level declines with age, and younger people do not seem to benefit from supplemental DHEA because their bodies are already making enough. Note, too, that DHEA is banned by many sports governing bodies.

DHEA is a hormone produced mainly by the adrenal glands. In men, it is also produced in the testes as an intermediate in testosterone production; and in women, it is also produced in the ovaries as an intermediate in estrogen production. DHEA seems to be a weak androgen (a steroid hormone that promotes masculine characteristics), and it has also been reported to induce growth of body hair in men and women. However, in a study using men between the ages of twenty and twenty-five, supplemental DHEA did not increase testosterone levels but did appear to help decrease body fat and increase lean body mass. Conversely, in another study, an increase in androgen levels was reported in postmenopausal women given supplemental DHEA, as was an increase in body-hair growth during the study period. Another study, this one using both men and women, did not report any significant changes in lean body mass or body fat but did report an

ON THE CUTTING EDGE

Creatine Benefits Performance and Body Composition

The effects of twenty-six days of creatine supplementation on high-intensity bench-press performance and body composition were evaluated in a study of eighteen male powerlifters. In an article published in the *Journal of Strength and Conditioning Research* in 1998, nine of the men were given creatine, while nine were given a placebo. Pre and post measurements of muscular strength, body mass, and percent of body fat were taken on days one and twenty-eight, respectively. The supplementation was divided into two periods—days two through six, during which 20 grams of creatine were given per day, and days seven through twenty-seven, during which 5 grams of creatine were given per day. The creatine supplementation significantly increased body mass and lean body mass with no changes in percent of body fat. In addition, significant increases in strength while bench pressing, both absolute and relative to body mass, occurred in both groups, but the increases were greater in the creatine group. The total repetitions that could be accomplished also increased significantly in the creatine group in absolute terms and relative to body mass, while no significant changes were seen in the placebo group.

Creatine Improves Anaerobic Power

To determine if creatine could help athletes who participate in sports that require both explosive bursts of power and endurance, a group of triathletes was given 6 grams of supplemental creatine for five days, according to an article published in *Medicine and Science in Sports and Exercise* in 1998. The subjects were then tested during an exercise regimen that alternated between anaerobic and aerobic training. The results showed that the athletes' power performance was increased by 18 percent during the anaerobic exercise, but that there was no effect on the endurance exercise. The supplementation had no effect on the cardiovascular-system oxygen-uptake or blood-lactate levels, although the fall in blood glucose during exercise was significantly reduced. The researchers concluded that anyone who takes part in a sport periodically requiring a high energy output, such as triathletes, could benefit greatly from taking 6 grams of creatine per day.

overall improvement in the feeling of well-being. This last study also reported a possible anabolic effect—an increase in the IGF-I level. IGF-I is an important growth promoter in muscles, especially in individuals undergoing intensive training. (For a discussion of IGF-I, see "Colostrum" on page 161.)

Studies with athletes have not yet been reported. Going by the results of the studies just mentioned, medically unsupervised DHEA use by young male athletes is not warranted, and use by female athletes and by male athletes over age forty may have some beneficial physical and physiological effects. Other reported benefits of DHEA include immune-system enhancement, anticancer activity, antidepressant action, enhancement of mental functioning, and longevity in laboratory animals. The amounts used in studies have varied, but benefits have been reported in the 25-to-100-milligram range. *A word of caution:* Do not take supplemental DHEA if you are a man who may have prostate cancer or a woman who may have breast cancer, a reproductive cancer, or a reproductive disorder.

Gamma Oryzanol and Ferulic Acid

Gamma oryzanol is a substance extracted from rice-bran oil that reportedly promotes a variety of metabolic effects. These metabolic effects include increased endorphin release, antioxidant activity, lipotropic action, stress reduction, GH stimulation, increased growth, and improved recovery. Ferulic acid (FRAC) is part of the gamma-oryzanol molecule and is also available as a supplement. The metabolic effects of FRAC include increased strength, improved recovery, reduced muscle soreness, reduced sensation of fatigue, and decreased catabolic effects by cortisol.

While research is sparse, athletes report beneficial results from the supplemental use of gamma oryzanol and ferulic acid. Daily dosages of 10 to 60 milligrams of ferulic acid and/or 300 to 900 milligrams of gamma oryzanol have been reported to have no toxic side effects. Ferulic acid appears to be about thirty times more bioavailable than gamma oryzanol, but some scientists believe that the sterol molecule to which the ferulic acid is bound is integral to the efficient transport of the ferulic-acid molecule.

For best results, take supplemental gamma oryzanol and/or ferulic acid before workouts on training days and in the morning on nontraining days.

Glucosamine

Glucosamine as a supplement is widely heralded as an effective treatment for arthritis. It is also beneficial to connective tissue. The body contains several types of connective tissue. These different types of connective tissue make up the tendons, ligaments, intervertebral discs, pads between the joints, cell membranes, and cartilage. Connective tissue has two components. The chief component is collagen, which is the most common protein in the body, making up one-third of the body's total protein volume. The other component is proteoglycan (PG), which forms the "framework" for collagenous tissue. PGs are huge structural macromolecules comprised mainly of glycosaminoglycans (GAGs), which are long chains of modified sugars. The principal GAG in PG is hyaluronic acid, of which 50 percent is glucosamine.

Over thirty years of research has gone into understanding how glucosamine acts as a precursor in GAG synthesis. Scientists have long known that ingesting purified glucosamine from connective tissue allows the body to bypass the step of converting glucose to glucosamine. Following are some of the findings from the research studies:

☐ Glucosamine is absorbed 95-percent intact through the gut wall.

☐ About 30 percent of orally administered glucosamine is stored by the body for later synthesis of more connective tissue.

☐ In human clinical trials, glucosamine given orally in doses of 750 to 1,500 milligrams daily initiated a reversal of degenerative osteoarthritis of the knee after two months. The normalization of the cartilage was documented through biopsies of the tissue.

☐ Of greater concern to athletes, glucosamine taken orally gives injured connective tissue the precursor that is the most critical in the rebuilding of its collagenous matrix.

☐ Glucosamine is the preferred substance in synthesizing PG, which forms the framework of connective tissue.

☐ According to in vitro research, glucosamine increases the production of GAG, the most important molecule in PG, by 170 percent.

Supplemental glucosamine clearly aids in the synthesis of connective tissue. All athletes need a supplement that can do this, as the repair and growth of connective tissue is never-ending. For this purpose, take 500 to 2,000 milligrams of glucosamine per day.

Glycerol

Glycerol is a three-carbon-atom molecule that is the backbone of triglycerides and phospholipids. Triglycerides consist of three fatty acids attached to a glycerol molecule, and phospholipids consist of two fatty acids attached to a glycerol molecule, with a phosphate-containing compound attached to the third carbon atom. (For discussions of triglycerides and phospholipids, see Chapter 3.) When glycerol is removed from these fats by hydrolysis, it is a clear, syrupy liquid. The liquid has been utilized in a variety of ways over the years, but it is especially popular as an emollient in skin-care products and cosmetics and as a sweetening agent in pharmaceuticals.

As a supplement, glycerol has been found by researchers to possibly help the body remain better hydrated. Studies have shown that athletes training for prolonged periods (more than one hour) are able to run cooler and longer when they ingest a water-glycerol mixture. Preliminary studies have suggested that glycerol acts like a sponge, absorbing water into the bloodstream and holding it there. However, researchers are still trying to determine appropriate dosages; the current estimates range from 10 to 60 grams, taken with the amount of water recommended for the activity, over a period of a few hours.

A word of caution: Some side effects, including bloating, nausea, and lightheadedness, have been reported with glycerol use. If you choose to try a glycerol-containing beverage, test it out at least several times before competition to see how your body reacts to it.

Inosine

Inosine is a naturally occurring substance found in all human tissues, particularly in the skeletal and cardiac muscles. It is involved in the regeneration of ATP, promoting its synthesis and replenishment. It also stimulates the production of 2,3 diphosphoglycerate (2,3 DPG), which is one of the substances essential in the transportation of oxygen molecules from red blood cells to muscle cells for cellular energy production. In addition, inosine is believed to enhance muscle growth, improve immune response and resistance to infection, and act as a vasodilator, increasing blood flow. It reportedly improves strength, resulting in the ability to lift more weight, finish more repetitions, and engage in better workouts. Endurance athletes have also reported benefits. However, because inosine contains nitrogen and can add to the production of uric acid, individuals with kidney problems or gout should not use inosine.

The recommended dosage of inosine is 5 to 10 milligrams for every 1 pound of lean body mass. For an individual with a lean body mass of 140 pounds, this works out to a total of 700 to 1,400 milligrams. When loading inosine before competition, take it in combination with creatine monohydrate and its cofactors for the best results. Furthermore, take it forty-five to sixty minutes before exercising. The form of inosine is also important. The best is inosine hypoxanthine riboside (inosine HXR), followed by betaglycosidic nucleoside of D-ribose and hypoxanthine, as well as hypoxanthine riboside. Do not use any other form, such as inosinic acid. Store inosine in a moisture-proof bottle in a dry location.

Inositol

Inositol is often classified as a member of the B-complex family. It is correctly called myo-inositol and is generally considered to be a nonessential vitamin because it is synthesized by most animals, including humans. Inositol is a lipotropic agent. It assists fatty-acid metabolism, carbohydrate metabolism, and calcium functioning. A deficiency of inositol can lead to a buildup of fat in the liver and may affect the nervous system. Inositol is not reported to have any effects on athletic performance.

Although no RDA value has been set for inositol, a PDI for men and women who are healthy and actively training has been established at 800 to 1,200 milligrams per day. Intake above 1,200 milligrams has not produced any toxic side effects in healthy individuals. The average adult diet supplies about 1,000 milligrams of inositol per day.

Inositol is found in foods such as heart, whole grains, fruit, milk, nuts, meat, and vegetables. It is available in supplement form as myo-inositol (pure inositol) and is also commonly included in multi-vitamin-and-mineral supplements and lipotropic supplements.

Lipoic Acid

See Lipoic Acid *on page 94.*

Melatonin

Melatonin is another substance produced by the body that has recently appeared in supplement form in health-food stores. Supplemental melatonin has not been shown in any tests to directly improve athletic performance, but it has been shown to indirectly improve performance by stimulating certain bodily processes. Melatonin's main function is improving sleep. According to studies, it helps people to fall asleep quicker, stay asleep, and enjoy a more restful sleep. Furthermore, it does this without causing sleep hangover, which is an aftereffect of most sleep medications.

Melatonin is the body's natural sleep substance. Researchers have determined that when the sun sets, the body's melatonin level begins to rise. At dawn, the body's melatonin level begins to drop again. There are times, however, when the body's natural melatonin production may be upset. Traveling across time zones disrupts melatonin production, causing what is commonly known as jet lag. Nervousness before a big athletic event affects melatonin production, as does the stress of training. Staying up late to study for a test can also be disruptive because, according to researchers, lamplight may be enough to suppress proper melatonin production.

Millions of people have been using supplemental melatonin during the past few years with no apparent side effects. The amounts used successfully in studies have ranged from 0.5 to 3.0 milligrams. However, until researchers determine the effects of long-term supplemental use of melatonin on the body's natural melatonin-production capabilities, the best advice is to be judicious in your selection of dosage and frequency. Do not use melatonin every night.

Octacosanol
Octacosanol is a component of wheat-germ oil and is used by athletes for its performance benefits. Some athletes take octacosanol as an individual nutrient, while others consume it as a part of wheat-germ oil, which also contains vitamin E, the essential fatty acids, and plant sterols. Among octacosanol's benefits are improved neuromuscular functioning, improved reaction time, improved endurance, improved muscle glycogen storage, and reduced effects of stress.

Supplementation with both octacosanol and wheat-germ oil on a daily basis is recommended during the season and preseason. Dosages of octacosanol of 1,000 to 2,000 micrograms and more per day have been used in studies with humans with no toxic side effects.

Pyruvate
Pyruvate is the byproduct of carbohydrate metabolism. It can also be obtained from the diet, with naturally ingested amounts ranging from 100 milligrams to 1 to 2 grams daily. Although pyruvate is found in a variety of foods, most of them contain less than 25 milligrams per serving. Foods high in pyruvate include certain fruits—most notably, red apples—and vegetables, most cheeses, and alcohol products, such as beer and red wine.

Some pyruvate products contain small amounts of dihydroxyacetone, which is a compound that can be manufactured by the body and also obtained from the diet. In the body, dihydroxyacetone is rapidly converted during glycolysis to pyruvate. Much of the early research conducted on pyruvate included dihydroxyacetone. The more recent studies have only used pyruvate.

In three studies conducted by Dr. Ronald Stanko at the University of Pitts-

ON THE CUTTING EDGE

Pyruvate Aids Weight Loss

A report on a recently completed six-week double-blind, placebo-controlled study presented at the 45th Annual Meeting of the American College of Sports Medicine, held in Orlando, Florida, in June 1998, detailed many significant findings about pyruvate supplementation. The object of the study had been to investigate the effects of a pyruvate-based product on weight loss, body composition, vigor, and fatigue levels in overweight adults. The group taking the pyruvate product lost 12 percent of their body fat and 4.8 pounds in absolute body fat, while gaining 3.4 pounds of lean muscle mass. All of these values were significant when compared to those of the placebo and control groups in the study. Furthermore, indirect calorimetry testing was conducted to determine the effects, if any, of pyruvate on the basal metabolic rate (BMR). The results indicated an average 2.2-percent increase in the BMR. Perhaps of greatest significance to this study was that these results were achieved with doses of only 6 grams of pyruvate per day. In the past, researchers used 30 grams of pyruvate per day to achieve the same results.

burgh, pyruvate was shown to improve endurance by enhancing the transport of glucose into the muscles. This process is commonly termed glucose extraction because it refers to the amount of glucose extracted by muscles from the circulating blood. A mixture of dihydroxyacetone and pyruvate, known as DHAP, increased glucose extraction by 150 percent after one hour of arm-cycling exercise, and 60 percent for leg-cycling exercise. DHAP also increases glucose extraction when the body is at rest, leading to a possible 50-percent increase in muscle glycogen stores. Research collected from Dr. Stanko's studies also showed that DHAP supplementation over seven days increased endurance in subjects' arms and legs by 20 percent—a very significant increase for athletes. The dosage used in these endurance studies was 100 grams of DHAP, containing 25 grams of pyruvate and 75 grams of dihydroxyacetone. (For a further discussion of these studies, see the special report on DHAP on page 173.)

All of this data suggests that DHAP supplementation can enhance muscle glucose extraction during and after exhaustive exercise. Since glucose is the body's high-energy fuel, increasing glucose extraction for immediate fuel could extend endurance, as well as enhance performance in high-intensity activities such as soccer and basketball. And, of course, enhanced glucose extraction can increase stored energy in the form of muscle glycogen, which will help to extend endurance in subsequent training sessions, or during competition.

According to Dr. Stanko, the most effective dosage of pyruvate is not actually 100 grams a day, but 3 to 5 grams a day, instead. The body does not use pyruvate in excess of these amounts, so results from 10 to 20 grams of pyruvate supplementation will be the same as those seen with 3 to 5 grams.

SPECIAL REPORT:

Dihydroxyacetone and Pyruvate Improve Athletic Endurance

Many athletes are forever searching for nutritional magic bullets to boost their performance. Sometimes, the remedies turn out to be fads and, like baseball caps worn backwards, don't have much practical purpose. Recently, pyruvate and its sister compound, dihydroxyacetone, have become popular dietary supplements in sports nutrition. Fortunately, these nutrients are backed by scientific evidence showing that they augment muscle-glycogen synthesis, fat loss, and exercise endurance.

Pyruvate and dihydroxyacetone are both three-carbon molecules that occur naturally in the body. The former is a byproduct of carbohydrate metabolism, the latter of both glucose and glycerol metabolism. Actually, the breakdown of glucose yields two molecules of pyruvic acid, not pyruvate. But, because pyruvic acid is chemically unstable, manufacturers stabilize it by combining it with sodium, calcium, potassium, or magnesium to form a pyruvate "salt." In the body, a series of enzymatic steps rapidly converts dihydroxyacetone to pyruvate. For this reason, more recent studies have used pyruvate alone, rather than pyruvate and dihydroxyacetone.

HOW DO DIHYDROXYACETONE AND PYRUVATE WORK?

The combination of dihydroxyacetone and pyruvate (DHAP) improves athletic endurance by enhancing glucose extraction—that is, the removal of glucose from the circulating blood by the muscle cells. The muscle cells can then burn the glucose for energy if exercising or store it as glycogen if resting.

In athletes engaging in intensive daily training, the muscle-glycogen stores undergo daily depletion and resynthesis. The amount and type of dietary carbohydrate that is consumed influences the muscle-glycogen synthesis. A study by David Costill,

PhD, director of the Human Performance Laboratory at Ball State University, Muncie, Indiana, assigned trained runners to three dietary regimes that varied in carbohydrate content. The first group consumed 25 percent (188 grams) of their total 3,000 kilocalories as carbohydrates, the second group 50 percent (375 grams), and the third group 70 percent (525 grams). To measure the glycogen content of the study participants, the researchers took muscle biopsies from the gastrocnemius in their calves immediately after exercising and again twenty-four hours later. The results showed that the subjects' muscle-glycogen synthesis increased in proportion to the amount of carbohydrate they consumed. Dr. Costill recommends that athletes whose daily training relies heavily on muscle-glycogen reserves, such as swimmers, runners, and cyclists, consume at least 70 percent of their calories in the form of carbohydrates.

In the past, experts advised athletes to consume their carbohydrates in complex form, stoking up on foods such as brown rice and whole-grain bread and pasta. Then, in the early 1980s, drinks made of glucose polymers (long chains of sugar molecules that stay connected in a solution) became commercially available to help replenish the glycogen stores without adding the bulk of whole grains to the intestinal tract. Recently, research showed that DHAP increases the muscle-glycogen stores without adding bulk even more effectively than do glucose polymers.

Two double-blind studies conducted by Ronald Stanko, MD, and colleagues at the University of Pittsburgh Medical Center showed that seven days of DHAP supplementation combined with either a normal or a high-carbohydrate diet significantly improved arm and leg exercise performance as compared to supplementation with a carbohydrate placebo. Muscular endurance in both the arms and legs rose by 20 percent. These results are supported by a third double-blind study, which assigned subjects to one of two dietary combinations. Both diets contained 15-percent protein, 30-percent fat, and 55-percent carbohydrate, with the treatment diet substituting 75 grams of DHAP for some of the carbohydrate. While cycling at the same exercise intensities, the subjects taking the DHAP reported a more than 20-percent decrease in the perceived level of exertion.

Researchers believe that DHAP improves exercise performance primarily by enhancing glucose extraction and also by increasing the glycogen stores. DHAP supplementation can increase glucose extraction by 150 percent while arm cycling and by 60 percent while leg cycling. DHAP also enhances glucose extraction at rest, leading to a 50-percent increase in the muscle-glycogen stores.

RECOMMENDED PYRUVATE INTAKE

Researchers have yet to determine the optimum pyruvate allowance. Total daily intake ranges from 100 to 2,000 milligrams. Although a variety of foods contain pyruvate, most have less than 25 milligrams per serving. Foods high in pyruvate include certain fruits and vegetables, as well as cheese. A red apple packs 450 milligrams of pyruvate, 12 ounces of beer contains 80 milligrams, and 6 ounces of red wine has 75 milligrams.

For athletes to get the full benefits of pyruvate, they usually need to take supplements. Many of the products on the market contain primarily pyruvate, while some also contain small amounts of dihydroxyacetone. Pyruvate is available in tablet, capsule, and powder form. It also appears in rehydration drinks and energy bars.

Early studies used 100 grams of DHAP, composed of 25 grams of pyruvate and 75 grams of dihydroxyacetone. Later, researchers realized that lower doses were just as effective. Dr. Stanko says that the optimum daily intake of pyruvate is 2 to 5 grams, divided into two doses and taken with meals.

SIDE EFFECTS AND CAUTIONS

In clinical studies, no major side effects have been associated with pyruvate or DHAP. In one study, the side effects associated with large doses (18 to 24 grams) of pyruvate administered according to caloric intake were gas and bloating, loose stools, and diarrhea. According to Med-Pro Industries in Westlake, California, a manufacturer of pyruvate, because the quality of raw pyruvate has increased tremendously, the intestinal side effects documented in the early studies are no longer seen. Notes Terry Newsom, director of marketing at Med-Pro, "Pyruvate is not only effective, but [as shown in Dr. Stanko's research] has no serious side effects." At this time, it is better not to use DHAP, since more research needs to be done to confirm its safety as a dietary supplement.

Since it has many metabolic effects, supplemental pyruvate is not recommended for pregnant women or children, unless monitored by a physician. Other people should consult a health-care practitioner before taking any supplement in pharmacological doses. As with all supplements and medications, unexpected side effects should be reported to a physician.

FUTURE RESEARCH

Research needs to be done on the effects of various dosages and forms of pyruvate on male and female athletes. For doses exceeding 5 grams a day, the impact of the minerals chelated with the pyruvate on the body's mineral and electrolyte balances needs to be determined.

In addition, more studies are needed to investigate the full range of pyruvate's benefits. Because it has been shown to increase fat loss, pyruvate may benefit people with obesity, diabetes, and hyperlipidemia (high blood fats such as triglycerides and cholesterol). Preliminary research also suggests that pyruvate may improve cardiac efficiency by increasing glucose extraction.

While the research described above is proof of pyruvate's performance-enhancing effects, it's important to note that these studies were conducted with subjects who did not train regularly. Data has not yet been collected about pyruvate's benefits for well-trained subjects. The preliminary research, however, is enough evidence of the advantages that pyruvate can offer athletes.

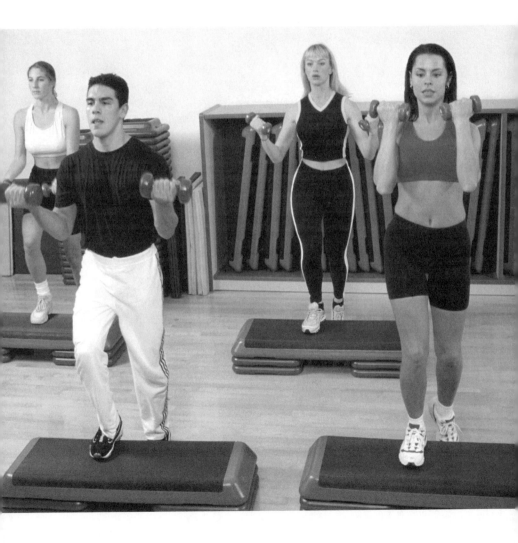

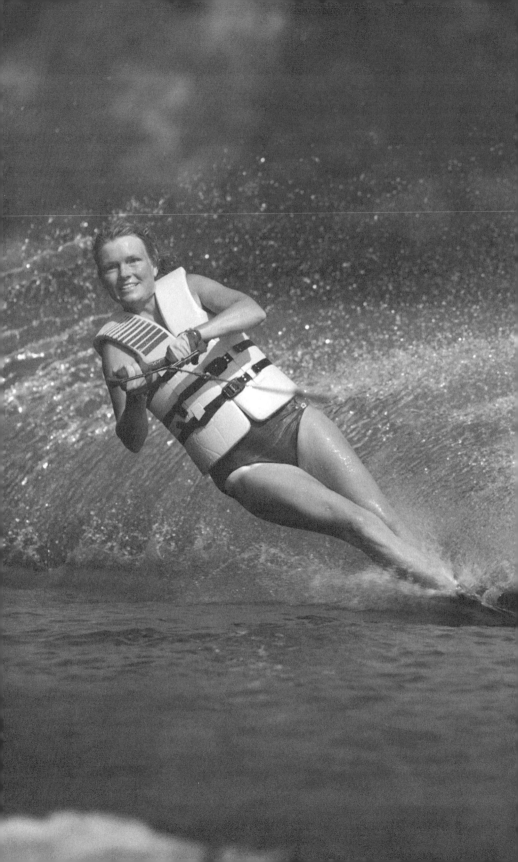

SCIENTIFIC
NUTRITION

9 MEAL REPLACEMENTS, PROTEIN POWDERS,
AND METABOLIC OPTIMIZERS

Nutritional intake plays a role in all phases of athletics, from precompetition training to postcompetition recovery. Many nutritional substances have been employed over the years to maintain and enhance physical performance. Among the most widely used of these performance foods are protein powders, sports drinks, and sports bars. More recently, nutritionally complete powder supplements have become popular and offer a multitude of benefits to athletes.

The appropriateness and effectiveness of these types of supplements, or of any nutritional substances intended to enhance physical performance, depend on a careful evaluation of the physical requirements of the sport and metabolic characteristics of the athlete. The metabolic characteristics include the rate of gastric emptying, ability to digest nutrients, taste preferences, and gastrointestinal tolerance. The sport-specific requirements may be for high-carbohydrate beverages to improve energy output and increase endurance; high-protein powders to assist muscle growth and recovery for strength and/or power activities; complete, high-quality meal-replacement products to aid weight loss or weight maintenance while maintaining peak physical performance; or metabolic optimizers, which offer the benefits of several supplements combined in a convenient and tasty nutrient-dense beverage. The appropriate nutritional product will contain ingredients that meet the specific demands of the athlete in question.

In this chapter, we will discuss the scientifically engineered sports-nutrition powders that are currently popular among athletes. These products include meal replacements, protein powders, and metabolic optimizers.

THE DEVELOPMENT OF SPORTS-NUTRITION POWDERS

The story behind the development of today's powdered sports-nutrition products is as compelling as those of the space program and computer technology in the last fifty years. In fact, the development of the first "meal in a can" can be traced back to post–World War Two nutrition research, during the early years of the space program. Exercise physiologists and nutritionists working closely together conducted pioneering nutrition experiments for the goal of finding a way to ensure the health and safety of the astronauts leaving the Earth's gravity for the first time in human history.

As information about the essential nutrients accumulated, nutrition researchers began to experiment with what came to be known as "chemically defined diets." Some of the researchers focused on creating a nutritionally adequate diet, made up of the known essential nutrients of the day. Their first subjects were laboratory animals.

In the early 1950s, after scientists figured out the correct formulas for animals, they diligently experimented to sort out exactly which nutrients were essential for humans to grow, develop, and maintain health and performance. For astronauts, they wanted to create a highly efficient meal that would keep the astronauts working at peak performance but that would also minimize the amount of waste products. Maintaining perfect health was considered to be essential for the astronauts' survival as they explored the unknown effects of zero gravity on the body.

One of the classic studies in this area, appearing in the May 1970 issue of the *American Journal of Clinical Nutrition,* reported on the history and interesting effects of chemically defined diets; it is required reading for anyone seriously interested in nutrition. In the article, Dr. Milton Winitz and his coworkers reported the results of their several-month-long study using chemically defined diets on human subjects. The composition of the completely defined chemical diet they used included the essential and nonessential amino acids, vitamins, minerals, carbohydrates, and essential fatty acids. This chemical nutrient concentrate was diluted in water and used as the sole source of nutrition during the experimental period. The total daily caloric intake of each subject was adjusted to match his or her specific metabolic demands.

While this pioneering nutrition research did not examine all of the intricate body-composition and physical-performance measurements typically used in today's medical studies, some interesting discoveries were made. First, it was found that the health of the subjects was maintained, and improved in some cases, during the twenty-five-week period. Second, cholesterol levels were reduced, along with blood pressure. Third, body-weight changes were observed, depending on the subject's starting condition. For example, overweight individuals rapidly lost fat tissue, underweight individuals showed healthy weight gains, and individuals considered to have normal starting weights did not experience any appreciable weight changes. Another interesting body-weight dynamic was also observed. The chemically defined diet was designed to exclude dietary fiber and other dietary bulk. As a result, during the first week of the study, all the subjects experienced an initial weight loss of up to 11 pounds. This lost weight was quickly restored during the first week after returning to a normal diet. The researchers attributed this abrupt initial drop in weight to the clearance of gastrointestinal bulk.

The significance of this research was multi-faceted and led the way to the development of new clinical therapeutic diets, weight-loss diets, and a vast array of sports-nutrition products. It also opened the minds of scientists to continue researching the intricate relationship among nutrients, body composition, health, and performance. Knowing about Dr. Winitz's early research makes it easy to understand how the different decades of research underlie the formulas of the various sports-nutrition products. The nutritional characteristics of the different sports-nutrition powders are the result of different nutritional strategies. But, this is only part of the powdered-sports-nutrition story.

The other side of the story involves developments in food technology that paralleled the discoveries made by nutrition researchers. These technological developments led to the invention of sophisticated experimental equipment and techniques, the identification of new and unique nutrients, and the creation of high-tech manufacturing techniques to turn these new ingredients into usable products. The advancements included technological developments that have resulted in better, more biologically active ingredients.

Another factor to consider in the food-technology story is the economics associated with the inclusion of these revolutionary new ingredients in sports-nutrition products. When new dietary ingredients are first made, they are usually very expensive due to the newness of their production process and their low market demand. In cases where the ingredients are protected by a patent, the producers can maintain the higher prices, due to the ingredients' patent-protected exclusivity. Eventually, as the market demand increases for these novel supplement ingredients and the manufacturers develop better and faster ways to produce them, the prices fall, and these savings are passed on to the consumer as a result of competition in a free-enterprise society. For example, several years ago, when creatine and isolated-whey-protein products were first introduced into the marketplace, they bore hefty price tags. Now, about double the amounts of these highly regarded sports-nutrition products can be purchased for less money than half the amounts cost several years ago. As manufacturing technology improves to meet increasing market demands, prices will continue to drop on some of the newer, more expensive sports-nutrition products that scientific research has recently brought to our attention.

MEAL-REPLACEMENT POWDERS

There is no doubt that when Dr. Winitz's research was originally published, the fast weight loss observed during the first week of his experiment influenced the weight-loss market to offer products that produced similar results. Millions of people turn to powdered meal-replacement drinks each year in their quests for slimmer bodies. When used properly, these products work. However, as already discussed, the rapid weight loss experienced with these products is caused mostly by the elimination of gastrointestinal bulk and water weight. While many of the meal-replacement powders currently available on mass-market shelves have long histories of being safe (when used properly, as part of a nutritionally balanced diet), the quality of the weight loss they facilitate and their total nutritional value are not necessarily the best for meeting the high-performance demands of athletic people. Athletes need to consider the amount of protein a meal-replacement product contains, as well as its total number of calories, different types of carbohydrates, fat content, and roster of vitamins, minerals, and other nutrients essential for promoting desirable body-composition changes and maintaining physical performance.

For example, athletes require two to four times the RDA of protein, but most mass-market meal replacements contain just very small amounts of this macronutrient, usually less than 10 grams per serving. It is extremely important for athletes to maintain an adequate protein intake all the time, to maintain their muscle mass and a healthy metabolism. Therefore, during this past decade, sports-nutrition companies have developed meal-replacement products specifically geared to athletes. As you shop around for a sports-nutrition meal replacement, you will notice that they are high in protein, containing usually 20 grams per serving or more, and include a comprehensive profile of essential nutrients.

These special sports-nutrition meals are also low in fat and contain customized blends of carbohydrates, mixtures of simple and complex carbohydrates, including dietary fiber. These special carbohydrate blends are designed to provide a sustained supply of energy to help maintain the blood-sugar level. Maintenance of the blood-sugar level is important for mental and physical performance, and appetite control. Dietary fiber also helps maintain the blood-sugar level, as well as control the appetite. Dietary fiber is nature's appetite-control substance and blood-sugar regulator.

Concerning the maintenance of the required daily caloric intake, athletes in intensive training and competition typically need to ingest 3,000 to 7,000 calories per day, depending on their activity level and body weight. Because of their hectic schedules, however, it is often difficult for them to consume enough calories and nutrients. This can lead to a nutritionally deficient diet, which can cause the muscle-glycogen level to decline and may impair the ability to train and perform adequately. Poor diets also often lack the protein, vitamins, minerals, and other nutrients needed for optimum training and performance.

Meal-replacement powders, which are also called "engineered foods," can enhance the nutritional value of athletes' diets tremendously. They provide carbohydrates, to supply energy to the working muscles; protein, to provide amino acids for muscle growth and repair; and vitamins, minerals, and metabolites, to satisfy nutritional requirements. In addition to using meal-replacement powders for weight loss, athletes have also found them to be convenient meal substitutes and high-quality snacks that increase the nutritional quality of the daily diet.

The Advantages of Meal-Replacement Powders

Meal-replacement powders can be used as follows:

☐ *As precompetition, postcompetition, or post-training meals, or as meals between events during tournaments.* Meal-replacement powders can serve as easy alternatives to solid food for athletes competing in day-long competitions or tournaments, or in multiple events. Solid food consumed before competition may cause stomach upset. The liquid and lactose-free formulations of many meal-replacement powders may help reduce gastric distress and nausea. Meal-replacement powders also can be consumed closer to competition time than regular meals, due to their shorter gastric-emptying time. This may help avoid precompetition nausea in athletes whose tenseness may delay gastric emptying. When using a meal-replacement powder as a precompetition meal, choose one that is high in total calories (450 to 650 calories), high in carbohydrates, moderate in protein (25 to 40 grams), and low in fat.

☐ *To maintain body weight.* Athletes' travel schedules and rigorous training regimens often do not allow time to consume an adequate diet. Meal-replacement powders can supply the calories and protein needed to prevent the loss of lean body mass.

☐ *To lose weight.* High-protein meal-replacement powders can help athletes lose fat weight without sacrificing muscle weight. They offer a balance of nutrients in place of high-fat, high-calorie foods. They also produce a low stool residue and thereby help keep the weight gain following a meal to a minimum, which may be of special benefit to wrestlers and bodybuilders, who always need to "make weight."

☐ *As a high-energy snack.* Meal-replacement powders can serve as convenient high-carbohydrate, moderate-protein snacks to maintain the energy level and enhance performance. They can also supply extra nutrition during heavy training, when the caloric requirements are greatly increased. They can provide a significant amount of calories and contribute to satiety without leaving the athlete feeling uncomfortably full.

☐ *To increase lean body mass.* In addition to a resistance-training program, consuming adequate calories and protein is essential for the development of muscle tissue. High-protein meal replacements can supply the calories and protein without the extra fat that usually is found in conventional food.

Meal-replacement powders can satisfy the requirements of pre- and postexercise food—they are palatable, have a high carbohydrate content, and contribute to both energy intake and hydration. They also have several advantages over conventional meals.

Meal-Replacement Powders Versus Conventional Meals

Does this mean that you should forgo conventional meals? Both conventional meals and meal-replacement powders help hydration, increase sub-optimum muscle-glycogen stores, and maintain the blood-glucose level during prolonged exercise. If an athlete has no difficulty with consuming conventional meals prior to exercising or with obtaining enough calories, meal replacements confer no advantage other than convenience, and they lack fiber. The ideal pre-exercise meal, whether a meal-replacement powder or solid food, is high in carbohydrates, tastes good, and does not cause gastrointestinal distress.

If you would like to try a meal replacement, there is a wide variety on the market. These days, high-quality meal-replacement powders are available for about two to three dollars a serving, which is a reasonable amount of money to pay for a nutritionally complete meal. And many of these products can be quite delicious and satisfying.

When shopping for a meal-replacement powder, the important things to consider when deciding which one is the best for you are taste and digestibility. Almost all meal-replacement powders are high in nutrients and low to moderate in calories. Some quality products are EAS Myoplex Plus Delux, TwinLab Rx Fuel, Weider Metaform, Nature's Best Perfect Rx, and MET-Rx, all of which supply high amounts of carbohydrate and protein, a low amount of fat, and additional nutrients required by athletes. Note that, no matter which specific brand you use, when you first use a sports-nutrition-quality meal-replacement powder, you may find your stomach slightly bloated or suffer gastrointestinal cramps or diarrhea. This is because your body needs time to adjust to the nutrient-dense character of these products. In some cases, there may be a certain ingredient you have trouble digesting. Don't fret; there are a good number of products from which to choose. If you have a problem with lactose, you may need to select a product that is lactose-free. You might need to try several products in order to determine which one works the best for you. The experimentation may be worthwhile, though.

PROTEIN POWDERS

Most people know that protein comes from a variety of sources and helps build and repair body tissues, especially muscle. The ancient Greeks didn't know about protein, but they did believe that if you ate the meat of a powerful animal, such as a lion, you would become strong yourself.

Of prime importance to proteins are the groups of hydrogen, nitrogen, carbon, and oxygen atoms called amino acids. Histidine, isoleucine, leucine, lysine, methionine, phenylalanine, threonine, tryptophan, and valine are the nine essential amino acids, the ones that you must obtain from food because they can't be made by your body. You also need cystine and tyrosine, which your body does make. Your body can also manufacture the remaining nine amino acids, for a total of twenty, but research indicates that ingesting both the essential and nonessential amino acids is best for peak performance. For a protein to do what protein is intended to do, it needs to be complete—that is, it must have a good balance of all nine of the essential amino acids. While meat has long been considered the primo source of complete protein, the humble egg white actually holds the distinction. Fish, milk, lean beef, and poultry follow. Contrary to antiquated arguments that meatless diets lack adequate protein, vegetarians can still ensure a complete protein intake by combining different plant foods that together provide all the essential amino acids. This is especially easy to do since the development of complete soy proteins, such as Supro.

Protein and More

As a category of food products, protein-powder supplements generically are dry powders, with 50 to 75 percent or more of their weight made up of essentially purified protein. All of these powders contain some moisture, so even though 100 percent of the calories in a product may come from protein, it's impossible for any product to be 100-percent protein by weight due to the moisture content and other nutrient, flavor, and excipient components. Quite often, ash (a noncaloric particulate matter) and small amounts of naturally occurring carbohydrates, such as the lactose associated with milk proteins, are present.

Carbohydrates are often intentionally added. This is because they are cheaper than protein, they can increase the caloric content of the product, and they seem to boost the efficiency of the protein, allowing it to be used to repair and build muscle rather than provide energy. Some protein products contain additional nutrients, such as vitamins, minerals, herbs, extra individual amino acids (such as L-glutamine), dietary fiber, flavorings, emulsifiers, artificial sweeteners, digestive enzymes, and metabolites, to improve the amino-acid profile or enhance the protein utilization.

Regardless of such additives, protein supplements, as a group, are not intended to serve as meal replacements, and many labels contain a disclaimer to that effect. (See "High-Protein-Content Warning Labels," below.) The reason disclaimers are printed on the labels of low-calorie, high-protein products is to caution consumers that these products are not intended for use as the sole source of calories. Using these products this way would be unhealthy. In addition, most protein supplements contain a "Supplement Facts" panel, which categorizes them as dietary supplements. Dietary supplements are intended to *supplement* the diet, not to serve as meals. Most protein supplements are potent, consisting of 85-percent

---

High-Protein-Content Warning Labels

The FDA's labeling regulations require that the following warnings appear on certain food and dietary-supplement products, including powdered products, that provide more than 50 percent of their calories from protein. The type of warning a particular product carries depends on whether the product is intended to be used for weight loss or not. Even further, weight-loss products that come with a written diet plan carry a different warning than weight-loss products without a plan. Altogether, there are three different types of warnings used on high-protein products:

☐ Sample warning for a weight-loss product that does not come with a written diet plan: *Warning:* Very-low-calorie protein diets (less than 400 calories per day) may cause serious illness or death. Do not use for weight reduction in such diets without medical supervision. Not for use by infants, children, or pregnant or nursing women.

☐ Sample warning for a weight-loss product that comes with a written diet plan or is intended for use as part of a nutritionally balanced diet plan: *Notice:* For weight reduction, use only as directed in the accompanying diet plan. Do not use in diets supplying less than 400 calories per day without medical supervision.

☐ Sample warning for a product not intended for weight loss: *Notice:* Use this product as a food supplement only. Do not use for weight reduction.

This label warning system was developed to ensure the proper use of high-protein products and to underscore the importance of using them with medical supervision.

or more protein. Many athletes use them between meals, adding them to other drinks or even to foods such as oatmeal and pancakes, or using them as high-protein, low-calorie snacks. However you choose to use your protein supplement, purchasing a high-quality product is the first step.

Protein Quality

Supplement manufacturers make numerous claims about their products, throwing around protein efficiency ratios (PERs) and processing nomenclature such as "micro-filtered, ionized-fractionated protein isolates" to bolster product intrigue. But, as a consumer, not a scientist, how are you to know exactly where the sources of protein—for example, soy, egg, meat, casein, and whey—rank in terms of quality? And how big are the differences between them? Consumers are constantly confronted with new "miracle" protein supplements claiming to be the best, with each one also purporting to have scientific literature backing it up.

Supplement manufacturers use various protein-rating methods to support the claims they make about their protein products. These methods, which are intended to determine protein quality (growth-promoting ability), include PER, net protein utilization (NPU), net protein ratio (NPR), biological value (BV), and protein-digestibility-corrected amino-acid score (PDCAAS). BV, which essentially is the amount of protein retained in the body relative to the amount absorbed, is the most often used method because it assesses digestibility as well as protein-utilization efficiency. When confronted with these methods in advertisements, in articles, or on product labels, keep two things in mind: First, the values were established at very low protein intakes. And second, there are significant differences between how humans and animals utilize protein, and many of these rating systems are based either on animal studies or just theoretical human-amino-acid needs.

Protein quality is also related to the amounts of the various amino acids contained in the product. Because athletes use more of certain amino acids, such as the BCAAs and glutamine, protein powders with higher amounts of these are considered to be of a higher quality for human performance. When comparing protein powders to food-source proteins, keep in mind that other nutrients, such as creatine and carnosine, found in high amounts in red meat, can affect muscle growth, recovery, energy, and strength, and may thus also influence the growth-promoting potential of the protein. In fact, it is interesting to note that the ancient Olympians, who were mostly strength athletes, apparently craved high-meat diets, as do today's power lifters, bodybuilders, and other strength athletes. We now know that, in addition to their higher protein needs, these athletes can boost their performance with a higher dietary intake of creatine, which is found mostly in red meat.

Additional Factors

Other factors contributing to a protein's nutritive value are the nutritional and metabolic status of the individual consuming it, and his or her total daily intake of calories and protein. The relative value or quality of any given protein is highly dependent on the total quantity of calories and protein being consumed. As either or both of these go up, the value of the given protein goes down. Metabolic status is itself influenced by the health of the individual, as well as by the physical (including training) and emotional stresses the individual is under. At this time, there is not a single published scientific study that has evaluated protein metabolism in athletes undergoing intensive training and consuming various quantities of calories, carbohydrates, and protein from specific sources. There are studies, however, that report improvements in body composition and performance with the use of certain protein supplements.

Certainly for athletes, the amount of the BCAAs consumed per day during intensive training affects the overall performance of the dietary proteins consumed. Accordingly, supplements that have a high BCAA content, either naturally or through the addition of extra BCAAs, may be more beneficial for athletes than those that don't.

Among the different sources of protein are soy, eggs, and milk. Milk provides two kinds of protein—casein and whey. For a discussion of these different sources of protein, see "Types of Protein in Powder Supplements" on page 189.

A further nutritional factor is the use of hydrolysates. Hydrolysates are proteins that have been partially digested by enzymatic hydrolysis. There are different degrees of hydrolysis, with the resulting hydrolysates containing small fragments of the original proteins, such as di- and tripeptides, which are quickly, easily, and completely absorbed. Hydrolysates are basically predigested and may offer the advantage of quicker assimilation. For athletes with high daily food intakes, speeding up digestion and absorption can leave more time for training and other activities.

Which protein product is best for you depends on many factors, including your health, training level, overall diet, taste preferences, and even pocketbook. Companies such as GNC, TwinLab, EAS, Champion, Weider, Designer Protein, and Universal are among the very best companies selling protein powders. It is always best to buy your supplements from the larger, well-established companies, since these companies are more likely to have substantial quality-control measures in place and superior manufacturing processes. Whichever brand of protein you choose, include its regular consumption in your daily diet and you'll be amazed at the beneficial results you will experience in a short period of time.

METABOLIC OPTIMIZERS

Metabolic optimizers are nutritionally complete powders that are used primarily during and after exercise. Their combinations of protein, fat, carbohydrate, vitamins, minerals, herbs, and metabolites are designed to not only replenish depleted glycogen stores, but to aid the recovery of muscle tissue after intensive exercise. They may also be used as liquid meal supplements or as nutritionally complete liquids, alternatives to solid food during and immediately after exercise. Their nutritional breakdown reflects a balanced approach towards nutrition for endurance athletes; they are approximately 60-percent carbohydrate, 15-percent protein, and less than 25-percent fat.

For people who have been around the sports-nutrition industry during the past fifteen years, the term "metabolic optimizer" is synonymous with a product called Metabolol, invented by Michael Zumpano. In the early 1980s, Zumpano, a bodybuilder, author of training and nutrition articles and books, and founder of Champion Nutrition, sought to create a comprehensive powdered supplement that would supply the essential nutrients as well as optimize the metabolism. This metabolic optimizer would rev the metabolism, improve muscle growth and recovery, and increase performance. In addition to including essential nutrients, Zumpano sought to provide ingredients with high bioavailabilities. When you take a close look at Metabolol, you see twenty-first-century sports-nutrition technology contained in a product that has been on the market since 1986, improved somewhat over the years as new ingredients became available. Metabolol uses an exclusive high-quality protein blend, a specialized carbohydrate system, highly bioavailable vitamins and minerals, and metabolic-enhancing ingredients such as carnitine, succinates, inosine, and the BCAAs. Metabolol, which is still the sports-nutrition industry's "gold standard" of metabolic optimizers, therefore provides scientifically engineered nutrition that improves your metabolism. Zumpano also was the first to include anticatabolic ingredients in his metabolic optimizer, as well as ingredients that help clear metabolic waste products, such as nitrogenous wastes and lactic acid. So, while metabolic optimizers may look like powdered meal replacements, they are not. They are several sports-nutrition products rolled into one, with very sophisticated formulas that offer athletes a convenient way to optimize their diets and performance.

Also for Endurance Athletes

One thing researchers in the field of sports nutrition often learn after years of work is that they not only need to know what they are looking for, but that they also need to understand what they have found. The development of metabolic optimizers is a perfect example of this phenomenon. Several years ago, while investigating diet drinks, a group of researchers from a major nutrition company discovered that the right balance of carbohydrate and protein would encourage a greater secretion of insulin into the blood than either carbohydrate or protein alone. A few years later, this group began to focus its attention in the area of sports nutrition. In their extensive investigation into the literature of biochemistry and physiology, the researchers realized that insulin is the body's natural biochemical trigger for the uptake of carbohydrate by the muscles, which aids recovery and muscle rebuilding after intensive exercise. It was at this point that the light bulb flicked on. The group realized that a food supplement could be developed that would not only provide the building blocks for recovery, but also flip the metabolic switches to hasten recovery and make optimal use of those building blocks. Based on earlier work with carbohydrate-protein combinations, the group hypothesized that a combination of these two macronutrients might stimulate the body's production of insulin and, by enhancing muscle-glycogen resynthesis, allow the body to restore muscle energy faster and thus recover faster after exercise.

Up until this point, much of the work on glycogen repletion after exercise had been conducted on the response to carbohydrate alone. It was at this time that

Dr. John Ivy from the University of Texas became interested in expanding the diet-drink concept into an actual exercise-recovery research project. He conducted an independent study comparing three 16-ounce, post-exercise drink supplements—a metabolic optimizer with a unique carbohydrate-protein combination formula (112.5 grams of carbohydrate and 40.5 grams of protein); a "protein" drink (40.5 grams of protein), and a carbohydrate drink similar to the "carbo-loading" products on the market (112.5 grams of carbohydrate). The subjects were nine trained cyclists, each of whom tested all three supplements on three separate occasions. Each athlete cycled to exhaustion under a protocol that reflected actual race conditions. After every session, the cyclists drank one of the three supplement drinks immediately and then again after two hours.

The results of the study confirmed that the carbohydrate-protein combination elicited a greater insulin response in the blood than did the carbohydrate or protein supplement alone. As a matter of fact, the metabolic optimizer's insulin response was greater than the sum of the other two products. The study also measured each cyclist's muscle-glycogen level—that is, the body's store of carbohydrate. As was hypothesized by Dr. Ivy, the greater insulin levels produced by the metabolic optimizer actually led to a greater increase in the rate of muscle-energy production in the four-hour period after exercise.

Build and Repair Muscle

Metabolic optimizers provide a unique protein-and-carbohydrate blend to help rebuild the muscles. These special nutrient combinations are formulated to increase the amount of the anabolic hormone insulin in the body for enhanced muscle rebuilding. Insulin is the body's principal anabolic "on-off" switch. It moves into the bloodstream and sets the muscle-building system into motion. Once the anabolic state is in high gear, metabolic optimizers play another muscle-building role. They provide the muscles with protein—specifically, amino acids—needed to rebuild existing muscles and lay down new muscle mass. Liquid metabolic-optimizer supplements also contain other essential nutrients, including chromium and creatine. These nutrients enhance insulin's anabolic, body-repairing activity. Research has shown that athletes who train intensively may be low in these essential nutrients.

The same as for standard high-carbohydrate drinks, individuals should consume 1.0 to 3.0 grams of metabolic-optimizer powder for every 1 kilogram (2.2 pounds) of body weight within thirty minutes of finishing an intensive exercise session. For example, a 150-pound cyclist should consume between 68 and 204 grams of powdered product after a long, hard training ride or race. This procedure should then be repeated two hours after finishing the exercise.

High-Energy Supplement

Dietary surveys of numerous groups of athletes have reported high intakes of carbohydrate, fat, and protein. The carbohydrate requirements of athletes in heavy training may be from 60 to 70 percent of total calories, but the consumption of bulky, high-volume carbohydrate diets is often restricted by gastric discomfort.

Long training sessions may further interfere with dietary intake by restricting the time available to prepare and eat meals, and by reducing interest in food due to fatigue or suppressed appetite resulting from the training.

Metabolic optimizers, as an adjunct to conventional food intake, offer the practical advantage of reduced bulkiness and easy preparation, as well as a calorie- and nutrient-dense intake. This may be of special interest to athletes with high daily caloric requirements or those in intensive training programs. In a recent research study, competitive weight lifters were shown to achieve significantly greater increases in lean body mass while using liquid meal/supplement products in addition to ad libitum (unrestricted) diets than a control group whose diets were unsupplemented. Metabolic optimizers may also be used to boost the caloric content of quick meals and snacks, a practice that may be particularly useful for traveling athletes whose training or competition takes them away from their normal food sources.

Pre-Event Meal

Pre-event meals should have no adverse effects on the body's carbohydrate stores and should even possibly increase the glycogen stores. They should allow the stomach to become relatively empty in time for the competition and should provide adequate hydration. They should not cause any gastrointestinal problems. Most coaches recommend the intake of a meal high in carbohydrates and low in protein and fat two to four hours before competition. To hone in on what works best for you, try experimenting with different types of foods and supplements, the amount of time pre-event that you consume them, and the amount of food that best provides you with energy nutrients for optimum performance.

In addition to determining your best pre-event meal, if your event or training session is longer than one hour, be sure to maintain the proper fluid intake. Your fluid intake can include beverages containing carbohydrate and electrolytes. Keep in mind that it may take your body several days or even weeks to adjust to sports beverages. So, if you have trouble tolerating the ingestion of a sports beverage during your activity, try using smaller amounts or diluting the sports drink until your body adjusts. Research has shown that the best energy carbohydrate your body can have during exercise is pure glucose. Some sports drinks contain glucose, along with glucose polymers and other complex carbohydrates, to provide a sustained supply of energy. Experiment to find out what works best for you.

Metabolic optimizers fit the criteria for a quickly digested, high-carbohydrate, practical pre-event meal, particularly for athletes whose nervousness may cause gastric problems. Two of the top-selling brands are Endurox R_4 and Champion's Metabolol. Most athletes should consume the supplement one-half to two hours before competition.

During Endurance Exercise

While being promoted primarily as a pre- and post-exercise nutritional supplement, metabolic optimizers may also have advantages during endurance exercise. "Cyclists are also experimenting with metabolic optimizers during long road races (120 miles plus) where it has been shown that not only is carbohydrate an important fuel, but that cyclists also begin to use amino acids (protein) for fuel after carbohydrate stores become depleted," says Steve Hegg, former U.S. Professional Road Cycling Champion. These products can help prevent the breakdown of muscle tissue by supplying protein during the later stages of exercise. Many of the newer optimizer powder drinks are easy to mix just with water, which makes them as convenient to use as standard powdered energy drinks at the race site. Remember to give your body time to adjust to these nutrient beverages during training and competition. Try using them during your practice sessions to see which products and dilutions work best for your digestive system.

WHY CHOOSE POWDER SUPPLEMENTS?

If you need extra protein, you may prefer the convenience of a protein powder. If you need extra calories and a quick meal, try a meal-replacement powder. However, if you'd like a mixed-carbohydrate-and-protein supplement during or immediately after exercising, reach for a metabolic optimizer. All of these come with all sorts of claims and in a variety of sizes, formulations, and prices. The important thing to keep in mind is to choose a nutrition product or dietary supplement that is complete for your training and competition needs, is low in fat and cholesterol, and contains both complex and simple carbohydrates, as well as all the essential amino acids. Use it strategically to enhance, rather than overwhelm, your diet and recovery. Keep in mind that any excess protein you consume will most likely be stored as fat and burden your body with the chore of clearing out extra nitrogenous waste products.

Following is a list of some essential criteria for selecting a high-carbohydrate drink:

☐ It should contain high-quality complex and simple carbohydrates.

☐ It should contain all nine essential amino acids, as well as non-essential amino acids.

☐ It should contain vitamins and minerals to fit your needs.

☐ It should be low in cholesterol.

☐ It should be low-fat or nonfat.

If you are going to go through the time and expense of purchasing a powdered sports-nutrition product, it is better to pay for quality. Make sure you get a complete carbohydrate mixture (both simple and complex) and protein-powder drink that is low in fat and cholesterol.

TYPES OF PROTEIN IN POWDER SUPPLEMENTS

Protein powders, meal replacements, and metabolic optimizers all are made from a variety of protein sources. The most common are whey, casein, soy, and egg. The particular product you choose should depend on your needs and personal preferences.

Whey Protein

Whey-protein supplements have been the most popular and talked-about protein supplements over the past few years. In the early 1990s, scientists discovered that whey was not simply a useless byproduct of cheese production and developed a number of methods to process it into a high-quality powder that is fat-free and lactose-free. Ion-exchange and microfiltration systems use cool temperatures to preserve the flavor of the whey and the natural configurations of the amino acids.

While whey is the most expensive of the primary protein sources used in protein products, it has some distinct nutritional advantages. It enhances the production of glutathione, one of the body's powerful natural antioxidants. It also has the highest levels of the BCAAs and has been shown to boost immune-system functioning. Another advantage of whey is that it dissolves easily in water, allowing you to mix your protein drink on the go, without excessive clumping. In comparison to the other protein sources, whey has less glutamine, arginine, and phenylalanine, but whey-protein products are often fortified with extra glutamine and other amino acids to boost their sports-nutrition quality. Lastly, whey protein exits the stomach much faster than proteins such as casein, and it is absorbed through the intestines more quickly, too. As a result, you get a large, quick rise in the blood amino acids, which is important during both exercise and recovery from exercise.

Casein Protein

Casein protein is also used in many sports beverages. In addition to whey, milk contains casein in varying proportions. As cheese is produced, the milk divides into a solid portion, which is the casein, and a liquid portion, which is the whey. The casein portion is higher in glutamine, while the whey portion is higher in the BCAAs.

Casein protein is hard to dissolve and requires a blender. Therefore, manufacturers sometimes use "instantized" casein, which dissolves better, but also drives up the cost of the protein supplement. Casein-protein products cost more than soy-protein products but are usually less expensive than whey-protein products. A big concern to many athletes is that casein contains lactose, which in many individuals can cause gastrointestinal upset and gas.

Soy Protein

Soy protein was the first protein on the market. Soy has a high BCAA and glutamine content. However, it is low in methionine, an essential amino acid. Some of the isoflavonoids in soy exert an estrogenic effect, which may be counterproductive for male athletes. For female athletes, however, it may be a benefit. Soy isoflavones can ease menopausal symptoms and promote bone density and other positive effects of estrogen. In scientific studies using Supro soy protein on male and female athletes, all the athletes had improved muscle mass, decreased body fat, and improved performance, metabolism, and health. So, while the various marketers of the different types of protein products present their promotional stories,

Supro brand protein is one of the few that has been clinically tested in adult Olympic athletes to provide measurable results in just a few weeks. The studies that showed the best results used about 60 to 70 grams per day of Supro in addition to a balanced diet. Many soy products require a blender, although the newer, top-of-the-line products are easier to mix.

Egg Protein

Egg protein does not provide high amounts of leucine (whey has double the amount), arguably the most important BCAA and an amino acid that is used by the body in large amounts during exercise, infection, trauma, and calorie restriction. For an athlete whose protein intake is marginal, this could be a negative factor in recuperation and growth. For an individual consuming adequate calories and protein throughout the day, egg protein is a good, lactose-free, high-quality protein choice.

Meal replacements, protein powders, and metabolic optimizers are scientifically prepared powdered supplements intended for use as or with meals or snacks, as pre- or postexercise meals or snacks, or as snacks during endurance activities. The better products offer nutrient ratios designed to match the metabolic require-

ON THE CUTTING EDGE

Whey Protein Boosts Immunity

Previously published research has shown that exercise causes a reduction in certain aspects of immunity in elite endurance athletes. Although moderate exercise has been shown to improve immunity, intensive physical exercise reduces the glutamine and glutathione levels, which are associated with immunosuppression. This negative effect on immunity correlates directly with the intensity and duration of the physical activity and the baseline immune status of the athlete. The glutamine level and the immune status, as measured by the incidence of illnesses such as colds, have been suggested as possible markers of overtraining syndrome. Research presented at the 1998 national meeting of the American College of Sports Medicine shows that whey-protein concentrate can dramatically improve both the humoral and cellular immune responses. Whey-protein concentrate appears to raise the glutathione level in animals and humans, which may be a mechanism for modulating immunity. Although the exact mechanism by which whey-protein concentrate affects immunity has not been fully elucidated, whey-protein concentrate is known to be rich in glutathione precursors, substances that support optimum immune function. Therefore, it would not be unwise for athletes to supplement their diets with up to 25 grams of whey protein per day during periods of moderate to hard training to help protect their immune systems.

ments of specific types of athletes. Some formulas are more suitable for strength and power athletes, while some are more suitable for long-distance endurance athletes. Some are suitable for all athletes looking to improve the nutritional quality of their performance diets. All these products are excellent performance foods for athletes training during the preseason, competing during the season, or recovering during the postseason.

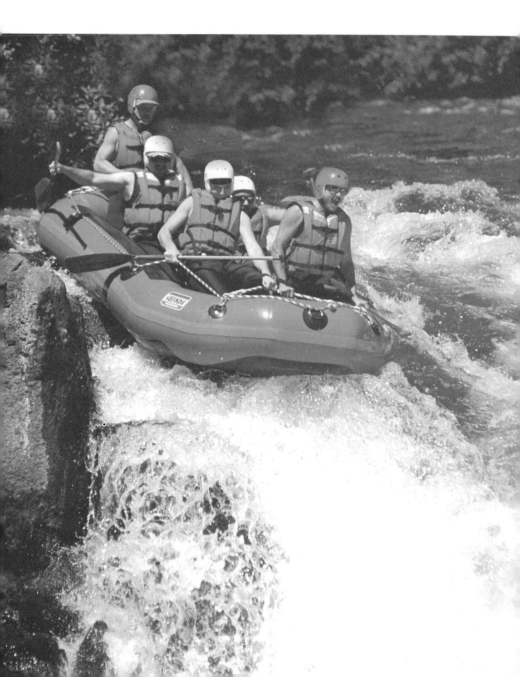

WINNING NUTRITION AND TRAINING PROGRAMS AND TIPS

In addition to being a science, the selection and consumption of sports-nutrition supplements is an art. While you have metabolic similarities with other people, you also have metabolic differences. By following the guidelines in this *Almanac,* you will not only learn how to get and stay on the right sports-nutrition track, but how to fine-tune your program to meet your specific needs. To give you a head start, this chapter offers the nutrition and training programs of some of the biggest and strongest champions in the worlds of bodybuilding and powerlifting. Among them is Lee Haney, eight-time winner of the Mr. Olympia title, and David Waterman, who lifted a whopping 620 pounds to capture the world record in the bench. This chapter also has a special report for women, who need to be aware of a devastating syndrome called the "female athlete triad."

NUTRITION AND TRAINING PROGRAMS OF SUCCESSFUL ATHLETES

Everyone is an individual. What works for one person may not work for another. As you read through the nutrition and training programs outlined in the following pages, remember that it took years of trial and error for the champions offering them to find their winning combinations. Also, keep in mind that these men and woman are *professional* athletes, and you will need to adapt their advice to your level of health and fitness. You will notice that these champions have tailored their programs to be as simple as possible. Two of the common themes are perseverance and concentration on the basics in both training and nutrition.

Gerard Dente—Bodybuilding's Entrepreneur

At age fourteen, Gerard Dente started bodybuilding to build muscle and strength to excel at football—and excel he did. He achieved state honors as a high school football player, then went on to play college football at Montclair State College, where he also studied intensively to prepare for a career combining athletics and business. In 1986, Gerard entered his first bodybuilding competition after following a special, twelve-week training, diet, and supplement program, and won the overall teenage Mr. New Jersey title. From there, Gerard continued to rack up wins, taking the Teen Nationals title in 1987 and the Collegiate Nationals title

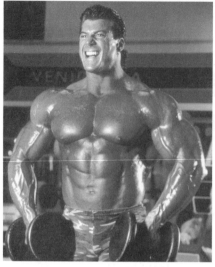

Gerard Dente

in 1988. His fame in bodybuilding led Gerard to many opportunities, including endorsement contracts, commercials, magazine covers, articles, and appearances on television talk shows.

Riding the wake of his bodybuilding success, Gerard next focused his efforts on merchandising the training, diet, and supplement program that had turned him into a champion. In 1997, he founded his own supplement company, Maximum Human Performance (MHP), with the unyielding goal of making top-quality sports supplements backed by real science. Launched with his invention and flagship product, Secretagogue-One, Gerard's business grew quickly and now offers a variety of innovative sports-supplement formulations. Today, MHP is one of the nation's fastest growing sports-supplement companies.

Diet and Supplement Program

Gerard's diet philosophy is high protein, moderate to low carbohydrates, and moderate fats. His goal is to eat six meals a day, with each meal approximately three hours apart. Following is a typical day's menu of food and supplements:

5:30 A.M. 2 ounces oatmeal; 5 strawberries; MHP BodyDesignRx shake with ½ banana; multi-vitamin-and-mineral supplement; MHP Daily Burn A.M. (fat burner); vitamin C; glucosamine and chondroitin; 3 grams glutamine; MHP Endo-Stak; MHP Nor-Stak

8:00 A.M. MHP Creatine Mixer

9:00 A.M. 10 egg whites and 2 egg yolks; 3 ounces oatmeal; 5 strawberries; MHP Whey Tocotriene; antioxidant supplement

Noon 12 ounces chicken breast; 1 cup rice; 1 cup broccoli; 1 teaspoon flaxseed oil; MHP Daily Burn A.M.; glucosamine and chondroitin; vitamin C

3:00 P.M. MHP BodyDesignRx shake; 2 ounces peanuts

6:00 P.M. 16 ounces top round steak; salad with 1 teaspoon flaxseed oil and vinegar; 1 cup green vegetable; MHP Daily Burn P.M. (fat burner and appetite suppressant); glucosamine and chondroitin; vitamin C

9:00 P.M. MHP BodyDesignRx shake; 2 servings Whey Tocotriene

11:00 P.M. Secretagogue-One

Gerard keeps his protein intake at around 2 grams per pound of body weight. To achieve this, he supplements with products such as Whey Tocotriene and BodyDesignRx, both manufactured by his company, MHP. He consumes most of his carbohydrates early in the day, before and after his morning workout, and then tapers down. His last two meals of the day usually consist of no complex carbohydrates, only fibrous green vegetables. His protein sources are also his fat sources, with additional fat coming from unsalted roasted peanuts or cashews, flaxseed oil, and, occasionally, olive oil.

Training Program

In his more than fifteen years of weight training, Gerard says that he's "tried just about every workout imaginable. I believe the biggest mistake people make when looking to gain muscle mass and strength is over-training. If your goal is strictly weight loss," he advises, "training 6 days a week is O.K. But if you're looking to pack on mass," he says, "you need to give your body a rest so you can build and repair."

The weekly training schedule that Gerard finds best is a four-workout rotation:

Sunday (Workout 1)		
Chest	Incline dumbbell presses	3 sets
	Flat barbell presses	3 sets
	Cable crossovers	2 sets
Biceps	Barbell curls	3 sets
	Preacher curls	2 sets
	One-arm dumbbell curls	2 sets
Calves	Standing toe raises	3 sets (25 reps each)

Monday (Workout 2)		
Legs	Leg presses	3 sets
	Squats	3 sets
	Extensions	2 sets
	Leg curls	3 sets
Abs	Crunches and leg raises (supersets)	3 sets to failure

Tuesday
Rest day

Wednesday (Workout 3)

Shoulders	Dumbbell presses	3 sets
	Lateral raises	3 sets
	Upright rows	2 sets
Triceps	Pushdowns	3 sets
	Dips	3 sets
Calves	Seated toe raises	3 sets (20 to 30 reps)

Thursday

Rest day

Friday (Workout 4)

Back	Seated rows	3 sets
	Bentover rows	3 sets
	Front pulldowns to chest	3 sets
Traps	Shrugs	3 sets (15 to 20 reps)
Abs	Crunches and leg raises (supersets)	3 sets to failure

Saturday

Rest day

In this four-week rotation schedule, Gerard works out each body part once a week, with the exception of his calves and abdominals (abs), which he works out twice a week. He also likes to vary his rep ranges so that he can recruit all the muscle fibers. He usually performs fifteen reps in the first set and ten reps in the second set. In the third set, he does six reps of the major exercises and fifteen reps of the secondary exercises.

David and Donna Waterman—A Winning Couple

Having dedication, following intelligent nutrition and training programs, and turning dreams into reality are ways of life for David and Donna Waterman. Dedicated health professionals, both David and Donna are living testimony of how the bodybuilding lifestyle can help facilitate achieving life goals.

Hailing from Utica, New York, David and Donna wake up each morning with a refreshed outlook on life. They greet each day with a healthy meal and vigorous workout, which have become important components not only in shaping their bodies, but also their destinies. Now in their late twenties, the Watermans have the energy and physiques of vibrant teenagers, which helps them breeze through hectic days. Working as nurses, their mental and physical abilities are continually tested to the extreme, with saving lives a part of their daily routines. On top of this, David Waterman has fashioned an outstanding championship powerlifting career, with endorsement contracts, interviews, articles, personal appearances, and seminars. Training partners, newlyweds, and the proud "parents" of two cats, Fred and Wilma, the Watermans are a force to be reckoned with.

David E. Waterman

At 187 pounds of body weight, most people would be happy to bench 310 pounds. But not David Waterman. Aggressive and goal-driven, David has completely shattered this goal with a new world record of a mind-blowing 620 pounds. Currently maintaining a lean, well-proportioned physique of 197 pounds, David's philosophy has been to keep his training and nutrition simple and scientific. As a health professional, he is fortunate to have a broad knowledge base from which to work. Because of this, you won't find David in the gym working long hours, since he knows first-hand how proper diet and supplementation are equally important for promoting maximum growth and quick recovery. David's world record in the bench

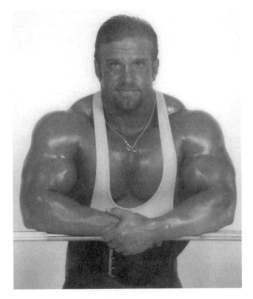

David Waterman

press stands as testimony to many things, including to what he considers a vital component of his success—perseverance. This unrelenting drive has earned David worldwide recognition, and all its glory, including sponsorship deals with major corporations, seminars, personal appearances, and an invitation to appear at the 1999 Mr. Olympia competition to demonstrate his championship powerlifting bench.

Diet and Supplement Program
David Waterman keeps his nutrition program simple and scientific. Following is a typical day's menu of food and supplements:

9 A.M.	MET-Rx Total Nutrition Drink Mix
10 A.M.	MET-Rx Mass Action Drink Mix
12 NOON	8 ounces steak; $\frac{1}{2}$ cup low-fat cottage cheese
2 P.M.	MET-Rx Total Nutrition Drink Mix
5 P.M.	1 pound chicken breast; 1 cup low-fat yogurt
8 P.M.	MET-Rx Total Nutrition Drink Mix; 2 small salt potatoes
10 P.M.	MET-Rx Mass Action Drink Mix; 8 egg whites and 2 egg yolks, scrambled

While David's breakfast consists of a meal-replacement powder, his lunch and dinner are composed of foods, primarily protein foods. He utilizes meal-replacement powders for his midmorning and midafternoon snacks, then combines them with foods for his two evening snacks.

Training Program One point that distinguishes David Waterman's training approach from most others is his avoidance of overtraining. In fact, David trains most of his body parts, including his chest, just once a week. The body parts he trains two or three times a week are the trapeziuses (traps), calves, and abs. And the most important ingredient of his program is his stick-to-itiveness. If you stick to your training and nutrition program, he says, the results will follow.

The weekly training schedule that David tends to follow is:

Monday	Shoulders, traps, and abs
Tuesday	Triceps and calves
Wednesday	Back, biceps, and abs
Thursday	Rest day
Friday	Rest day
Saturday	Chest, traps, and abs
Sunday	Legs and calves

In general, for the first exercise, David utilizes heavy weight and high resistance, for strength. He does three sets, one to three reps per set. For the second through fourth exercises, David utilizes moderate weight and moderate resistance, for shaping and sculpting. Again, he does three sets, this time of ten reps per set, with a one-minute rest in between each set. He does both aerobic and anaerobic work, to shape and pump the muscles and increase the heart rate to burn fat.

ON THE CUTTING EDGE

Training May Compromise Chromium Status

The body's chromium requirement increases during strength training, researchers at the U.S. Department of Agriculture (USDA) have reported. Unfortunately, the American diet is notorious for providing only a marginal amount of chromium, which increases the chances of poor chromium status in people involved in muscle-building athletic activities. According to an article published in the *Journal of Nutrition* in 1998, chromium absorption, use, and excretion were tracked in ten men participating in a sixteen-week resistance-training program. In this group of exercising men, the increased chromium need induced by the exercise was met by the body's enhanced absorption of chromium from the diet. This increased absorption may partially explain why exercise improves insulin sensitivity— chromium is needed for insulin action. On the downside, the researchers caution that the poor chromium intake in the United States puts many exercisers at risk of compromised chromium status. To combat this, supplement your diet with up to 200 micrograms of chromium daily to ensure an adequate chromium intake.

Donna M. Waterman

Donna Waterman has perfected her training and nutrition program to yield impressive results. At 120 pounds, she has sculpted her body into an attractive 34-22-34 figure. Her training program combines intensive weightlifting five days a week as David's training partner and aerobic exercise classes twice a week. Her nutrition program, like her husband's, is high in protein and loaded with sports-nutrition supplements and high-calcium foods.

Diet and Supplement Program Donna Waterman follows husband David's philosophy and keeps her nutrition program simple and scientific. Following is a typical day's menu of food and supplements:

9 A.M.   MET-Rx Total Nutrition Drink Mix

10 A.M.   MET-Rx Mass Action Drink Mix

12 NOON   4 ounces steak; 2 small salt potatoes

2 P.M.   4 ounces Cheddar cheese; $\frac{1}{2}$ cup fruit

5 P.M.   4 ounces chicken breast; $\frac{1}{2}$ cup cottage cheese

8 P.M.   MET-Rx Total Nutrition Drink Mix combined with MET-Rx Mass Action Drink Mix

10 P.M.   Small salad including tuna fish and hard-boiled eggs

Midnight   3 egg whites and 1 egg yolk, scrambled, with melted cheese or low-fat yogurt

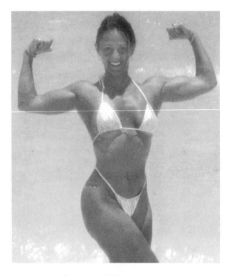

Donna Waterman

The same as her husband's, Donna's breakfast consists of a meal-replacement powder, while her lunch and dinner are composed of foods, primarily high-protein and high-calcium foods. She also utilizes meal-replacement powders for her midmorning and midevening snacks, but in the midafternoon and late evening, she enjoys some more protein- and calcium-rich foods.

Training Program
Again like her husband, Donna Waterman does not believe in overtraining. She trains most of her body parts once a week, working only her abs, hamstrings, and calves twice a week.

The weekly training schedule that Donna follows is:

Monday   Shoulders, traps, and abs; cardio kickboxing class

Tuesday   Back and biceps

Wednesday   Gluteals, hamstrings, inner and outer thighs, and calves

Thursday   Rest day

Friday   Quadriceps, hamstrings, and calves; cardio kickboxing class

Saturday   Chest, triceps, and abs

Sunday   Rest day

In general, for the first exercise, Donna utilizes heavy weight and high resistance, for strength. She does three sets, one to three reps per set. For the second through fourth exercises, Donna utilizes moderate weight and moderate resistance, for shaping and sculpting. Again, she does three sets, this time of twelve to fifteen reps per set, with a one-minute rest in between each set. She does both aerobic and anaerobic work, to shape and pump the muscles and increase the heart rate to burn fat.

TIPS FROM TOP ATHLETES

Glimpses at some more nutrition and training programs—this time from such greats as eight-time Mr. Olympia Lee Haney and top fitness model Sherry Goggin-Giardina—are offered in the following pages, as well as tips that may help you reach your optimum performance level. Note, again, that no two of the highlighted athletes follow exactly the same diet, supplement, or training program—each has determined his or her own specific needs and tailored the best plan to meet them.

Joe Young

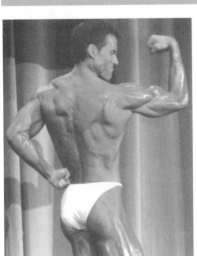

Joe Young

Joe Young is a nutritionist and director of research and product development at M.D. Labs in Tempe, Arizona. In addition to owning his own personal training studio, Young has competed successfully in the Arizona Natural Bodybuilding Championships. Earlier this year, he also won the NGA Western States Natural in the middleweight class. At age 42, Young plans to continue practicing what he preaches.

Nutrition Tips

☐ Drink plenty of water.

☐ Eat cleanly, consistently.

☐ Maintain 40-30-30 ratio of carbohydrates-protein-fat.

☐ Use whey protein for principal protein source.

☐ Cycle lower carbohydrate days with extra cardiovascular exercise to reduce body fat.

☐ Strictly limit saturated fat intake.

☐ Include lots of healthy fats—Omega-3, DHA, GLA, CLA, MCT.

☐ Cycle all nutritional supplements.

☐ Keep food records when trying to be strict.

☐ Enjoy what you eat—cheat once in a while.

Training Tips

☐ Never work out longer than one hour.

☐ Two or three weekly workouts produce better results than five or six workouts.

☐ Dwell on eight to 10 basic movements.

☐ Never totally exclude cardiovascular work.

☐ Don't let body fat drift over 10 percent, even in the off season.

☐ Slower the better as far as exercise speed of motion.

☐ Vary routines (sets, reps, exercises) to shock the body into growth.

☐ Make mind-muscle connection—visualize the muscle contracting.

☐ Keep expectations realistic.

☐ Avoid injuries at all costs.

Favorite Supplements

☐ PRO-BLEND 55—great tasting whey protein drink

☐ CM5000—creatine monohydrate

☐ ProHGH—growth hormone releaser

☐ 19-NORAN-19—norandrostenedione

☐ 5-ANDRODIOL-5—androstenediol

☐ ANDROS-DT 600—androstenedione, chrysin, tribulus, DHEA, avena sativa and saw palmetto

☐ GLX-37,5—vanadyl sulfate complex

☐ Thermadrene-ECA—thermogenic stack

☐ NFA 500—neuro-focusing formula

☐ CLA-tonalin brand

Lee Labrada

Lee Labrada is founder and president of Labrada Bodybuilding Nutrition in Houston. He is also a former professional bodybuilder and a past winner of the IFBB Mr. Universe competition.

Nutrition Tips

☐ The answer to maximum fat-free muscular weight gain is a diet ratio of 60 percent carbs, 30 percent protein and 10 percent fat.

☐ Common bodybuilding wisdom dictates 1 g to 1.5 g of protein per pound of body weight.

☐ Carbohydrate calories should come primarily from complex carbohydrates such as rice, potatoes, vegetables, etc.

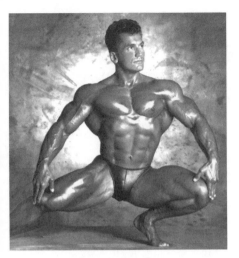

Lee Labrada

☐ Avoid cake, pie and other sugar laden foods.

☐ Two to three tablespoons of flax seed oil per day is recommended for muscle growth.

☐ Combine all three macronutrients in roughly the same proportions at each meal.

☐ Eating six meals a day is necessary to ensure that your muscles are constantly bathed in nutrients such as amino acids.

☐ No athlete should be without a multivitamin and multimineral supplements.

☐ Creatine monohydrate is another beneficial supplement proven to build strength. Take 5 g, four to five times per day the first week, followed by 5 g, twice per day thereafter.

☐ Supplements are great, but food is still the most anabolic substance you can ingest.

Training Tips

☐ Train intensely with heavy weights 4 to 5 times per week.

☐ Train each body part no more than twice per week, and for no more than 20 to 30 minutes.

☐ Use as much weight as you can handle on each exercise for 8 to 12 "reps." Decrease the weight you use as you work through your sets.

☐ Take each set of an exercise to exhaustion.

☐ In between exercises, rest only long enough to catch your breath.

☐ Allow your body enough time to recover in between workouts—48 to 72 hours is optimal.

☐ Use basic exercises, as they stimulate more muscle and have a more profound effect on your body.

☐ Limit aerobics to 30 to 45 minutes, 3 times per week.

☐ Work is what causes muscles to grow.

☐ Concentrate on that which you are doing.

☐ Be patient. Rome was not built in a day, and your body won't be either.

Favorite Supplements

☐ Creatine Cooler—a sugar-free and near calorie-free creatine transport product.

☐ Lean Body—takes the guesswork out of constructing a nutritious diet.

☐ Kwik Size XXXL helps put on quality lean muscle mass.

Lee Haney

Lee Haney has captured and held the bodybuilding world's most coveted title, Mr. Olympia, for eight consecutive wins—breaking Arnold Schwarzenegger's seven-title record. As an amateur, Haney held both the Mr. America and Mr. Universe titles and in 1983, earned his first professional title. Today, Haney focuses much of his attention on his two fitness centers, located in Atlanta and Stone Mountain, Georgia.

Nutrition Tips

☐ Whether to gain or lose weight, eat every few hours. Lighter, more frequent meals are the ticket to staying lean or adding lean muscle.

☐ Eat for what you are about to do, not for what you've done.

☐ If you can't flex it, don't carry it. Stay lean and in shape all the time, even when your interest is to gain size.

☐ Lean protein is the key to balancing blood chemistry and building lean muscle.

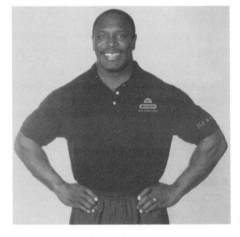

Lee Haney

☐ The timing of food intake is as important as the quantity and ratio.

☐ Eat carbohydrates with breakfast, early in the day and after training.

☐ Divide protein throughout all meals.

☐ Don't go to bed on a full stomach. Allow about one hour after training before eating the post workout meal, which consists of a balanced protein and carbohydrate meal.

☐ Eat a diet of 60 percent to 70 percent carbohydrates for weight gain; about 30 percent for weight loss.

☐ Keep a journal of what you eat, and a chart to calculate calories and grams of fat, carbohydrates and protein.

Training Tips

☐ Motivation provides the energy needed until success is achieved.

☐ It is permissible to miss a workout if you are physically under the weather. However, if you have had a long day, just cut back on the intensity and number of sets.

☐ Muscle responds to resistance and stimulus, so train the muscle by using proper form and technique.

☐ In order to stimulate muscle mass, basic, explosive training of the muscle groups must be performed.

☐ Many people use too heavy a weight during an exercise, resulting in imprecise, sloppy form.

☐ It's the quality not the quantity. Short intense workouts are more beneficial.

☐ It's smart to vary your training routine to keep the muscles stimulated.

☐ Recuperation is key to results. Be sure to incorporate balanced rest periods into your training program.

☐ Put in perspective the philosophy, "No pain, no gain." The aim should be to train or stimulate, not annihilate.

Sherry Goggin-Giardina

One of the industry's top fitness models, Sherry Goggin-Giardina has appeared in countless covers and issues of *Ironman Magazine, Muscle & Fitness, Muscular Development* and *Oxygen*. Currently, Goggin-Giardina is a spokesmodel for Bodyonics/ Pinnacle, Power Board, Yamaha Watercraft, American Power Products and Power Bar, and is the fitness editor for *Total Health Magazine*. Additionally, she maintains a Web site at www.sherryg.com, where visitors can purchase her own CD-Rom entitled "Health & Fitness."

Nutrition Tips

☐ Never be afraid to drink water, especially during your workouts.

☐ The body does require a small amount of fat, about 2 g to 4 g of linoleic acid, which can be obtained from a large bowl of oatmeal.

☐ Set a realistic goal to lose your body fat.

☐ Graze. Eat smaller, more frequent meals.

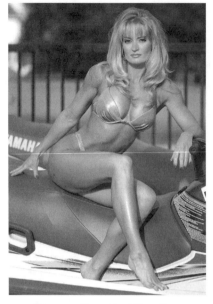

Sherry Goggin-Giardina

☐ Watch out for the "low-fat" foods, where the fat is hidden.

☐ You do not have to starve yourself to lose weight.

☐ In order to lose weight, you have to use up more calories than you take in to burn the fat.

☐ Get the proper amount of protein and carbohydrates in your diet.

☐ On the days you are unable to get enough protein in your diet, take a good protein powder supplement.

Training Tips

☐ Proper warm-up and cool down are essential to any exercise program.

☐ Stretching is most effective after an initial warm up.

☐ Quality is more important than quantity.

☐ Proper form is the key to results.

☐ Do not throw or swing your weights.

☐ Always concentrate on the muscle being used for each exercise.

☐ Never sacrifice technique for heavier weights.

☐ Never be afraid to try a new exercise.

☐ Use full range of motion on all exercises.

☐ Rest a minute between sets and two minutes between exercises.

☐ Do variations of different exercises to keep the muscle stimulated.

Favorite Supplements

☐ Pinnacle Pyruvate—helps promote greater weight and fat loss and promotes ATP production for endurance.

☐ Pinnacle's Whey Ahead—a high protein drink that contains no fat or carbohydrates.

☐ Pinnacle's Crea-Glutide—contains glutamine, an essential amino acid that is one of the building blocks of protein.

Michael Matarazzo

Since earning the title of Mr. USA in 1991, Michael Matarazzo has consistently enjoyed the distinction of being one of the Top 5 professional bodybuilders competing in the Night of Champions and the Toronto Grand Prix.

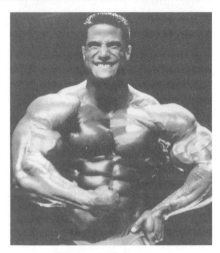

Michael Matarazzo

Nutrition Tips

☐ Eat a ton of protein. Try and get as much protein as you can.

☐ Take Weider supplements, especially the new Metaform products.

☐ Eat plenty of greens for proper digestion.

Training Tips

☐ Go to the gym to train. Do your job, don't socialize.

☐ Train hard on every exercise until you can't do anymore.

☐ Keep it consistent. Shorts periods of rest while you train.

☐ When you finish training, leave the gym. Get on with your life.

☐ As soon as you get home, feed your body. Your muscles don't grow in the gym, they grow when you feed them.

☐ Keep a positive mental attitude. Especially in your workout, at your job and in your life.

☐ Maintain a healthy lifestyle.

☐ Always maintain a proper workout regimen.

☐ Plenty of rest. Your body needs rest to grow.

☐ Follow all the Weider principals when it comes to training.

Favorite Supplements

☐ ABB Pure Pro Protein drink

☐ ABB Glutamine Caps

☐ ABB L-Carnitine caps

☐ Metaform Megabolan packs

☐ Metaform Ultra Performance powder

☐ Metaform Lean Mass powder

☐ Metaform Proton powder

☐ Metaform Hyperdrive

☐ Metaform Neurodrive

Laurie Vaniman

In addition to winning several fitness competitions including Ms. Fitness USA in 1996, Laurie Vaniman has graced the pages of several fitness magazines including *Muscle & Fitness, Ironman, Oxygen* and *Flex*. She has also appeared in *Whatever It Takes*, a movie featuring Don "The Dragon" Wilson and *Bodywaves*, a fitness show on FIT-TV.

Nutrition Tips

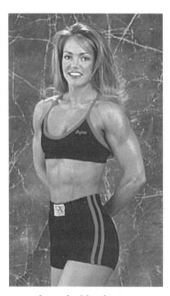

Laurie Vaniman

☐ Drink plenty of water—at least 8 to 10 8oz glasses per day.

☐ Do not "diet." Make eating healthy a lifestyle.

☐ Eat small meals frequently throughout the day.

☐ Stick to whole foods such as chicken and fish and avoid too many processed foods.

☐ Balance your diet with moderate protein and carbohydrate levels and keep fat intake to 20 percent or below.

☐ Eliminate excess sugar and salt from your diet.

☐ Allow yourself to indulge in your favorite foods occasionally.

☐ Remember—Nutrition is No. 1 in determining how your body feels and looks.

Training Tips

☐ Combine weight training and cardio work for the best overall results.

☐ Find a good trainer to teach you proper technique.

☐ Maintain a high intensity level throughout your workout.

☐ Find a training partner with similar goals for motivation purposes.

☐ Make your workouts fun and interesting by crosstraining.

☐ Set goals for yourself. Motivate yourself during your training sessions by visualizing what you want to look like.

☐ Consistency is the key to success.

☐ Patience is a virtue.

Favorite Supplements

I am a strong believer in supplements. Most importantly:

☐ Good whey protein (I use Metabolic Response Modifiers')

☐ A multi-vitamin

☐ Creatine (Again, Metabolic Response Modifiers')

☐ Vitamin C

☐ Calcium supplement (especially for women)

☐ Antioxidants

ON THE CUTTING EDGE

Diet, Exercise, and Bone Status

The amount of bone attained by early adulthood is a major determining factor of bone mass in later life, which in turn is related to fracture risk. Accordingly, achieving optimum bone mass during the growing years should decrease the risk of fractures due to osteoporosis in later life. Although genetic factors are the primary determining factors of peak bone mass, other modifiable factors, including nutrition (mainly calcium intake) and exercise, may make important contributions. A review article published in the *International Journal of Sports Nutrition* in 1998 examined how nutrition and exercise affect the status of bone-mineral accumulation during growth and assessed whether they interact with each other. The authors recommended that children take part in weight-bearing exercises and sports with diverse movements, such as gymnastics, and that they start an exercise program on a continuous basis before puberty. The authors also recommended that children eat a well-balanced, nutritious diet that supports the energy demands of normal growth as well as of physical activity, and that supplies an adequate amount of dietary calcium.

SPECIAL REPORT

FAQs About the Female Athlete Triad

Recent findings indicate that while female athletes require nutrition similar to that of male athletes on a pound-for-pound basis, they are at a higher risk for developing nutrition disorders. Medical professionals noticed that as the number of female athletes increased during the 1980s and 1990s, so did the number of injuries and ailments among them. A frequently observed set of symptoms among female athletes is called the "female athlete triad," and it can have devastating effects on individuals who fall victim to it. Being aware of the reasons for, cure of, and prevention of this syndrome can be critical for all female athletes.

Q. Exactly what is the "female athlete triad"?

A. The female athlete triad is a set of health problems that occurs in female athletes. It is characterized by disordered eating and menstrual irregularities, and can eventually lead to osteoporosis. The triad's early diagnosis is critical for preventing severe health problems. Menstrual irregularities are the first warning sign. These have been common among female athletes and have historically been thought of as trivial occurrences. Medical researchers now consider them to be more serious, however.

Q. What causes the female athlete triad?

A. Poor nutrition combined with strenuous training is the root cause of the female athlete triad. Inadequate nutritional practices create deficiencies in energy and essential nutrients. These lead to a poor state of health, which is typically associated with a loss in body weight. The reduced body weight triggers menstrual irregularities to develop, which should be considered early warning signs of overtraining and inadequate nutrition. Then, if the condition is allowed to persist, osteoporosis develops, which leads to an increased risk of bone fractures.

Q. Who is at risk for the female athlete triad?

A. It seems that the female athletes who are at the highest risk for the female athlete triad participate in sports in which nutritional deficiencies are common—for example, distance sports and sports in which body weight or appearance is important. These sports include gymnastics, diving, figure skating, triathlon, dancing, rowing, martial arts, and long-distance running, cycling, and swimming.

Q. What is disordered eating?

A. Disordered eating should not be confused with eating disorders, such as anorexia and bulimia, which are psychiatric in nature. Eating disorders do occur among female athletes and are another serious problem of which to be aware. However, disordered eating involves abnormal eating patterns. It includes poor nutrition habits, eating the wrong foods (junk foods), undertaking unneeded or extreme dieting, and using purging or laxatives for weight control. Disordered eating leads to an energy deficit, decreased metabolic rate, and reduced structure and function of the body. When it is combined with intense athletic training, it can lead to health problems, the first ones of which are menstrual irregularities.

Q. What are the specific causes of the menstrual irregularities of the female athlete triad?

A. There are many factors that can cause menstrual irregularities. However, the primary triggers of the menstrual irregularities associated with the female athlete triad are poor nutrition and intensive training, which deplete the body's nutrient stores and alter its function. Eventually, ovarian function becomes impaired and can even lead to a shutting down of the production of estrogen and other hormones. While amenorrhea (lack of menstruation) is also observed in a small percentage (less than 5 percent) of non-athletic females, it occurs in 40 percent or more of athletic females. There are two types of amenorrhea observed in the female athlete triad—primary and secondary. *Primary amenorrhea* is the absence of menstruation in females sixteen years old or older who have already developed secondary sex characteristics. It is very important to prevent the triad from ever occurring in teenaged female athletes. Any type of menstrual irregularity in teenaged females should be given serious attention and prompt treatment. *Secondary amenorrhea* is the absence, not caused by pregnancy, of three to twelve consecutive menstrual periods after menarche. This condition also warrants medical attention.

Q. I thought exercise helps prevent osteoporosis. Is this belief wrong?

A. Osteoporosis is a condition marked by decreased bone mass and an increased risk of bone fracture. It has several causes and is most often thought of as occurring in older females. It can be prevented and treated with a program of exercise and proper nutrition. However, doctors recently made a connection between secondary amenorrhea and osteoporosis in young adult athletic females. Secondary amenorrhea causes weak-

ening of the bone tissue and leads to an increased risk of bone fractures. For example, amenorrheic female runners have lower bone densities than normally menstruating runners. If the secondary amenorrhea is allowed to persist, researchers believe that normal bone formation may not be able to be restored and the triad's osteoporosis may not be able to be reversed.

Q. What measures can I take to prevent the female athlete triad?

A. First and foremost, you should strictly adhere to a sound performance nutrition program. This means eating the proper amounts of carbohydrates, protein, and fats, divided among five to seven daily meals; maintaining an adequate fluid intake; and taking supplements to ensure intake of the essential nutrients, such as the essential fatty acids, protein, vitamins, and minerals, especially calcium and magnesium. The major cause of osteoporosis is poor nutrition. In fact, the FDA has approved a health claim for foods and supplements high in calcium (over 200 milligrams) as being able to help prevent osteoporosis. It is also a good practice to keep a training journal, documenting your training, competitions, medical exams, health problems, medications, diet, supplement intake, sleep patterns, menstrual periods, and behavior patterns. Keeping a training journal takes just minutes a day and will prove to be extremely beneficial, resulting in improved performance and optimum health.

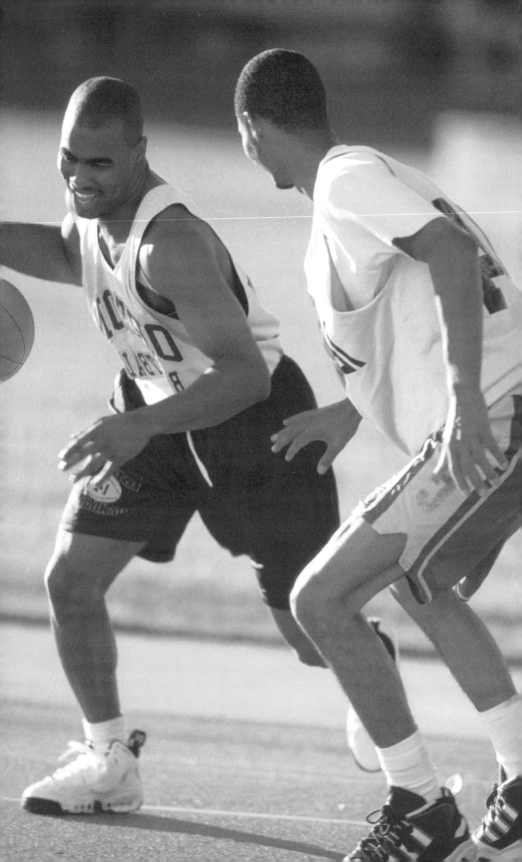

NEW ON
THE MARKET

11

The last couple of years have seen many new supplements, as well as improved versions of existing supplements, come to market. Several new forms of creatine, presented as more effective than the original form, hit the shelves. Other supplements, such as androstenedione and tribulus terrestris, were introduced with much fanfare but backed by little science, and, more important, accompanied by many issues about their safety. New protein supplements and metabolic optimizers also made debuts, and supplements that have been in use for health purposes, such as nicotinamide adenine dinucleotide (NADH) and phosphatidylserine (PS), used in the areas of cognition and disease states, found new applications in the sports-nutrition field.

In this chapter, we will take a look at some of these new sports-nutrition products and attempt to separate the hype from the facts.

Androstenedione
The admission of Mark McGwire, record-breaking batter for the St. Louis Cardinals, that he takes supplemental androstenedione to improve his athletic performance has spurred unprecedented sales of the bottled testosterone precursor. Purported to increase muscle mass and strength, androstenedione, however, remains controversial because of its hazy relationship to steroids and the stigma associated with them.

Androstenedione's popularity among athletes and bodybuilders is easily understood—it is a metabolite of the well-known "youth hormone" dehydroepiandrosterone (DHEA) and a hormonal precursor to testosterone, the hormone responsible for making the male body masculine. Androstenedione has about one-seventh the activity of testosterone and is directly converted to the hormone by a single reaction. It is naturally produced in the body from either DHEA or 17-a-hydroxyprogesterone.

Does Androstenedione Work?

Androstenedione's research history is brief. It was first synthesized in 1935. One year later, Charles Kochakian, an expert on steroid hormones, discovered that androstenedione has both androgenic (masculinizing) and anabolic (tissue-building) properties. These hormonal effects were ignored by the scientific community until 1962, when Drs.V. B. Mahesh and R. B. Greenblatt from the Medical College of Georgia at Augusta investigated the effect of androstenedione on the testosterone level. Four nonathletic women were given either 100 milligrams of DHEA or 100 milligrams of androstenedione, and the results indicated that both hormones elevated the testosterone level, but the androstenedione-induced increase was more than double the DHEA-induced increase. The testosterone levels of the women who took the DHEA rose from less than 199 nanograms per deciliter (ng/dl) to 280 nanograms per deciliter within sixty minutes. The testosterone levels in the androstenedione group rose to as high as 660 ng/dl—three times the normal level—during the same time period. The androstenedione-induced testosterone increase lasted several hours but remained at a peak level for just a few minutes.

The results of this single study that is almost four decades old remain the basis for androstenedione being marketed as a muscle-building supplement for professional male athletes. This is despite the facts that the data were gleaned from four untrained females and that the study examined transient changes in testosterone levels, not changes in muscle mass or muscle strength. To date, there are no published studies indicating that supplemental androstenedione increases human muscle mass or strength. Androstenedione's claimed benefits are extrapolated from the findings that supplemental androstenedione briefly increases the testosterone level and testosterone increases muscle mass. (To get around this, a time-release form of androstenedione is now being marketed. There is no scientific proof, however, that such a formulation is effective.)

Furthermore, there is no scientific evidence to support using androstenedione to improve athletic performance. It was used by athletes from the former German Democratic Republic as an anabolic, energy-enhancing supplement, but few details are available. Androstenedione has a short half-life (the amount of time it takes for a substance to be degraded by the body to half its concentration). The shorter a substance's half-life is, the less time it spends in the body. Androstenedione thus may not lend itself to a long-term regimen. An athlete would need to take the supplement several times a day on a nearly continuous basis to maintain a substantial blood level of it.

Is Androstenedione Safe?

Athletes should use anabolic-androgenic supplements such as androstenedione cautiously. A review of the "doping" program used in the former German Democratic Republic details a litany of adverse effects in male and female athletes who used other androgenic-anabolic supplements, including anabolic steroids and growth hormone. Anabolic steroids are synthetic analogs of testosterone. Their side effects include muscle tightness and cramping, weight gain, acne, gastrointestinal problems, changes in libido, and liver damage, as well as amenorrhea in women and stunted growth in adolescents.

A review of anabolic steroids in the journal *Clinical Chemistry* adds decreased HDL cholesterol and increased risk of prostate disease, liver cancer, and psychological problems, including dependence on the steroid, to the list of side effects.

The author of the review stresses that the therapeutic index, the ratio of the dosage required for supposed beneficial effects to the toxic dose, is unclear, adding, "The long-term consequences and disease risks of androgenic-anabolic steroids to the sports competitor remain to be properly evaluated."

In fact, Richard Weindruch, MD, of the University of Wisconsin at Madison stated in a prostate-cancer research-grant proposal to the National Institute of Aging that "epidemiologic data suggest that diet and serum androstenedione levels may influence the progression of latent forms of prostate cancer into more aggressive prostate cancer." He further stated, "One prospective study linked high androstenedione levels with the later development of prostate cancer." He concluded that selling androstenedione may be irresponsible due to the potential risks associated with its long-term use.

Excessive testosterone, naturally present in some people and produced as part of the conversion of androstenedione in others, may be further metabolized to dihydrotestosterone (DHT) by the enzyme 5 alpha-reductase. There is no benefit to high levels of DHT, as it has no muscle-building effect. It is, however, linked to male-pattern baldness, lowered HDL cholesterol, increases in facial and body hair, and abnormal prostate growth. Researchers hypothesize that taking large amounts of androstenedione could certainly trigger such side effects. High DHT levels may also cause enlargement of the breast tissue in males, called gynecomastia, through a process known as aromatization, during which testosterone is converted to the estrogen estradiol.

The Estrogen Angle

Androstenedione's conversion to testosterone, which in turn is converted to various forms of estrogen, may be responsible for the increased cancer risk among premenopausal and postmenopausal women, according to a 1996 study. Nancy Potischman, PhD, of the National Cancer Institute, reported that high circulating levels of androstenedione were associated with a 3.6-fold and 2.8-fold, respectively, increased risk of endometrial cancer among sixty-eight women. Dr. Potischman measured the circulating hormone levels of the women who were not taking androstenedione as a medication or supplement. (Some people have naturally high levels of androstenedione.) According to Dr. Potischman, the increased cancer incidence could have been caused by androstenedione or by other factors, such as increased levels of estrone or estradiol, diet, or lifestyle.

In another study investigating androstenedione's estrogenic effects, James Harper, PhD, of Imperial Chemical Industries, Cheshire, England, reported that androstenedione administered to rats interfered with pregnancy. In the rats, the androstenedione was metabolized to estrogen, which in turn accelerated egg transport, limiting the time for fertilization.

To prevent androstenedione from forming estrogen, some manufacturers are combining it with aromatase inhibitors. Aromatase naturally converts testosterone to estrogen. Chrysin, a bioflavonoid also known as flavone X, is being widely promoted as such an inhibitor. When combined with androstenedione, it seems to enhance testosterone formation. Very little data, however, support chrysin's new use as an anti-estrogen compound. Although research in this area continues, conclusive evidence has yet to be published. At the very least, the claims that chrysin works in humans distort the existing data. For example, a 1984 study by James Kellis and Larry Vickery indicates that chrysin and other aromatase inhibitors successfully inhibited estrogen synthetase in human placental cells. This effect, however, was achieved in a test tube, not in a human.

Male Andropause

Androstenedione may have a useful application quite apart from sports—it promises to help prevent male andropause. Andropause is the gradual decrease in mens' normal levels of circulating testosterone. A normal testosterone range is defined as 350 to 1,000 ng/dl, but levels as low as 200 ng/dl have been found in fifty-year-old males. Supplemental androstenedione and DHEA may restore the testosterone balance in men whose hormone levels are unhealthy.

The Final Verdict

Although it has been noted that many adverse effects from androgenic and anabolic agents are reversible and that few severe incidents occur with moderate use, men who use androstenedione for extended periods of time should confirm their prostate health with regular prostate-specific-antigen (PSA) blood tests. They should also discuss their use of the supplement with their health-care practitioner.

The efficacy and mechanisms of action of androstenedione and other androgenic-anabolic supplements currently remain unknown. Until there is scientific evidence supporting its long-term safety, androstenedione should not be sold as either an effective or safe ergogenic aid. Clearly, it should not be used by adolescents or women of child-bearing age. The ethics of using androgenic-anabolic sports supplements are also debatable. In 1998, androstenedione was added to the list of substances banned by the International Olympic Committee. It is also banned by several professional and amateur sports organizations, including the National Collegiate Athletic Association and the National Football League.

Creatine
The objective of creatine supplementation is to increase creatine intake, which in turn increases the creatine stores in the muscles. Therefore, supplemental creatine basically serves to supply energy. In this capacity, it allows the performance of more work and increases the performance effects of training. The finding that the body's creatine stores can be increased has led to further research exploring the potential of supplemental creatine to enhance exercise performance.

If all of the protein you ate could be efficiently broken down into amino acids, and then all of the resulting arginine, glycine, and methionine efficiently converted to creatine, your body still would not produce more than approximately 2 to 3 grams of creatine, the amount needed daily to replace what is lost in the urine. The same would be true if you merely took supplements of arginine, glycine, and methionine. The best way to increase the amount of creatine in the muscles is to take creatine in supplemental form. Luckily, the last couple of years have seen the introduction of a whole bevy of new forms of the popular sports supplement.

Micronized Creatine

Creatine recently became available in a micronized particle size. Structurally, it is the same as the creatine monohydrate that has been available for years; it differs only in the size of the particle. This might seem like a minor difference, but as users of the traditional product know, creatine rapidly settles to the bottom of the glass and is known for its gritty texture. Micronized creatine reduces this problem by staying suspended in solution for a longer period of time. There is no real difference in absorption, however. Theoretically, the longer the creatine remains suspended, the less of it will remain in the glass, and the more will be ingested and absorbed into the bloodstream. However, when using standard creatine monohydrate, swirling the glass to keep the particles in suspension can produce a similar result. Micronized creatine is convenient more than anything else.

Liquid Creatine

Recently, several liquid creatine products arrived on the market. These new supplements contain creatine monohydrate suspended in liquids that contain carbohydrates and other ingredients, such as glycerin. By suspending the creatine in solution, the problem of the creatine settling at the bottom of the glass is eliminated. One manufacturer also claims that the liquid delivery system "increases absorption by 600 percent" and reduces the number of creatine nonresponders (individuals who do not experience the benefits) to less than 10 percent. Nonresponders to powdered creatine have been estimated at 20 to 25 percent. Gastrointestinal distress is also said to be reduced with the liquid creatine products.

It should be noted, however, that no studies supporting these claims have been published to date. Another important issue regarding liquid creatine products is the stability of the creatine in the liquids. While creatine monohydrate can be safely kept in liquid for a few hours, it starts to destabilize soon after that. Creatine largely degrades to creatinine and other byproducts within days if left in solution. At this time, it would probably be wise to forgo purchasing creatine in liquid form.

Creatine Citrate

Creatine citrate is a newly patented form of creatine. According to the patent, creatine citrate is more rapidly absorbed into the bloodstream than creatine monohydrate. Recent research done at the University of Milano (but unpublished in the scientific literature) suggests that creatine citrate reaches its peak concentration in the blood within one hour, while creatine monohydrate can take up to three hours to reach its peak level. The manufacturer contends that this is what makes creatine citrate more effective for athletes who want to take it right before an event and could even eliminate the need for a loading phase.

Creatine citrate dissolves more easily in water than the monohydrate form, which may allow it to be absorbed faster. However, no study has yet determined whether a single dose of creatine citrate (or creatine monohydrate, for that matter) can produce a performance benefit. Athletes usually take creatine for long periods of time, during which the concentration of the nutrient in the muscle cells is increased. Creatine citrate appears to be as effective as creatine monohydrate in this regard, although research needs to be conducted.

Twice as many grams of creatine citrate as creatine monohydrate need to be consumed to get the same amount of the active ingredient. Creatine citrate is 40-percent creatine and 60-percent citrate, while creatine monohydrate is 90-percent creatine and 10-percent monohydrate.

Creatine Phosphate

Creatine is stored in the muscle tissue as creatine phosphate. Because of this, some people believe that supplementing with creatine phosphate is more effective than supplementing with the more popular creatine monohydrate. A recent study conducted at Truman State University in Kirksville, Missouri, attempted to determine which form of supplemental creatine was superior for strength and muscle gains during a six-week training cycle. Thirty-five males in excellent physical condition were divided into three groups. One group was given creatine monohydrate, another group was given creatine phosphate, and the last group was given a placebo. Prior to administering the supplement, the researchers tested the subjects' bench-press and leg-press strength, arm-curl endurance, and amount of lean body mass. The subjects were then loaded with 20 grams of supplement per day (5 grams four times daily), then given a 10-gram daily maintenance dose for the remainder of the six weeks.

In the sixth week, both of the creatine groups demonstrated increases in their bench-press and leg-press strength, arm-curl endurance, and lean body mass. The placebo group, however, showed no changes. The researchers concluded that supplementation with creatine, whether monohydrate or phosphate, may be more effective than resistance training alone for improvements in strength and muscularity.

This is the first study to compare both types of creatine and their effectiveness. Some supplement companies commonly claim that one form of creatine is superior to the other, but this study showed the monohydrate and phosphate forms to be equally effective. Binding phosphate or monohydrate to creatine only serves to stabilize the creatine so that it doesn't convert to creatinine, a waste product that has no performance-enhancing benefits. It really doesn't matter which form of creatine is used. If you follow the typical loading practice of taking 5 grams four times a day for five days, then 3 to 5 grams once a day as a maintenance dose, you will experience the same muscle and strength gains. Creatine monohydrate has probably been more popular to this point because creatine phosphate is less stable and simply tastes a lot worse.

Effervescent Creatine

An effervescent creatine that recently reached the market is a combination of creatine monohydrate, potassium bicarbonate, and citric-acid powder. Once that combination hits water, the reaction between the bicarbonate and the citric acid produces an effervescent effect. The effervescent effect then causes the creatine to disassociate from its salt, the monohydrate, resulting in a free-ionized creatine.

Free-ionized creatine is soluble and dissolves completely in water. This means no grit, and the creatine is more efficiently absorbed once it enters the gastrointestinal tract. Other advantages of the effervescence include a possible reduction in stomach distress by the buffering action. Effervescent creatine also has 20 grams of dextrose to further speed the transport of the creatine to the muscles. In simple terms, it uses effervescence to enhance the delivery of the creatine to the bloodstream.

Jeff Stout, PhD, performed a study involving effervescent creatine at Creighton University's Exercise Science Research Laboratory in Omaha, Nebraska. Using a test that simulated weight training, he compared the anaerobic work capacity of subjects taking creatine monohydrate, creatine monohydrate plus carbohydrates, the new effervescent creatine, and a placebo. (According to other studies, creatine monohydrate plus carbohydrates is currently the premier creatine transport solution.) The preliminary findings showed an increase in anaerobic work capacity of 9.0 percent in the creatine-monohydrate group, an increase of 15.0 percent in the creatine-and-carbohydrate group, and an increase of 28.3 percent in the effervescent-creatine group.

While the results of this study are intriguing, more research on effervescent creatine needs to be conducted to confirm them.

Creatine Combined With Pyruvate

Some manufacturers are now combining creatine with pyruvate. Glucose is an important fuel in the production of energy in the muscles during exercise, and pyruvate has been shown to assist in the delivery of glucose into the muscles. The assumption is that creatine is taken up better and in greater amounts by the muscle tissue when it is combined with pyruvate.

As part of a diet and exercise program, creatine combined with pyruvate has been reported by one manufacturer to contribute to a reduced gain of body fat without reducing muscle protein, which is an important factor in increasing lean muscle mass. A study reported by one company showed that athletes taking creatine combined with pyruvate had an approximately 7-percent decrease in body fat and an approximately 4-percent increase in lean body mass.

However, the same as for the other unproven forms of creatine, it should be noted that no studies supporting these claims have been published in the scientific literature to date. Other studies would assure that the above claims were reviewed by individuals outside the company selling the product.

Creatine With Protein

Combining creatine with good-quality protein and/or the amino acids prevalent in muscle tissue is a good idea. These amino acids include glutamine, the BCAAs (valine, leucine, and isoleucine), and taurine.

Studies have suggested that glutamine helps regulate the synthesis of protein in skeletal-muscle tissue, plus may help protect muscle tissue from breakdown. The body always has a need for glutamine, but this need is especially great during physical stress such as exercise. When the dietary intake of glutamine is low, the body turns to its glutamine stores. When stored glutamine is pulled from muscle tissue, that tissue may suffer degradation. Consuming glutamine during exercise helps spare the glutamine stored in the muscle tissue. There has also been some indication that glutamine may function in cell volumization—that is, increase in size of the muscle cells.

Some creatine-powder supplements also contain the amino acid taurine. It has been reported that taurine is the second most abundant amino acid in human skeletal muscle. Animal studies suggest that taurine may also potentiate the action of insulin. The same as for glutamine, there is a weak suggestion that taurine may be anticatabolic and cell-volumizing.

Creatine Precursors

To increase your creatine levels naturally, you need to consume large gram amounts of arginine and glycine daily. You could do this to a point by consuming a good protein powder, which is more economical than supplementing with large doses of pure arginine and pure glycine.

Other precursors of creatine are the methyl donors choline and betaine (pronounced *BAY tah-een*), folate, and vitamins B_6 and B_{12}. Whether supplementing with these precursors would improve your creatine synthesis hasn't been studied yet, but it makes for interesting speculation.

Another possible synergistic nutrient is phosphatidylserine (PS), a normal component of cell membranes. When taken as a supplement at dosages of 400 to 800 milligrams daily for ten days, PS has been shown to lower the exercise-induced rise in cortisol and adrenocorticotropic hormone (ACTH). This means that PS may have anticatabolic actions, which are vital for maximum muscle growth. Since creatine and protein enhance muscle-protein synthesis, the addition of PS to creatine supplements may mean a further boost to maximizing muscle gains.

There are also creatine products that combine creatine with chromium, sodium, alpha lipoic acid, and dextrose under the assumption that these insulin and glycemic-index enhancers will accelerate creatine uptake. Again, while the advertisements for these products seem packed with information, no scientific papers have been published on this form of creatine supplementation.

Methylsulfonylmethane (MSM) Recently, a form of sulfur—more specifically, organic sulfur, the kind the body can absorb and use—has been shown to help relieve inflammation and muscle cramping. This form of sulfur is called methylsulfonylmethane, or MSM for simplicity.

MSM is a member of the sulfur family but should never be confused with sulfa drugs, to which some people are allergic. MSM has been used as a dietary supplement for several years, with no reports of intolerance or allergic reaction. Acute, intermediate, and long-term studies indicate that MSM exhibits very low toxicity no matter how it is administered. How low? Its profile is similar to that of water! Within limits, you cannot overdose on MSM because your body will take and use whatever it needs and, after a twelve-hour period, flush any excess amounts.

One of the most significant applications of MSM is as a pain reliever, due to a demonstrated ability to alleviate the pain associated with systemic inflammatory disorders. People with arthritis report substantial and long-lasting relief while taking supplemental daily dosages of MSM ranging from a low of 100 milligrams to a high of 5,000 milligrams. This beneficial effect is due in part to the ability of MSM to sustain cell flow-through, allowing harmful substances such as lactic acid to flow out while permitting nutrients to flow in, thereby preventing the pressure buildup in the cells that causes inflammation in the joints and elsewhere.

In one study, eight people suffering from various forms of intractable pain were given MSM by mouth in differing amounts for periods of up to nineteen months. All reported reduced levels of pain. If you suffer from joint pain or swelling, you might want to try MSM and glucosamine.

The nerves that sense pain are located mainly in the soft tissues of the body, such as the muscles. Many types of pain can be attributed to a pressure differential involving the cells that make up these tissues. When the outside pressure drops, the cells become swollen and inflamed. The nerves register the inflammation, and pain is experienced. Often, contributing to the pain are rigid fibrous tissue cells, which lack flexibility and permeability. MSM has been shown to restore flexibility to the protein layer of cell walls, allowing fluids to pass through more easily. This softens the tissue and helps to equalize the pressure, thereby reducing, if not totally eliminating, the cause of the pain. MSM, by equalizing the cell pressure, treats the cause of the inflammation, unlike aspirin, which treats the symptom by shutting off the nerve.

MSM has demonstrated the remarkable ability to reduce the incidence of or entirely eliminate muscle soreness, and leg and back cramps, particularly in geriatric patients who have such cramps during the night or after long periods of inactivity, and in athletes after high physical stress.

Marathon runners and other athletes who compete or exercise vigorously can learn from the trainers of million-dollar racehorses. Many trainers administer MSM to their prize horses both before a race, to prevent muscle soreness, and afterwards, to lessen the risk of cramping. Delayed-onset muscle soreness, which may last for many days after intense exercise, was gone in two to three days in individuals who had taken 1,000 to 2,000 milligrams of MSM per day in split dosages for the preceding six months.

Nicotinamide Adenine Dinucleotide (NADH) *NADH* is an acronym for *nicotinamide adenine dinucleotide,* a coenzyme. This coenzyme's other name, coenzyme 1, reflects its pivotal role in cellular-energy production. Coenzymes are essential components of the enzymes that drive our metabolic reactions. The same as coenzyme Q_{10}, NADH is involved in the synthesis of ATP, the intracellular currency of energy. Much of the food we eat eventually winds up as ATP, making it the most elemental form of energy.

Every living cell, from bacteria to human cells, contains NADH. Human heart cells contain a whopping 90 micrograms of NADH in every 1 gram of tissue. To keep up with this demand, the body continuously synthesizes NADH.

The process involves nicotinamide, or niacin, a B-complex vitamin. In other words, niacin is required for energy production.

NADH and Energy Production

NADH is actually the reduced form of coenzyme 1. When NADH is oxidized, energy is released and made available to the cells. This oxidation process takes place within the mitochondria, the energy-producing compartments of the cells.

In a cascade of reactions, NADH and oxygen combine to form water and energy. The energy is preserved in the form of ATP. Every one of the body's energy-consuming reactions requires ATP. The more NADH a cell has available, the more energy it can produce. The organs that use the most energy—the brain and the muscles, including the heart—have the highest NADH contents.

Again, NADH occurs naturally in all cells, plant and animal. The highest concentrations are found in red meat, poultry, and yeast. Vegetables are not as rich in NADH as animal tissues. However, most NADH present in food is destroyed during processing and cooking, and it is also degraded by the gastric acids of digestion. Therefore, you may be better off eating raw fruits and vegetables, and sprinkling yeast on foods, to increase your NADH intake.

NADH in Mental and Physical Functioning

A growing body of scientific research is suggesting that supplemental NADH can improve mental and physical health. For example, studies show that NADH dramatically boosts the production of the neurotransmitter dopamine. Neurotransmitters are the chemical messengers of the brain and nervous system. Dopamine is vital for short-term memory, involuntary movements, muscle tone, and spontaneous physical reactions. It also mediates the release of growth hormone and dictates muscular movement.

Without sufficient dopamine, your muscles become stiff, an effect exemplified by Parkinson's disease. In fact, Parkinson's disease is a disorder caused by the destruction of the cells in the brain that synthesize dopamine.

Preliminary data suggest that NADH may be able to help ameliorate the symptoms of Parkinson's disease. J.G.D. Birkmayer, MD, of the Birkmayer Institute for Parkinson Therapy, Vienna, Austria, gave 885 people with Parkinson's NADH as medication in an open-label trial. About half of the patients were given 12.5 milligrams of NADH by intravenous (IV) infusion, while the remaining half were given the same dosage orally, by capsules. About 80 percent of the patients displayed a beneficial clinical effect. Specifically, 19.3 percent of the patients showed a very good (30- to 50-percent) improvement in their disabilities, and 58.8 percent showed a moderate (10- to 30-percent) improvement. The remaining patients, or 21.8 percent, did not respond to the NADH. Statistical analysis of the improvements in correlation with the disabilities prior to treatment, the duration of the disease, and the ages of the patients revealed that all three of these parameters had a significant although weak influence on the patients' improvement. The disability before treatment had a positive regression coefficient. In addition, the duration of the disease had a negative regression coefficient, as did age. In other words, the younger patients and patients with shorter durations of the disease had better chances to gain marked improvements than the older patients and patients with longer durations of the disease. The orally applied form of NADH yielded an overall improvement in the disability that was comparable to that of the IV form.

NADH also enhances the rate of synthesis of another neurotransmitter, norepinephrine (noradrenaline). Norepinephrine contributes to alertness, concentration, and mental activity. Serotonin, dopamine, and noradrenaline are the feel-good brain chemicals. When you have low brain levels of them, you feel depressed. Drugs that raise the brain levels of dopamine and noradrenaline elevate the mood to the point of euphoria, as illustrated by cocaine, which blocks the breakdown of these two chemicals in the brain.

As you might expect, NADH, by boosting the synthesis of both dopamine and noradrenaline, appears to ease depression. A recent study by Dr. Birkmayer used NADH in an open-label trial as medication in 205 patients suffering from depression with various clinical symptoms. The NADH was given orally, at a dosage of 5.0 milligrams; intramuscularly, at a dosage of 12.5 milligrams; or intravenously, at a dosage of 12.5 milligrams. The duration of the therapy ranged from 5 to 310 days. About 93 percent of the patients exhibited a beneficial clinical effect. The overall improvement was 11.5 points on a test that measured the degree of severity of the depression.

Other preliminary studies showed that NADH may aid in the treatment of Alzheimer's disease. NADH was used as a medication by Dr. Birkmayer in an open-label trial done with 17 patients suffering from dementia of the Alzheimer's type. In all the patients evaluated so far, improvement in cognitive dysfunction was observed. Based on a minimental state examination, a psychological test to determine cognitive state or level of awareness, the minimum improvement was 6.00 points and the maximum improvement was 14.00 points, with a mean improvement of 8.35 points. The improvement, measured with the global deterioration scale (GDS), was a minimum of 1.00 point and a maximum of 2.00 points, with a mean improvement of 1.82 points. The duration of the therapy was eight to twelve weeks. No side effects or adverse effects were reported by the patients during the observation period, which in some patients was more than a year. This open-label trial represented a pilot study from which no definitive conclusion could be drawn. A double-blind, placebo-controlled study is necessary to demonstrate the clinical efficacy of NADH.

One theory about the aging process postulates that the cells begin to age when DNA repair becomes inefficient. DNA repair requires NADH. Furthermore, much of the constant attack on cellular DNA comes from free radicals, renegade byproducts of normal oxygen metabolism. As a potent free-radical scavenger, NADH helps ensure cellular integrity.

NADH and Athletic Performance

Investigators are just beginning to look at NADH's possible applications for athletic performance. Theoretically, the physiologic functions promoted by NADH could have beneficial effects for athletes. The results of research conducted by Dr. Birkmayer with competitive athletes does indicate that NADH has a work-enhancing effect. The study measured improvements in reaction time, physical performance, and performance quality in 17 competitive cyclists and long-distance runners. Physical performance was measured on a bicycle ergometer. Performance quality was determined by measurements of continuous attention.

The athletes underwent these tests before and after taking 5 milligrams of NADH (specifically, of ENADA, a stabilized form of NADH) before breakfast each morning for four weeks. During the test period, the subjects kept constant the frequency and intensity of their training and exercise programs, as well as lifestyle factors.

After four weeks of NADH supplementation, the reaction times in the majority of the athletes were significantly decreased, dropping up to 10 percent in 5 athletes, 10 to 20 percent in 8 athletes, and over 20 percent in 3 athletes. Overall, the reaction times improved considerably in 16 of the 17 subjects.

Compared to the baseline measurements, the parameters for physical performance also improved. For 2 of the athletes, the maximum work performance increased by more than 10 percent, with another 7 athletes showing increases of up to 10 percent. Similar improvements were made in maximum exercise capacity.

The researchers hypothesized that the improved reaction times in some of the athletes may have been the results of a correction of NADH deficiency or of an increase in dopamine production, leading to an increase in alertness and vigilance. The latter explanation is further supported by studies in which NADH supplementation was shown to increase dopamine production in rats.

The researchers went on to say that stimulation of cellular ATP production by NADH may enhance athletic performance. Theoretically, the more NADH a cell has available, the more energy it can produce. Conversely, an NADH deficit results in reduced strength, power, and performance.

Safety and Continued Research

NADH is now available as a dietary supplement for anyone whose lifestyle demands increased energy, vitality, and mental activity. NADH is a safe substance, nontoxic even in high concentrations. No adverse effects have been reported. NADH research is continuing both in the United States and abroad. Current studies and clinical trials are exploring NADH's full potential for improved health and athletic performance.

Phosphatidylserine (PS)
Most athletes wonder if intensive training can have a detrimental effect upon muscle growth. Can the stress of intensive exercise slow muscle growth by affecting the growth equation? Muscles grow when anabolism (muscle building) is greater than catabolism (muscle breakdown). Intensive training increases the release of cortisol, a hormone that, at the cellular level, plays an important regulatory function in the metabolism of protein, fat, carbohydrate, sodium, and potassium. However, cortisol is a catabolic hormone, and since it is elevated during and after intensive training, it has a negative impact

upon muscle growth and strength. Therefore, lowering the cortisol level may effectively improve performance.

Now, a new supplement may prove to be even more effective than anabolic steroids at suppressing cortisol—and without anabolic steriods' detrimental effects. This supplement may also improve the effectiveness of high-calorie drinks. Phosphatidylserine (PS), a phospholipid found in cell membranes and derived from soybeans and bovine cerebral cortex, has been shown to weaken cortisol's response to exercise. PS helps promote homeostasis within the body's cells. It not only supports the proteins that manage membrane function but seems to anchor many of the proteins in the matrices of cell membranes, allowing them to function optimally. Among the activities facilitated by PS are the entry of nutrients into cells and the exit of waste products from cells, the movement of ions into and out of cells, and cell-to-cell communications.

PS and Cortisol

Three clinical studies have suggested that supplemental PS may be effective at suppressing the cortisol level. These human studies found that PS can actually inhibit exercise-induced increases in cortisol. Two of the studies were published in scientific journals, while the third study, which was conducted in the fall of 1997, was presented at the national meeting of the American College of Sports Medicine in June 1998. The first study, by Palmiero Monteleone and his colleagues at the University of Naples, Italy, found that an intravenous injection of PS significantly reduced cortisol production at both a 50-milligram and 75-milligram dosage. Eight healthy, nonathletic males had blood samples taken before, during, and after an exercise session of bicycling to near-exhaustion. As expected, their ACTH and cortisol levels rose after the exercise session, but the increases were approximately 33 percent and 45 percent, respectively, less than the placebo.

In the second study, Dr. Monteleone and his colleagues conducted the same experiment using 400 milligrams and 800 milligrams of PS taken orally. They found that the plasma-cortisol response to the exercise was lowered by 16-percent and about 30-percent, respectively. These findings show that PS can soften the severity of the stress response in healthy individuals during exercise.

The most recent study was conducted by Thomas Fahey, EdD, of California State University at Chico. In this double-blind, cross-over study, eleven weight-trained college students were given 800 milligrams of oral PS daily and then, four times a week, were put through a vigorous, whole-body weight workout intentionally designed to overtrain them. Half of the athletes were given the PS for two weeks, were allowed to rest for three and a half weeks, and then repeated the workout program for another two weeks with a placebo. The other half of the athletes were first given the placebo for two weeks, allowed to rest for three and a half weeks, and then given the PS for two weeks. The three-and-a-half-week rest period was to give the PS time to wash out of the athletes' systems.

Fifteen minutes after the eighth workout, the point at which overtraining was at its peak, blood samples were taken, and the cortisol levels were found to be 20-percent lower in the individuals taking the PS. Also, the individuals taking the PS did not have suppressed testosterone levels, whereas the individuals not taking PS had 20-percent drops in their levels of this important anabolic hormone. The exit interviews showed that the subjects taking the PS felt better and that their perceived exertion (how difficult they perceived the exercise session to be) also dropped.

Blood samples taken twenty-four hours after the workouts provided additional information about cortisol and exercise. Overtraining did not affect the long-term elevation of the cortisol levels in either group. This part of the study suggested that individuals may reach homeostasis during the twenty-four hours after intensive training and that intensive training does not cause an extended increase in the cortisol level. Dr. Fahey's research suggested that up to 800 milligrams of PS will be effective at suppressing cortisol and reducing muscle soreness.

Reducing cortisol to the degree accomplished in these studies could dramatically improve the way athletes train and use supplements for recovery. After an intensive workout, rather than suffering from high cortisol levels and muscle breakdown, athletes could use PS to shorten their recovery time and decrease their muscle soreness. Because cortisol can halt protein synthesis, PS may increase athletes' postworkout absorption of amino acids. In other words, PS may improve the effectiveness of the carbohydrate and protein-powder drinks used in athletes' recovery programs, perhaps making these supplements as effective as they were originally designed to be.

Dosing and Safety

PS is not found in many foods. According to rough estimates, all the PS coming into the body from food sources (mostly from meat) amounts to barely 80 milligrams per day, while the clinical doses are in the range of 200 to 500 milligrams per day. In addition, the body can make PS only through a complex series of reactions, with a high energy cost to the body. Because of this, PS is sometimes referred to as a "semi-essential" nutrient—that is, a nutrient the body cannot make in sufficient amounts when under stress or during periods of intensive training.

Recent breakthroughs in technology have allowed PS to be made available commercially in a concentrated form. Until recently, vegetable-derived phospholipids such as lecithin contained PS only in trace amounts. Concentrated PS was available just as a bovine-derived product with potential safety problems, now outmoded because of the danger of mad-cow disease. The new, concentrated PS is derived from soybeans and is a safe, effective source of PS.

Safety and toxicology studies have shown that PS is safe. A large clinical study reported that PS has a remarkable lack of side effects. PS has been proven safe in standard toxicology tests; dogs, for example, survived oral dosages of 70 grams per day for one year. Out of the large number of human studies conducted with PS has come a flawless safety record. The new, concentrated form of PS derived from soy phospholipids has a history of safe use in dietary supplements and foods.

Since PS is a nutrient that is not found readily in common foods, supplementation with concentrated PS should prove welcome to athletes in intensive training. When used in combination with a proper diet, concentrated PS taken in dosages of 400 to 800 milligrams daily should be prudent and well advised for athletes in intensive training. There is no indication of potential problems from long-term supplementation with PS.

Profile Protein Substrate

Profile Protein Substrate is a product developed for GNC based on over twenty years of scientific studies by the world's leading expert on muscle-protein metabolism, Robert Wolfe, PhD, of the University of Texas at Galveston. The purpose of Profile Protein Substrate is to supply the most important amino acids used to make the skeletal muscles. Furthermore, these amino acids are provided in a combination, or profile, that accurately reflects the way the body uses them to synthesize these muscles.

The science of muscle development is no longer limited to just making protein available to the muscles in the hopes of supporting muscle development. Today, science has evolved to such a level of sophistication that we know which amino acids at what specific levels and in which specific combinations must be provided. Because Profile reflects the amino-acid profile of skeletal muscle, it promotes a significantly higher rate of muscle synthesis and improved muscle strength. The net result, when using the optimum intake level, is a more effective muscle gain. In fact, scientific studies conducted by Dr. Wolfe and his associates have shown that when Profile is taken as directed, it is more effective than 100 grams of protein. This formulation is so effective and unique that patents have been developed, and exclusive manufacturing rights are now in place.

Profile couples the anabolic action of amino acids with the direct stimulatory effect of insulin. This combination results in maximum stimulation of muscle-protein synthesis. When other protein supplements are taken after a workout, some of the amino acids may stimulate the effects of exercise on muscle synthesis. These effects are limited, however, since any excess amino acids consumed will be excreted as urea, as well as increase the excretion of calcium. By selecting the right amino acids, in the right combination and levels, Profile specifically and maximally stimulates protein synthesis. Additionally, the specific combination of amino acids promotes an increased availability of amino acids in the blood. Profile actually increases the blood flow to the muscles.

In addition to muscle synthesis, the combination of amino acids in Profile stimulates an increase in the body's hormones, which act to directly increase the synthesis of skeletal-muscle tissue. This synergistic effect results in a 50-percent gain in muscle synthesis compared to the individual effect of each response. Profile is able to stimulate the uptake of amino acids into the muscle tissue while also increasing the efficiency with which the amino acids can be made into skeletal muscles—and it does so even more effectively than whey protein.

While Profile clearly increases muscle synthesis, it has the additional benefit of supporting the rebuilding of the muscle-glycogen stores following exercise. Not only does it increase muscle synthesis, it also helps make sure that the working muscles have the needed energy reserves to continue working. This effect is a result of Profile's ability to increase the blood flow to the muscles. The increased blood flow improves the delivery of energy reserves to the muscle, plus facilitates the removal of waste products, which are produced during intensive exercise.

Additional studies are currently underway testing the use of Profile to avoid muscle atrophy in the elderly. The preliminary results look promising. This is a potentially important benefit for senior citizens who are unable to consume nutritionally sound diets.

In summary, Profile is a unique, proprietary formulation supported by a number of scientific studies and endorsed by the world's leading expert in protein metabolism. This product currently may prove more effective than any others at building muscles, avoiding fatigue and overtraining, and supporting resynthesis of the energy reserves. No other product on the market at this time can provide this demonstrated level of nutritional support for athletes.

Tribulus Terrestris
Until the September 1996 issue of *Muscle & Fitness,* very few Americans knew of puncture vine, more commonly known by its Latin name, *Tribulus terrestris.* Used by Eastern European Olympic and world-champion strength and power athletes since the mid-1990s, the herb is purported to enhance muscle mass by increasing testosterone production. Even today, only a small group of scientists, herbalists, and doctors trained in Oriental and Ayurvedic medicine know of the plant, and little research has been conducted on it. Nonetheless, it is increasingly popular among athletes.

The arguments for the herb's effectiveness are largely based on its traditional uses. The ancient Greeks employed it as a diuretic, mild laxative, and general tonic. Ayurvedic physicians have long valued the plant for its diuretic and aphrodisiac properties, and include it in rejuvenative formulations for treating sexual deficiencies. In China, the herb is frequently used to treat a variety of diseases affecting the liver, kidneys, urinary tract (including urinary stones), and cardiovascular system.

Cross-culturally, tribulus is most often used to treat infertility in women, and impotence and libido problems in both sexes. It was the search for safe, nonhormonal treatments for infertility and other reproductive disorders that inspired scientists at the Chemical Pharmaceutical Research Institute, in Sofia, Bulgaria, to investigate tribulus over two decades ago, based on its seemingly successful historical use.

Early Studies

Reports and articles by supplement companies state that tribulus boosts the blood level of luteinizing hormone, a pituitary hormone responsible for regulating the testosterone level. Luteinizing hormone actually "turns on" natural testosterone production in humans. The supplement companies are also promoting tribulus's ability to decrease fatigue, basing these claims on some rather weak science.

Indian researchers investigated the tonic effects of tribulus in 1993. They used a preparation of tribulus to treat fifty male and female subjects who complained of fatigue and a lack of interest in performing their daily activities. The results showed a 45-percent improvement in symptoms for the group after taking the herb. This study was a clinical trial, with all the subjects receiving the tribulus and the changes measured through a series of clinical tests.

Another study, reported by Dr. J. Wright in *Muscle & Fitness,* involved a group of men suffering from impotence and infertility. The subjects were given a standardized extract of tribulus, administered for thirty to sixty days in doses ranging from 750 to 1,500 milligrams per day. The article reported that the subjects' testosterone levels were increased and libidos improved. However, nothing was reported regarding increased muscle mass or strength.

These two early chemistry and pharmacology studies, as well as reports in layman's magazines, suggested that tribulus might have clinical applications, and in as early as 1981, Eastern European pharmaceutical companies released standardized tribulus preparations for treating various sexual disorders. However, it should be noted that the two studies, reported in European scientific journals and layman's articles, should be viewed with caution. A couple of vague studies don't qualify as extensive research, and these studies don't speak to improved muscle mass or muscular strength.

Plant Chemistry

Tribulus is an attractive sports supplement because it contains steroid saponins such as terrestrosins, dioscin, gracillin, kikuba saponin, protodioscin, neohecogenin glucoside, and tribulosin. These saponins may be responsible for the aphrodisiac properties of tribulus, according to a report by Dr. W. Yan in the journal *Phytochemistry* in 1996. Several steroidal sapogenins and three flavonoid glycosides also have been isolated from the tribulus plant.

Tribulus on Trial

Some supplement-company researchers are beginning to wonder if the increase in testosterone produced in the aforementioned studies and reports is significant. Would this increase have either an acute or long-term impact upon muscle mass? In addition, it isn't clear how long the serum testosterone was elevated and how much variation in elevation there was among the subjects—that is, did some men have large increases, while others had just small increases? Or, did all the subjects enjoy the same increase?

Unless an individual reaches pharmacological, or above-normal, levels of serum testosterone, the increase in the testosterone level after taking tribulus may not mean anything. It has also been shown that serum testosterone levels rise after an intensive power workout or weight session in the gym. Tribulus may not have the physiological punch to have a significant, long-term effect on the testosterone level. To get around this enormous obstacle, manufacturers are combining tribulus with other hormones that purportedly enhance testosterone production.

Do DHEA and Androstenedione Help?

DHEA and androstenedione are promoted as testosterone enhancers, but they work differently than tribulus. Both DHEA and androstenedione provide the raw material for testosterone formation, while tribulus purportedly increases the level of luteinizing hormone and therefore may affect testosterone production.

Assuming that a combination of the three will work better than any one ingredient on its own, several supplement companies are producing "stacked" products—that is, products that combine DHEA, androstenedione, and tribulus. They claim that the testosterone-related effects of each of these substances have been studied separately, and all have been shown to potentiate testosterone production to a varying degree and by various mechanisms. This is a stretch of science by the supplement companies selling these products, since there is currently no research on stacked products in the scientific literature. Whether stacked products yield better results remains to be seen.

DHEA and androstenedione are potent male hormones, and customers should be cautious about using them. Anyone taking either DHEA or androstenedione should have regular blood tests and discuss their therapy with their healthcare provider. The assumption that DHEA, androstenedione, and tribulus are effective aids for bodybuilding and fitness training is, at this point, sheer speculation. Additional studies are needed before the use of tribulus terrestris—and, for that matter, DHEA and androstenedione—can be recommended for improved athletic performance.

Dosing and Safety

No significant adverse effects have been noted in any of the clinical trials or human research studies on tribulus. Toxicity has been extremely low in both acute and long-term animal studies in which rats were given more than 10 grams of tribulus for every 1 kilogram of body weight, as reported by C.A.B. Enterprises, an importer of the herb. No negative effects have been reported by people using tribulus. However, neither children nor women who are pregnant or lactating should use this product, since it has the potential to significantly alter hormonal chemistry. Men with enlarged prostates or other medical conditions also should not take the herb without first consulting a physician.

Dr. James Wright, in an article in *Muscle & Fitness,* said that a reasonable intake of tribulus is 250 to 750 milligrams a day, taken in divided doses with meals. Try to find tribulus standardized to provide 40-percent furostanol saponins, which is considered the active ingredient in the herb.

What's the bottom line? Despite the anecdotes of athletes, there is no conclusive evidence that tribulus enhances muscle growth. For now, its use is merely a fad. More research must be conducted on healthy people who have no libido or hormonal problems to see if tribulus truly affects the muscle tissue. It must be evaluated alone and in combination with other supplements. And finally, the study results must be published in peer-reviewed journals, not in layman's magazines.

There is no substitute for scientific data—something to remember when buying sports supplements.

(For more on tribulus terrestris, see page 152.)

TRENDS FOR THE FUTURE

12

As we enter the new millennium, the scientific community has a whole new batch of products under investigation. Many companies are looking for the next "super supplement," the one that will be as successful as creatine. A number of products with the potential to improve athletic appearance that may reach the market will be discussed in this chapter. These products with promise include huperzine A, lactic-acid clearance products, rhodiola, ribose, and 7-keto dehydroepiandrosterone (7-keto DHEA).

Only time will tell if any of these products becomes a hot-selling supplement that stands the test of time. Only time will tell if any of these products survives the scientific community's scrutiny and athletes' perception of improved performance. All of these factors play a role in a supplement's success.

Huperzine A

Huperzine A is a natural compound isolated from the club moss, *Huperzia serrata*. It is a Chinese folk medicine, called *qian ceng ta,* and has been used for centuries to improve memory, focus, and concentration, and to help alleviate memory problems in the elderly. Reports from China, where an estimated 100,000 people have been treated with the compound, indicate that huperzine A is safe and effective. In addition to its effects on memory, huperzine A seems to protect the nerve cells from toxic substances and from the damage generally caused by strokes and epilepsy. It is also used to treat Alzheimer's disease and myasthenia gravis. Based on laboratory studies, some researchers believe that huperzine A may additionally serve as an ergogenic aid by improving muscle performance and reducing fatigue.

Huperzine A and Muscle Contraction

Huperzine A has been shown to increase skeletal-muscle contractions in rats. It has also been clinically shown to significantly improve muscle weakness, as well as to boost memory in patients with impaired memory. Because it prevents the selective degeneration of the acetylcholine-producing neurons in the brain plus enhances the availability of acetylcholine in the brains of patients suffering from neurological disorders such as Alzheimer's dementia, huperzine A also improves the functioning of the connections between the nerves and muscles. This improvement in neuromuscular transmission leads to an improvement in the general condition of the patient.

Huperzine A and Myasthenia Gravis

In a clinical trial conducted by Y. S. Cheng and his associates in China in 1986, huperzine A was shown to significantly improve the muscle weakness associated with myasthenia gravis. Myasthenia gravis is a neuromuscular disease characterized by weakness and marked fatigability of the skeletal muscles. The defect caused by the disease involves the nerve transmission at the neuromuscular junctions, the areas in the body where the nerves meet the muscles. When a nerve "fires" and activates a muscle at a neuromuscular junction, the muscle should contract, or move. Although patients with myasthenia gravis can move their muscles initially, they cannot maintain muscle movement, since repeated activation of the muscles causes diminished responses.

Acetylcholine is a neurotransmitter that is essential for normal learning and memory, as well as for muscle contractions. Neurotransmitters carry chemical messages from one nerve cell (the presynaptic nerve) to another, causing the receiving neuron (the postsynaptic nerve) to fire its neurotransmitters. Because the nerve cells are close together, separated only by a miniscule space called a "synaptic cleft," the released neurotransmitter, such as acetylcholine, will activate the next cell in the sequence. It will bind to a receptor on the postsynaptic nerve.

In human and animal brains and muscle cells, the enzyme acetylcholinesterase (AChE) normally breaks down acetylcholine, keeping it from repeatedly firing the nerve and thus regulating the availability of this neurotransmitter at the receptor site. Acetylcholine function is deficient in patients with memory impairment or Alzheimer's dementia, probably due to the selective degeneration of acetylcholine-producing neurons in the brain. It has been demonstrated in Alzheimer's patients that acetylcholinesterase inhibitors (AChE inhibitors) reduce the breakdown of acetylcholine and thus increase its availability. This can conceivably lead to an improvement in the patient's condition. Huperzine A is a potent AChE inhibitor and thus helps to increase the levels of acetycholine in the brain and muscles.

AChE inhibitors, by keeping the acetylcholine level high, can increase muscle response. Dr. Cheng and his associates also compared the clinical effects of huperzine A to those of prostigmine, another AChE inhibitor. The 128 patients with myasthenia gravis experienced as good an improvement with huperzine A as has been shown in the scientific literature for prostigmine. The duration of the action of the huperzine A was about seven hours.

Sports Applications of Huperzine A

Several supplement manufacturers are looking at huperzine A as a potential product for increasing muscular performance and reducing muscular fatigue. Currently, however, dosing recommendations still need to be established.

Lactic-Acid-Clearance Products   Lactic-acid (lactate) buildup and its effects on exercise capacity is a training issue faced almost universally by

athletes. Lactic-acid buildup causes muscle soreness and stiffness, and results in decreased performance and endurance. Products that help clear lactic acid from the system thus would be a boon to athletes and, in fact, may be a developing trend—the first such product, 2nd Wind by Metaflex, has already hit store shelves.

Lactic acid is constantly produced at all levels of exercise intensity—and even while at rest—but little appears in the bloodstream at rest or at low-intensity exercise. This is because, under aerobic conditions, lactic acid is readily metabolized by the muscle cells. As you exercise harder, however, your body is less and less able to metabolize lactic acid, and it builds up in your system. The fitter you are aerobically, the harder you are able to exercise before your body goes into oxygen debt, which is when the muscles draw fuel from anaerobic (nonoxygen) energy sources. This is when the lactic acid starts to build up. When the lactic-acid buildup reaches its maximum capacity, the muscles stop working.

A normal resting blood-lactate level is less than 2.0 milliliters per liter of blood. Exercise scientists use blood measurements because they are easy to do. They are an indirect but reliable indication of the lactate level in the muscle cells.

As the intensity of the exercise effort is increased, progressively more and more lactic acid is produced than can be metabolized within the muscle cells, and the excess diffuses into the bloodstream. This increasing accumulation of lactic acid in the muscles causes pain and fatigue. During high-intensity exercise at maximum levels, the lactic acid accumulates rapidly in the muscles, fatigue sets in quickly, and the blood levels of lactic acid climb rapidly. If the high exercise intensity is maintained, a maximum level of lactic acid is reached. The tolerance to high levels of lactic acid varies from individual to individual and increases with training.

Lactic acid is often called a waste product. It isn't. Lactic acid is neither wasted nor excreted by the body. It is chemically processed and converted into other compounds. Contrary to popular belief, lactic acid is itself a fuel for the production of energy.

Lactic acid produced in muscle cells has several fates. Some of it is used as a fuel in the muscle cell in which it is produced. A significant portion diffuses out of the cell and is shuttled to other tissues that have an affinity for it and can more easily convert it into a usable energy source. These tissues include the liver, kidneys, heart, and other inactive muscle tissues. The heart is exceptionally efficient at processing lactic acid and converts large quantities of it into fuel for cardiac contraction.

It is well known, however, that the accumulation of lactic acid in muscle cells will hinder and eventually inhibit exercise performance. This is due to lactic acid's characteristics as a weak acid. In a muscle cell's water medium, the lactic acid ionizes (gives off hydrogen ions) and increases the cell's acidity. This inhibits the cell's ability to break down carbohydrates and fat into energy. Therefore, it is the acidic property of lactic acid, not the lactic acid itself, that causes the decline in exercise.

Benefits of Lactic-Acid Clearance

One of the biggest problems faced by athletes is designing a training program that uses lactic acid more efficiently or finding a way to help clear lactic acid more effectively from the muscle cells and blood system. Faster clearance of lactic acid from the blood following exercise indicates enhanced energy production. This enables:

☐ Faster recovery of the muscle tissue, allowing for continued energy production and increased work and exercise performance.

☐ Increased exercise capacity and more intensive training sessions due to shortened recovery periods.

☐ Increased use of lactic acid as a fuel, conserving the other energy sources, such as glycogen, for extended exercise performance.

Additionally, speeding the clearance of lactic acid from the muscles may help reduce postexercise muscle soreness and fatigue.

Research on Lactic-Acid-Clearance Products

Recently, a peer-reviewed study was performed on 2nd Wind, a special blend of herbs, at the Sports Research Institute at Beijing Medical University. The study subjects were twenty male first-year university students, who were randomly divided into two groups. Group A was given 1,000 milligrams of a placebo each morning, while group B was given 1,000 milligrams of the herbal formulation each morning. The capsules were given to the subjects on a double-blind basis under the direct observation of a laboratory assistant. The treatment was continued for two weeks for both groups, and for an additional two weeks for group B. (After the first two weeks, the study was "unblinded.")

An exercise-challenge test using a treadmill programmed to be increasingly difficult was the exercise protocol in the study. The subjects exercised for fifteen minutes at a workload level that doubled their resting heart rates. The subjects performed the test before ingesting the supplement or placebo, after two weeks of treatment with either the supplement or placebo, and, in the case of group B, after four weeks of treatment with the supplement.

The subjects' lactic-acid levels were measured from blood samples taken from their earlobes thirty minutes before exercising for the resting level, immediately upon finishing the exercise for the maximum level, and fifteen minutes after finishing the exercise for the end-point reading.

The results of this trial revealed that 2nd Wind produced a statistically significant improvement in lactic-acid clearance after the exercise was stopped, as well as a trend of increasingly better lactic-acid clearance the longer the product was taken. The lactic-acid-clearance levels in the supplement group after four weeks were more than 200 percent of the levels at the beginning of the trial, before taking the product. The two-week levels were 180 percent of the beginning levels. In the placebo group, the rate of lactic-acid clearance actually declined over the test period. One benefit of having a placebo group in this study was that the normal variations and changes in lactic-acid clearance could be assessed, and more weight given to the improvements seen in the supplement group.

Safety of Lactic-Acid-Clearance Products

The ingredients in 2nd Wind include herbal extracts and mushrooms that have been used in natural medicines in China for centuries. The researchers in the aforementioned study suggested that long-term daily intake of this formulation would produce optimum results. Therefore, in order to develop additional safety data on the formulation, the liver enzymes of the study subjects taking the supplement were evaluated. No negative side effects could be detected. The research team also asked the study participants about subjective side effects, and no one reported any.

Sports Applications of Lactic-Acid-Clearance Products

As noted earlier, increased lactic-acid clearance can significantly improve muscle performance and lead to reduced muscle soreness. The research on using a formulation of herbal extracts and mushrooms to help clear lactic acid from the system is very promising, indicating that natural products may be available that can be used by athletes in conjunction with various training methods to improve their training and athletic performance. Simply put, 2nd Wind is an all-natural sports supplement that improves the lactic-acid-clearance mechanism and helps lactic acid to be converted into a fuel that can be used quickly by the body during exercise or recovery.

Rhodiola

A native of Russian and Asian territories, rhodiola is an alpine plant growing 2,000 to 3,400 miles above sea level. *Rhodiola rosea,* also known as golden root and arctic root, is one of the most fascinating plant species in the world. Until recently, it was largely unknown in the United States, possibly due to the fact that, because of its extraordinary medicinal benefits, the places where it grew were always kept secret.

Although rhodiola has been used in folk medicine for more than 3,000 years, serious scientific research on it was not started until 1945. Soviet scientists from the USSR Academy of Sciences reported that extracts from the Siberian indigenous plant helped to increase the body's natural resistance to environmental stresses. In the early 1990s, after many years of research and the fall of the Communist system, information on the extraordinary benefits of rhodiola was finally released from the Soviet Union.

Many scientists feel that rhodiola is not just another adaptogen. This is because it possesses several unique properties. Its most active phytochemicals are the phenylpropanoids, with the most important being salidrosid, rosavin, rhodiolin, rosarin, and rosin. These chemical constituents have been shown to have performance-enhancing applications.

Rhodiola, Performance, and Endurance

Adaptogens can help provide the foundation on which an energy reserve is built for use by the body when it needs it the most—under extreme physical conditions and during recovery from fatigue. Test subjects administered adaptogenic extracts displayed improved indicators of energy and endurance, and athletes were able to greatly improve their athletic endeavors.

In one study, it was shown that rhodiola extract increased the activity of proteolic enzymes and also significantly increased the levels of protein and RNA in the skeletal muscles. In another study, it was revealed that when *Eleutherococcus, Rhaponticurn carthamoides,* and rhodiola were administered to people performing physical labor, all the test subjects showed improvements in their general, physical, and mental states. They also displayed improvements in their functional indicators (pulse, arterial pressure, vital capacity, back-muscle strength, hand endurance, and coordination of movement) and reductions in the duration of their recovery periods. In yet another study, ingesting rhodiola extract for three weeks prior to demanding, prolonged, and tense mental activity was found to prevent mental burnout in students, doctors, and scientific workers aged nineteen to forty-six years old.

Rhodiola has been shown to increase the amount of the basic beta-endorphin in the blood plasma that helps prevent the hormonal changes indicative of stress. In addition, it has been observed to enhance memorization and concentration for prolonged periods. For example, after ingesting rhodiola, test subjects showed an 88-percent decrease in the quantity of mistakes on proofreading tests in comparison to a control group.

Sports Applications of Rhodiola

Look for rhodiola to appear in multi-adaptogen formulas intended to help improve mental performance and adaptation to stress. Time will tell if it is as effective as other adaptogens at increasing exercise performance.

Ribose
To stay healthy and active, to keep your heart functioning properly, and to maintain peak levels of muscle performance, you need to keep your pool of adenosine triphosphate (ATP) at its highest possible level. This pool of ATP is absolutely vital for your heart and skeletal muscles to have all the energy they need to provide maximum strength and endurance.

Researchers have learned that a simple sugar, ribose, stimulates the body's production of ATP. In fact, ribose is the essential molecule required to make ATP and to maintain high levels of it in the heart and skeletal muscles. Whether you are young or old, healthy or ill, a serious athletic competitor, a weekend athlete, or just concerned about your normal well-being, you should understand the role of ATP in your body and its contribution to your health, fitness, and well-being.

A Natural Sugar

When you exercise, some of the ATP that your body uses for energy is lost from your cells and must be replaced. Ribose is the only compound the body uses as a starting point to replace these energy-producing molecules. However, ribose production in the heart and skeletal muscles is a slow process and cannot keep up with the loss of energy during ischemia (insufficient blood flow) or strenuous, intensive exercise. Under normal conditions, it may take several days to completely replace the energy molecules that are lost due to ischemia or intensive exercise.

While it is not important to understand all of the complicated biochemistry that is involved, you should know that supplemental ribose bypasses the slow, rate-limiting steps the body uses to make ribose from glucose. Supplemental ribose can be directly applied to rebuilding the energy-producing molecules as they are used up by the cells. As a result, your body can quickly rebuild its energy supply, making it available for peak performance.

While all living cells contain ribose, there is not enough in food to get the beneficial effects needed to keep the energy level high during strenuous exercise or ischemia. Most of the ribose in meat is lost during cooking. In fact, ribose reacting with amino acids initiates the chemical process that turns meat brown and gives it its characteristic aroma and flavor when cooked.

Although ribose is found naturally in all the cells of the body, the heart and the skeletal muscles cannot make it very quickly. During times of metabolic stress, such as strenuous exercise or diminished blood flow, the cells are not even able to form enough ribose to replace nucleotides as they are used. Nucleotides are compounds such as ATP that form the basic constituent of DNA and RNA. Furthermore, there is no known food source that supplies a sufficient amount of ribose to be metabolically significant. Therefore, ribose supplementation is essential to quickly replace the ATP, adenosine diphosphate (ADP), and adenosine monophosphate (AMP) used by the cells.

Loss of Nucleotides

Although our heart and muscle cells have developed very elaborate mechanisms for forming, recycling, and conserving energy-producing molecules, they are not always successful at keeping sufficient levels of ATP, ADP, and AMP available. Both intensive exercise and ischemia can cause significant losses of nucleotides, leaving the cells starving for energy. Obviously, when this happens, the functioning of the cells may be compromised. If you are a weight lifter, you may not be able to generate the powerful contractions you need to lift your barbell, and the weight you lifted only a day or two ago may be impossible to move today. Your heart may not pump enough blood to supply your tissues with adequate amounts of oxygen.

When exercising at maximum capacity, there is a substantial decrease in the total stores of ATP, ADP, and AMP in the skeletal-muscle cells. In fact, research has shown that decreases in these nucleotides can be as much as 20 percent to 28 percent after periods of high-intensity exercise. Both the fast-twitch and slow-twitch muscle fibers use ATP for energy to contract. During strenuous exercise, the ATP is broken down rapidly, causing AMP to build up in the cell. Some, but not all, of the AMP formed by either the fast-twitch or slow-twitch fibers can be converted to other compounds that give the cell the ability to conserve energy-producing molecules to continue to fuel its work. A substantial portion of the AMP, however, is broken down and washed out of the cell. It is this breakdown of AMP, and the loss of the breakdown products, that depletes the cell of its energy-producing compounds.

Nucleotide Loss During Exercise

Is the amount of ATP, ADP, and AMP lost during exercise really significant? The simple answer to that question is *yes!*

The skeletal muscles are very efficient at conserving energy. However, when they are called upon to perform exercise at maximum capacity, the number of energy-producing and energy-conserving molecules that are lost can be significant. As long as there is a sufficient amount of oxygen present for aerobic metabolism, muscle cells are able to recycle energy virtually without losing any adenine nucleotides. Nevertheless, during periods of extremely intensive exercise, when there is not enough oxygen present in the bloodstream to fulfill the demands of the cells, a large percentage of the total pool of ATP, ADP, and AMP can be lost.

A considerable amount of research has been done to show that the losses of adenine nucleotides by the skeletal muscles can be severe during periods of intensive exercise or ischemia. One very important study was performed at the Karolinska Institute in Stockholm, Sweden, one of the foremost centers for skeletal-muscle research in the world. In this study, eleven healthy male volunteers underwent six weeks of high-intensity training three times a week, followed by one week of two training sessions a day. A second group of nine healthy volunteers rested for the first six weeks, but trained twice a day along with the first group during the final week. A small amount of muscle tissue was taken from the thigh of each of the subjects to analyze the amount of adenine nucleotides present following these periods of exercise and during the three days following the final day of training. Muscle-tissue samples were also taken before the exercise was begun as a point of comparison.

This research showed that the ATP levels in the thigh muscles of the first group dropped 13 percent during the six weeks of training. The ATP levels in the muscle tissues of this group did not go down further during the final week of training. This indicates that, after a period of intensive exercise, ATP, ADP, and AMP all dropped to well below their pretraining levels. More significant, however, is the fact that, even after the three days of rest following the last exercise session, the ATP levels in this first group still did not recover to the pretraining levels. In fact, the ATP in the muscle cells of these subjects was still almost 10-percent below the pretraining levels. In other words, even after the three-day rest period, the thigh muscles were not able to fully replace their lost ATP.

In the second group, the results were even more dramatic. This group did not have a period of training before beginning the high-intensity exercise in the final week. In fact, the members of this group went from being sedentary to performing two exercise sessions a day for one week. In this group, the ATP levels in the thigh muscles dropped by 25 percent immediately after the last exercise session. Even after three days of rest, this group still had ATP pools that were 19.5 percent less than they were initially. This means that the total energy currency in the thigh muscles of this group dropped by 25 percent after the intensive exercise and was still almost 20-percent lower than normal even after three days of rest.

These dramatic results show that the cells lose their energy-producing compounds during exercise and do not recover even after three days of rest. In their paper, the researchers concluded that "repeated high-intensity intermittent exercise caused a decrease in resting levels of skeletal muscle adenine nucleotides [ATP]." They added, "The decrease was greater when exercise was more frequently repeated."

In a similar study, a group of researchers from Victoria University in Australia showed that, after seven weeks of sprint training, thigh-muscle ATP levels fell by 19 percent. These researchers concluded that, because of exercise, these muscle cells lost the molecules necessary to recharge their energy.

Dosage Recommendations for Ribose

On average, the human body contains 1.6 milligrams of ribose in every 100 milliliters of blood at any given time. Some people do not have any free ribose in their blood, while others have as much as 3.6 milligrams per 100 milliliters. There are no foods that provide enough ribose to be helpful. Of course, since all living cells contain ribose, we do take in a small amount whenever we eat. However, taking ribose as a dietary supplement is required to rapidly increase the level of ribose in the blood to make it available to the cells to build up the stores of 5-phosphoribosyl-1-pyrophosphate (PRPP). PRPP is the compound that is the starting point for the production of the energy-producing compounds in the heart and skeletal muscles. When taken as a supplement, ribose is absorbed very quickly into the blood, with much of the absorption occurring before the ribose is even swallowed.

Research has shown that about 3 to 5 grams of ribose taken every day should put enough in the bloodstream to ensure that the heart and skeletal-muscle cells have an adequate supply. Serious athletes and people concerned about their circulation may want to take more. In fact, these people may require 10 grams or more per day. A good course of action would be to start out with about 5 grams of ribose per day. If you feel you need more, increase your dosage by about 2 to 3 grams per day. However, do not take more than 15 to 20 grams per day. If you are in serious physical training or have concerns about the circulation to your heart or extremities, you may want to take up to 10 grams per day to start. If you are not in training but just want to maintain healthy levels of energy in your heart and skeletal muscles, 3 to 5 grams per day should be an adequate maintenance dose.

Taking this amount of ribose will ensure that all of your heart and skeletal-muscle cells are able to get enough of the compound to maintain peak levels of PRPP and energy. Ribose must circulate in the blood for several minutes to give all the cells an opportunity to take it in. If there is ribose left over after all the cells have absorbed their share, it is either converted to glucose or passed in the urine.

If your muscles become sore or cramped after even mild exercise, you may want to modify your supplementation regimen. Try taking 10 grams of ribose before beginning any physical exercise and then supplementing with additional doses of 4 grams every thirty minutes during and then at the conclusion of the exercise. If this works, you can cut back the amount of ribose you take until you find your proper individual dosage level.

Safety of Ribose

Scientific research with ribose has been going on for several years. In some of these studies, very high doses of ribose are being administered. In one study, Dr. Wolfgang Pliml, a cardiologist at the University of Munich, Germany, gave ribose to patients with severe coronary artery disease in doses of 60 grams per day for three days. In these patients, there were no lasting side effects. In still another study, ribose was given in 60-gram doses for seven days to patients with a skeletal-muscle-enzyme disorder called myoadenylate deaminase deficiency disease (MADD). Some of the patients taking these very high doses developed minor cases of diarrhea, while others had occasional mild and asymptomatic hypoglycemia. In a third study, which went on for over one year, ribose was given to a patient with MADD in doses of 60 grams per day without side effects. This study reported that doses of up to 50 or 60 grams per day could be well tolerated.

It should be noted, however, that the first two studies just mentioned using high doses of ribose were short in duration. The third study cited went on for over one year, but there was only one patient involved. There have not been any long-term studies with large numbers of subjects done to really determine what the effects of large doses of ribose might be over a long period of time. However, there is no reason to think that there should be a problem. Ribose is a natural sugar produced by the body that is easily excreted in the urine if there is too much in the blood. Certainly, in the doses thus far discussed, there should be no noticeable side effects.

Sports Applications of Ribose

If you are a serious competitor or a hard-charging weekend athlete, ribose might be beneficial. Athletes' hearts and skeletal muscles use energy faster than it can be replaced. Ribose is effective at rebuilding these critical energy stores to keep the heart and skeletal muscles at their peak.

No one can say, however, that taking ribose will definitely make you feel more energetic. Nor can anyone say that your athletic performance will improve. The scientific evidence is clear, however, that ribose will help your heart and skeletal-muscle cells maintain their energy charge and normal function, and that taking ribose before, during, and after periods of high-intensity exercise will increase your exercise effectiveness.

7-keto Dehydroepiandrosterone (7-keto DHEA)

During the past few years, many individuals have taken DHEA for a variety of reasons—primarily to fight the effects of aging, but also to bolster the immune system, build muscle, and enhance memory. Now, there is 7-keto dehydroepiandrosterone (7-keto DHEA), a natural derivative of DHEA that is more potent than DHEA and is found in all our bodies. But, unlike DHEA, 7-keto

DHEA will not convert to testosterone or estrogen, which is especially good news for women. While 7-keto DHEA may not be looked upon as a testosterone builder, it may help athletes to protect their immune systems and lose weight.

Benefits and Risks Associated With DHEA

Research has documented many health benefits from DHEA supplementation, including an increased life span, improved immune system, greater insulin sensitivity, and prevention of atherosclerosis. Additionally, some recent research has shown that DHEA accelerates weight loss and leads to higher blood-DHEA levels correlated to higher HDL levels.

The problem with DHEA, if there is one, is that taking it "in high doses or for long periods of time will result in a higher incidence of adverse reactions," according to John Zenk, MD, in his book *BoomerAge*. You also risk the androgenic-related side effects when taking higher doses.

Unlike DHEA, 7-keto DHEA is not converted to testosterone or estrogen in the body. The National Institute of Aging last year warned against the excessive use of DHEA because high blood levels of testosterone can increase prostate-cancer growth in men and high levels of estrogen can speed up the growth of breast cancer in women.

A Scientific Solution

A derivative of DHEA that is more potent and has the same therapeutic benefit but none of the adverse side effects would clearly be an answer to this problem. This derivative would allow individuals to essentially take a higher dosage of DHEA for a longer period of time and not have to worry about the adverse side effects of virilization, prostate enlargement, and cancer. As Dr. Zenk noted in his book, many people in the medical community have pointed out that, in order to receive the health benefits of DHEA, you must take DHEA for a long time and probably at a high dosage level.

The other reason that derivatives of naturally occurring substances are important is the action of hormones in the body. In order to be classified as a hormone, a substance must have a receptor on a target tissue somewhere in the body. DHEA, as a parent compound, does not have its own receptor. Therefore, for DHEA to have an action in our bodies, which it clearly does, it must have the action via a metabolite or a derivative of the parent compound that does have a receptor.

Researchers such as Dr. Henry Lardy, professor emeritus of biological sciences at the University of Wisconsin in Madison, realized this long ago and have been actively searching for DHEA derivatives that are biologically more active but cannot be converted to sex steroids. Dr. Lardy is renowned for his research on DHEA derivatives.

Derivative Research

Dr. Lardy and his team have isolated over 150 DHEA derivatives. In the process of isolating these derivatives, they have found one compound to clearly stand out because it provides greater benefits than DHEA but does not exhibit the unwanted side effects. This derivative is 7-keto DHEA.

According to Dr. Lardy, 7-keto DHEA is more potent than its parent, DHEA, and cannot be metabolized to estrogen or testosterone, hence the fewer side effects. It is clearly much more beneficial than DHEA and can be taken long-term without the risk of serious side effects. Interestingly, 7-keto DHEA is also a naturally occurring substance and can be found in many of our body tissues. Like DHEA, 7-keto DHEA is associated with human functions supporting the immune system, increased thermogenesis, and improved memory.

The human body has many different enzymes that perform specific metabolic sequences. These enzymes react uniquely with the chemicals in our bodies to provide different end products. Certain enzymes within our bodies convert DHEA into three substances—7-keto, androgens (testosterone), and estrogens. Since 7-keto DHEA is a downstream metabolite, it cannot be converted into testosterone or estrogen.

Safety of 7-Keto DHEA

The safety of 7-keto DHEA has been evaluated in both preclinical studies and human clinical trials. The preclinical toxicology studies were quite favorable. These included a mutagenicity assay to demonstrate the effects of 7-keto DHEA on genetic material, an acute rat study, and an escalating-dose primate study to evaluate short- and long-term exposure and tolerance. These studies showed no mutagenic activity and no adverse effects connected with 7-keto DHEA taken in doses of up to 2,000 milligrams per kilogram of weight in rats and 500 milligrams per kilogram of weight in primates. It should be noted that 500 milligrams per kilogram of weight would be a dose of approximately 3.5 grams for the average 70-kilogram (150-pound) human, which is seventy times greater than the recommended daily dose of approximately 50 milligrams for humans.

A human clinical trial was also conducted to assess the effects of 7-keto DHEA on several endocrine and safety parameters in healthy adult men. The compound was found to be safe and well tolerated at doses of up to 200 milligrams per day for a twenty-eight-day period. It was found to lack the clinically significant hormone-elevating action reportedly possessed by DHEA.

Laboratory safety results also indicated that 7-keto DHEA did not affect hematology, serum chemistry, or urine values any differently than a placebo. In addition, 7-keto DHEA did not have any detrimental effects and may have had beneficial effects on vital signs and body weight.

The results of these preclinical and clinical safety trials indicate that 7-keto DHEA is a safe and well-tolerated DHEA metabolite that may potentially be used as a supplement for the myriad medical conditions for which DHEA is currently being used.

Efficacy Studies

Dr. Lardy has been the principal researcher investigating the effects of 7-keto DHEA. Based on his research, he has been granted several patents for uses of

DHEA derivatives, including to enhance and modulate immune function and weight loss.

Pilot animal studies conducted at the University of Wisconsin at Madison suggest that 7-keto DHEA can be used by persons infected with human immunodeficiency virus (HIV) to combat the chronic symptoms of the disease and boost the immune system. In the animal studies, the 7-keto DHEA increased T-cell counts five-fold to six-fold in primates chronically infected with simian immunodeficiency virus (SIV). T-cells are a type of lymphocyte made in bone marrow whose role is to fight viruses and some cancers. The test animals' levels of total white blood cells also increased, as did their total T-cell counts. Additionally, these SIV-infected primates demonstrated reversals in their disease-wasting, increases in weight, and improvements in overall behavior and overall clinical condition.

In a paper published in the *Annals of the New York Academy of Sciences* in 1995, Dr. Lardy and his associates described 7-keto DHEA as a compound that also activates thermogenic enzymes in the livers of rats. In fact, the induction potential of 7-keto DHEA seems to far exceed that of any of the other DHEA derivatives they tested, indicating an increased potency when compared to DHEA. Activation of these thermogenic enzymes is not only an effective assay for the activity of DHEA derivatives and a standard of activity for use when testing new compounds, it also causes animals to lose weight without an alteration in their food intake.

Sports Applications of 7-Keto DHEA

The initial data presented by Dr. Lardy and other researchers point to 7-keto DHEA being a potent immune-system stimulator, memory enhancer, and anti-obesity agent. Used long-term, it may ameliorate the effects of aging, which is good news for master's athletes. Since 7-keto DHEA is a safe second-generation DHEA derivative, it offers the potential of worry-free long-term use as a dietary supplement.

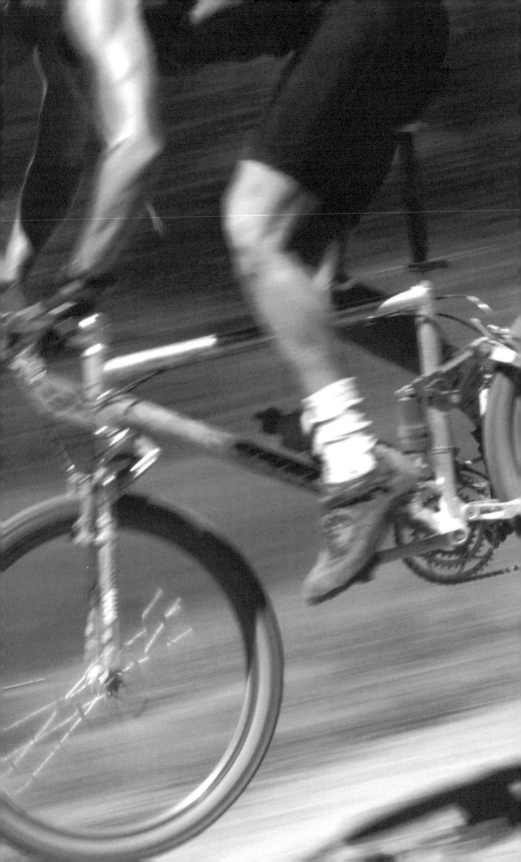

PART THREE

FACTS AND RESOURCES

Parts One and Two of *Avery's Sports Nutrition Almanac* presented detailed descriptions of individual nutrients and supplements, and their effects on athletic performance. Part Two additionally provided the winning nutritional and training programs of a number of accomplished athletes to guide you in designing your own program. Current and future trends in sports-performance enhancers were also detailed.

Part Three now pulls together the who-what-and-where of sports nutrition and offers it in one convenient package. Included is a biographical listing of who's really who in the field of sports nutrition to help you weed the true experts from the wannabe's—and the true expert information from the hype. A directory of addresses and phone numbers will help you track down sports-nutrition companies and websites for more information on specific products and topics. Finally, a dictionary of health and training terms defines key words and phrases, and a compendium of books and software, as well as a listing of reference sources, will point you toward helpful reading and viewing matter.

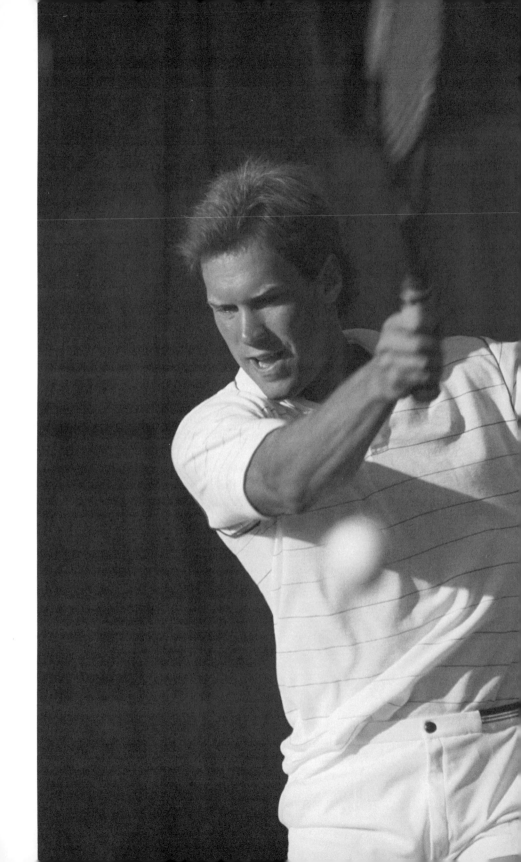

WHO'S REALLY WHO IN SPORTS NUTRITION

13

T he way athletes train, the way they eat, and the supplements they take are all the result of decades of effort by experts in human health, nutrition, sports nutrition, and physiology. Following is a listing of some of the people who have made significant contributions to these fields in the twentieth century. Some are scientists, some are the captains of industry, some are authors, and still others are the founders of important organizations. All of the people on this impressive roster have dedicated their lives to the advancement of athletics and sports nutrition.

Sal Arria   Sal Arria, DC, MSS, is the cofounder of, and director of sports medicine for, the International Sports Sciences Association (ISSA). He was a team doctor for the U.S. track-and-field team at the 1984 Olympic Games and at three U.S. Powerlifting Federation world championships. A three-time California State powerlifting champion himself, he was ranked among the top three in the United States in the 220- and 242-pound divisions. Dr. Arria was director of the Santa Barbara Chiropractic and Sports Medicine Clinic for two decades. He was appointed a Special Advisor to the (California) Governor's Council on Physical Fitness. As a cofounder of the ISSA, Dr. Arria has traveled around the world to personally educate fitness trainers, strength coaches, doctors, and other health professionals on the proper use of physical conditioning and nutrition for improvement in sports performance and rehabilitation of sports injuries.

George A. Brooks   George A. Brooks, PhD, is an internationally acclaimed exercise physiologist from the University of California at Berkeley. He is a coauthor of the classic textbook *Exercise Physiology: Human Bioenergetics and Its Applications,* as well as the author of numerous scientific research reports. Dr. Brooks has conducted innovative sports-nutrition research on exogenous carbohydrate metabolism, searching for a better understanding of which energy substrates are used by the human body during exercise. He is also a contributing author to popular fitness and nutrition magazines.

Nancy Clark   Nancy Clark, MS, RD, is an author and consulting nutritionist specializing in nutrition for athletes. She is the author of two highly acclaimed sports-nutrition books: *The Athlete's Kitchen* and *Nancy Clark's Sports Nutrition Guidebook*. She is a frequent contributor to scientific journals and magazines, writing articles on a variety of sports-nutrition topics, and has also developed educational materials on sports nutrition that are used by coaches, trainers, and athletes in high schools and colleges around the world. Ms. Clark is herself an athlete. In addition to running marathons, she has biked across the United States and trekked through the Himalayas.

Michael Colgan
Michael Colgan, PhD, CCN, is the founder of the Colgan Institute, a consulting, education, and research facility concerned with issues relating to nutrition, athletic performance, and aging. He was a senior member of the science faculty of the University of Auckland, New Zealand, and has conducted research on human aging and physical performance. However, he may be most noted in the sports-nutrition industry for his book *Optimum Sports Nutrition*.

A. Scott Connelly
A. Scott Connelly, MD, is the founder of the leading performance-food company, MET-Rx USA, Inc. His work as a critical-care metabolic physician and sportsman led him to develop one of the first "engineered nutrition" products, a protein powder manufactured by MET-Rx. He is also credited with inventing other products produced by MET-Rx. In addition, Dr. Connelly writes and lectures on sports nutrition, and directs medical research to prove the effects of his products on body composition and performance.

David Costill
David Costill, PhD, has dedicated decades of effort to studying how fluid, electrolyte, and carbohydrate intake affect athletic performance, and his research contributions have helped shape the many sports-nutrition beverages used by millions of athletes to boost performance and increase endurance. He is a pioneer and leader in sports nutrition, and is the author of many scientific articles reporting on his important research discoveries.

Mauro G. Di Pasquale
Mauro G. Di Pasquale, MD, MRO, MFS, is a licensed physician in Ontario, Canada, specializing in sports medicine. He is an assistant professor at the University of Toronto and holds a master of fitness science degree from the International Sports Sciences Association. Dr. Di Pasquale has written many books and articles on a number of sports-nutrition topics, and his most recent scientific reference book, *Amino Acids and Proteins for the Athlete,* is a "must-read" for all health professionals involved in sports nutrition. He also writes regular columns and articles for several fitness magazines, including *Muscle & Fitness, Men's Fitness, Flex, Iron Man, Muscle Mag International,* and *Powerlifting USA.*

Thomas D. Fahey
Thomas D. Fahey, PhD, is an internationally acclaimed exercise physiologist and the coauthor of the classic textbook *Exercise Physiology: Human Bioenergetics and Its Applications.* He is also the author of numerous scientific research reports and a contributing author to popular fitness and

nutrition magazines. Dr. Fahey's most recent research involved the development of diagnostic home test kits for athletes, including a saliva test to measure the testosterone-to-cortisol ratio.

Frederick Hatfield

Frederick Hatfield, PhD, has specialized in sports nutrition and fitness for over thirty years. The cofounder and president of the International Sports Sciences Association, he is a world-champion power lifter and has trained hundreds of professional and elite athletes and their trainers. Dr. Hatfield has taught sports psychology, strength physiology, and physical education at the University of Wisconsin, Newark State College, Bowie State College, the University of Illinois, and Temple University. He has acted as a consultant to the U.S. Olympic Committee, West German Body Building Federation, Australian Powerlifting Federation, and CBS Sports. He has coached the U.S. National Powerlifting Team and served on the executive committees of the U.S. Olympic Weightlifting Federation and U.S. Powerlifting Federation. In addition, Dr. Hatfield is the founding editor of *Sports Fitness* and *BodyCraft* magazines, and has written over sixty books and hundreds of articles on fitness and nutrition. He also has developed hundreds of products for athletes, including sports-nutrition products, weightlifting equipment, and athletic-performance products. Due to his frequent world-record-breaking performances in the power squat, Dr. Hatfield has come to be known as Dr. Squat in powerlifting circles.

James F. Hickson, Jr.

James F. Hickson, Jr., PhD, RD, is the co-editor of the outstanding professional reference book *Nutrition in Exercise and Sport,* as well as the co-editor of the entire *Nutrition in Exercise and Sport* series. He is a retired professor from the University of Houston, where he spent many years researching nutrition and sports nutrition. He has made significant research contributions and discoveries, most notably in the areas of protein metabolism and exercise.

Jack La Lanne

Jack La Lanne is a fitness and nutrition expert who brought the bodybuilding lifestyle into American homes via the first (and longest running) fitness show on television. The author of numerous books, he also created a number of exercise videos and developed the Three-Point Plan, designed to help people become fit and trim. And they have. Millions of people have benefited from Mr. La Lanne's fitness and nutrition programs. Now in his eighties, he himself has the vitality and vigor of a teenager as a result of practicing what he has been preaching for more than sixty years—a lifestyle of exercise and proper nutrition. The Three-Point Plan consists of regular exercise, scientific instruction, and an improved diet including more hunger-appeasing high-protein foods and essential vitamins. This plan shows that Mr. La Lanne was far ahead of traditional nutrition science, advocating—decades ago—a low-fat, moderate-protein, and moderate-carbohydrate diet with whole foods and plenty of vegetables. One of his more famous quotes is, "If man made it, don't eat it." Another is, "If you don't use it, you'll lose it."

Bill Phillips
Bill Phillips is best known as the founder of the popular strength-training magazine *Muscle Media*. His "tell-it-like-it-is" approach to publishing, and aggressive marketing and business savvy have won him national acclaim from both his industry peers and extensive, loyal readership. Mr. Phillips started publishing in 1990, the year he came out with the first edition of his *Natural Supplement Review*. Being a weight lifter and bodybuilder, he knows firsthand the kind of information about training and nutrition that strength athletes want, which is a key to his publishing success. Through his sports-nutrition company, EAS, Mr. Phillips has consistently dedicated financial resources toward supporting ongoing sports-nutrition research studies.

Ben Weider
Ben Weider, CM, PhD, is the cofounder of Weider Nutrition International; Weider Publications, Inc.; Weider Health and Fitness; and the International Federation of Bodybuilders. Together with his brother Joe Weider, he has had a tremendous impact on twentieth-century culture and society. While both Ben and Joe Weider have contributed to the growth of their health and fitness products empire, Ben Weider is best known as the president of the International Federation of Bodybuilders (IFBB), which he founded in Montreal, Canada, in 1946. Since its beginnings, the IFBB has grown to include over 170 countries as members, making it one of the largest sports organizations in history. In 1998, the organization was granted official recognition by the International Olympic Committee. Nominated for the Nobel Peace Prize in 1984, Dr. Weider's list of awards and accomplishments can fill an entire book. Included are the Silver Medal of Paris; the Distinguished Service Award, United States Sports Academy; and the Order of Canada, the highest award bestowed by the Canadian government on a citizen. He also holds three honorary doctorate degrees; was appointed to the International Council of Sports and Physical Education, Research Committee; and has been inducted into the Maccabea Sports Hall of Fame. Dr. Weider's career has been marked by a commitment to the advancement of science, education, business, society, health and fitness, and humanity. He attributes his success to setting visionary long-term goals, then following up with hard work, dedication, and a relentless drive. (For an interview with Dr. Weider, see "Words of Wisdom From Ben Weider" on page 251.)

Joe Weider
Joe Weider has been a true pioneer in bringing fitness and health consciousness to the American public. As the cofounder of Weider Nutrition International; Weider Publications, Inc.; Weider Health and Fitness; and the International Federation of Bodybuilders, he has had a very strong impact on twentieth-century culture and society. From his headquarters in Woodland Hills, California, he has helped to build a fitness empire that reaches throughout the world. Bodybuilders everywhere utilize Weider Nutrition's state-of-the-art sports-nutrition products as essential parts of their training programs. The weightlifting newsletter that he started with seven dollars at the age of seventeen has blossomed into a publishing empire that today is a dominant force in the health and fitness

Words of Wisdom From Ben Weider

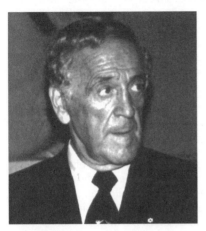

Bodybuilding, powerlifting, weightlifting, and sports nutrition signify different things to different people. To some, they represent goals. To others, they are roads to health and happiness. Following is an interview with Ben Weider, a man who is synonymous with the sport of bodybuilding. Dr. Weider was generous enough to share some of his thoughts, philosophy, and insights on how living the bodybuilding lifestyle has helped him attain success.

Avery's Sports Nutrition Almanac: What tips can you offer our readers for turning a dream into reality and success?

Ben Weider: The key to turning a dream into a reality is perseverance and belief in your goals. You must never give up and, regardless of how much opposition and rejection there is, you must always plan to find a way to get around it. Perseverance and confidence will "win the day."

ASNA: How does living the bodybuilding lifestyle fit into the life/career success model?

BW: Aristotle, the Greek philosopher, once said, "A sound mind and a sound body." This is exactly what is required to have a healthy life and successful career. What Aristotle meant by making this statement was that an individual should practice bodybuilding, in order to strengthen his body, and eat properly, so his body will be very healthy. Combine this with good education and you have the formula for a healthier and longer life and successful career.

ASNA: Your crowning lifelong accomplishment of getting the sport of bodybuilding into the Olympics was thought to be an impossible goal by many critics. Can you share with us some of the key milestones and major goals of getting bodybuilding into the Olympics?

BW: It took exactly fifty-two years of "blood, sweat, and tears" to obtain Olympic recognition. I had six meetings with Avery Brundage, eight meetings with The Lord Killanin, and fourteen meetings with President Juan Antonio Samaranch before Olympic recognition was granted. Obtaining recognition by the International Olympic Committee meant informing and educating various members around the world about the importance of bodybuilding. It took patience, diplomacy, and intelligent planning to make this lifelong goal happen.

ASNA: What do you consider the key breakthroughs in bodybuilding science during the twentieth century?

BW: The key breakthrough in bodybuilding was to get the coaches of athletes in any sport to accept the fact that an athlete requires strength, and not only technique, in order to become an elite athlete. This took numerous years of education and information to succeed. To complete the formula to become an elite athlete, the athlete also needs energy, and energy is derived from intelligent nutrition, which results in improving performance, growth, and recovery. We have pioneered nutrition for athletes during the past fifty years. Therefore, I consider these the two key breakthroughs in this century—accepting bodybuilding as a method to increase strength for athletic performance, and to eat intelligently and supplement your diet with protein, vitamins, minerals, and other natural factors to obtain energy necessary to succeed in sports.

ASNA: What are your thoughts about the future of fitness, nutrition, IFBB, and humanity in the twenty-first century?

BW: Fitness and nutrition are not a fad. They are a lifestyle and, therefore, they will become a part of everyday life. The humanity aspect that the IFBB brings is to consider all people as equals. Since I believe in the Napoleonic philosophy, which states, "Fraternity, liberty and equality," I believe that every person, regardless of his race, religion, or political determination, is equal and deserves the utmost respect.

ASNA: Do you have any favorite quotes you would like to share with your bodybuilding fans?

BW: My favorite quote is, "A sound mind and a sound body." Aristotle.

ASNA: Do you have any other thoughts you think will keep people on the right track in business and life that you have found contributed to your success?

BW: To keep on the right track in business and in life, here is what a person has to do: Do not wait until things will happen. Make them happen. Do not wait until people will come to you. You go to them, if you have a project that you wish to follow through on. Perseverance and belief in your goals always bring results.

industry. Weider Publications now publishes eight magazines—*Muscle & Fitness, Flex, Shape, Men's Fitness, Prime Health and Fitness, Living Fit, Natural Health,* and *Fit Pregnancy.* In 1983, Mr. Weider was named Publisher of the Year by the Periodical and Book Association. In 1992, the United States Sports Academy presented him with the Dwight D. Eisenhower Fitness Award. And in May 1995, he was given the Lifestyle Achievement Award by the (California) Governor's Council on Physical Fitness. But the honor of which Mr. Weider is the proudest is the Distinguished Citizen award, which was presented to him by the Boy Scouts of America in 1991 and refers to him as "the father of fitness."

Ira Wolinsky
Ira Wolinsky, PhD, is a professor of nutrition at the University of Houston. He is the co-editor of the outstanding professional reference book *Nutrition in Exercise and Sport,* as well as the co-editor for the entire *Nutrition in Exercise and Sport* series. Dr. Wolinsky is currently involved in researching issues concerning sports nutrition, as well as the nutrition of bone and calcium.

Michael Zumpano   Michael Zumpano is the founder of Champion Nutrition. During the past two decades, he has also taught college classes on bodybuilding, written articles for *Muscle & Fitness* magazine, conducted original medical research with athletes, lectured, and acted as a consultant for many famous athletes and bodybuilders, including the San Francisco 49ers and the Los Angeles Lakers. However, he is best known for inventing the first metabolic optimizer, Metabolol. Mr. Zumpano's driving mission has been to create scientifically based sports-nutrition products to give athletes effective drug-free choices. He has clinically tested his hypothesis that there are effective nutritional ways to optimize muscle growth, decrease recovery time, and increase athletic performance. He calls his approach the "science of metabolic optimization." Mr. Zumpano continues to fund original university research projects using Champion Nutrition products.

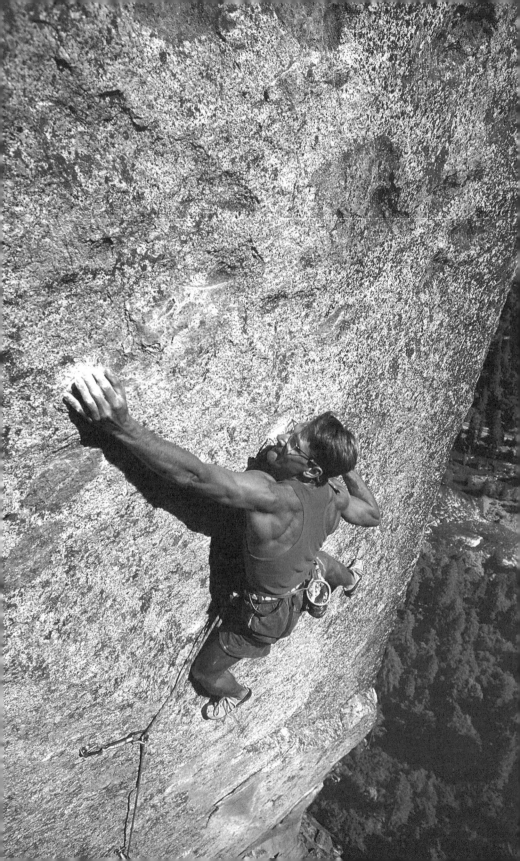

ADDRESSES AND WEBSITES

14

Many people feel that "surfing the Web" is an Olympic-quality sport. However, it can also be a tremendous time-waster if you have a general area of interest in mind but don't have specific addresses or websites. Make your time on the computer productive and educational. Following are the addresses, phone numbers, and websites of many of today's leaders in fitness and sports nutrition, for answers to questions, help with problems, and tons of useful tips and facts.

All Natural Muscular Development Magazine
http://www.musculardevelopment.com
A website offering information on nutrition, training, and supplementation for strength and power athletes, as well as reprints of articles and information from *All Natural Muscular Development* magazine.

Amazon Books
http://www.amazon.com
A convenient website for locating and ordering books on sports nutrition and other topics.

Avery Publishing Group
120 Old Broadway
Garden City Park, NY 11040
800–548–5757
http://www.averypublishing.com
The publisher of this *Sports Nutrition Almanac*. Avery has also published hundreds of books on health and fitness topics, available online and from health-food stores and bookstores nationwide.

Bodyonics Ltd.
140 Lauman Lane
Hicksville, NY 11801
516–822–1230

http://www.pinnaclebody.com
Manufacturer of the fine Pinnacle sports-nutrition product line.

Will Brink
http://www.brinkzone.com/
A website developed by Will Brink, author of *Priming the Anabolic Environment* and columnist for *MuscleMag International,* to provide information on cutting-edge supplements.

Champion Nutrition
2615 Stanwell Drive
Concord, CA 94520
510–689–1790
http://www.champion-nutrition.com/
A leading sports-nutrition company. Its website offers product information, as well as training and nutrition information.

Cybergenics America
http://www.cybergenics-america.com/
Home site of Cybergenics America, a leading manufacturer of sports-nutrition products. It is a "virtual gateway" to the competitive advantage through nutrition and training.

Designer Protein
PO Box 2469
Carlsbad, CA 92018
http://www.designerprotein.com/
A leading sports-nutrition company. It offers an FAQ section, recipes, and a newsletter on its website.

Dr. Squat
http://www.drsquat.com/
Fitness and nutrition expert Dr. Fred Hatfield's personal website. Filled with useful information on powerlifting, fitness, and sports nutrition.

ESPN
http://www.espn.go.com/
The home website of one of the leading television sports networks. The site covers all sports and is packed with facts, figures, stories, and more. It features "Headline News," "Today's Best," a listing of events, online ticket purchasing for sporting events, and links to the websites of the NBA, NASCAR, and NFL.

Cory Everson
http://www.coryeverson.com/
The personal website of the six-time Ms. Olympia. In addition to daily fitness tips, it features a "Guide to Working Out," "12 Rules of Motivation," "5-Week Motivator Program," "Cory's Guide to Eating Right," healthy recipes, and links to other fitness sites.

Fitness America Pageant
http://www.fitnessamerica.com
The home website of the Fitness America Pageant, one of bodybuilding's premier contests.

Fitness Magazines
http://www.fitnessonline.com/newsstand/
A site that offers links to the websites of such fitness magazines as *Shape, Muscle & Fitness, Men's Fitness, Prime Health & Fitness, Flex, LivingFit, Natural Health,* and *Fit-Pregnancy.*

Fitness Pros BodyBuilding
http://www.fitnesspros.com
A website loaded with all types of information on sports nutrition. It also provides links to companies, magazines, and individuals involved in the sport of bodybuilding.

Flex Magazine
Weider Publications, Inc.
21100 Erwin Street
Woodland Hills, CA 91367
http://www.flexonline.com/
The official magazine of the International Federation of Bodybuilders. Its website has plenty of great articles, such as "How to Get Huge" and "Eat It Up," and the results of IFBB contests.

Gatorade Sports Science Institute
http://www.gssiweb.com
A website loaded with useful articles and information concerning sports nutrition.

General Nutrition Centers
921 Penn Avenue
Pittsburgh, PA 15222
412–288–4600
http://www.gnc.com

The world's largest dietary-supplement retailer. Its website offers information on nutrition, supplements, and sports-nutrition products.

Gold's Gym
http://www.goldsgym.com
The home website of Gold's Gym. It has a search engine to locate the Gold's Gym nearest you by zip code, state, or city. It also offers information on training and nutrition, and has a calendar of events.

Health and Nutrition Breakthroughs Online
www.hnbreakthroughs.com
The website of *Health and Nutrition Breakthroughs* magazine. It's a no-nonsense website created to educate consumers. It presents the research and facts behind vitamin, mineral, herbal, and other supplements.

HealthNotes
www.healthnotes.com
A website containing articles on all aspects of health, nutrition, and wellness. You can obtain the full page by subscription only.

Healthwell.com—Natural Search
www.naturalsearch.com
A search engine for the natural-products industry. Visitors to this site can search for information about natural products and the companies that make them.

Human Kinetics
PO Box 5076
Champaign, IL 61825
http://www.humankinetics.com/
The developer and publisher of over 100 books, 23 journals, 12 video tapes, and numerous audio tapes and software programs for professionals in the sports profession. Also check out its website for the *International Journal of Sport Nutrition* at http://www.humankinetics.com/infok/journals/ijsn/intro.htm.

International Bibliographic Information on Dietary Supplements
http://www.nal.usda.gov.fnic/IBIDS/overview.html
A website with a search engine that accesses the abstracts of more than 250,000 scientific articles on dietary supplements.

International Federation of Bodybuilders
2875 Bates Road
Montreal, Quebec
Canada H3S 1B7

http://www.ifbb.com

The largest sports organization around today. Its website offers quick access to information on training, nutrition, and upcoming events. It is a must-see for anybody interested in bodybuilding. Also check out its website on IFBB cofounder Ben Weider at http://www/ifbb.com/ben.html.

International Sports Sciences Association

1035 Santa Barbara Street
Suite 7
Santa Barbara, CA 93101
805–884–8111

http://www.issaonline.com/

A fitness and sports-nutrition education and certification organization. Its website provides up-to-date information on sports nutrition and training.

Ironman Magazine
http://www.ironmanmagazine.com/

The home website of *Ironman* magazine. It contains information on training and nutrition, articles, and links to other sites related to sports nutrition.

Journal of Nutrition
http://www.nutrition.org/

The home website of the American Society for Nutritional Sciences' comprehensive *Journal of Nutrition*. You can search through recent issues for scientific articles on nutrition.

Labrada Bodybuilding Nutrition

403 Century Plaza Drive
Suite 440
Houston, TX 77073
281–209–2137

http://www.labrada.com/

A sports-nutrition company. Its website offers information on training, supplements, and nutrition.

Maximum Human Performance

1376 Pompton Avenue
Cedar Grove, NJ 07009
973–857–6474
973–857–5866 (fax)

http://www.maxperformance.com/

Gerard Dente's sports-nutrition company. Its website includes online ordering, a newsletter, information, and links.

Men's Fitness Magazine
Weider Publications, Inc.
21100 Erwin Street
Woodland Hills, CA 91367
http://www.mensfitness.com/
A popular men's fitness publication. Its website offers information on fitness, sports nutrition, and bodybuilding.

Men's Health Magazine
http://www.menshealth.com/
The home website of *Men's Health* magazine. It contains information on fitness, sex and relationships, health, nutrition, money, career planning, and more.

Mesomorphosis Interactive
http://www.mesomorphosis.com
A great site loaded with information on training, sports nutrition, and sports-related people, companies, and events.

MET-Rx
2112 Business Center Drive
Irvine, CA 92612
949–930–4400
http://www.metrx.com/
One of the leading sports-nutrition companies. Among the offerings on its website are product information, FAQs, and an internet search engine.

Ms. Fitness Magazine
PO Box 2378
Corona, CA 91718
908–371–0606
http://www.msfitness.com
The magazine for today's active woman, published quarterly. Its website provides information on nutrition, exercise, and contests.

Muscle & Fitness Magazine
Weider Publications, Inc.
21100 Erwin Street
Woodland Hills, CA 91367
http://www.muscle-fitness.com/
A popular bodybuilding magazine published by the Weider empire. It is loaded with information on bodybuilding, training, nutrition, supplements, sex, fitness, and much more. It also includes a very useful muscle-meal planner, which is a four-week-long meal plan, along with training guidelines.

Muscle Media Magazine
http://www.musclemedia.com/
Home site of *Muscle Media* magazine. It offers information on bodybuilding, products, and nutrition.

MuscleMag International
21555 Clifford Drive
Fairview Park, Ohio 44126
http://www.musmag.com
A leading bodybuilding magazine. Its website includes information on bodybuilding events, training, and sports nutrition.

National Library of Medicine
http://www.nlm.nih.gov/
A website whose free Medline search engine can be used to conduct searches through more than 3,000 medical-related scientific journals. It's a great place to go for quick access to the scientific articles referenced in other articles and books. You will get only abstracts online; you can order the full-text articles.

NPC News
National Physique Committee
PO Box 3711
Pittsburgh, PA 15230
412–276–5027
The national amateur bodybuilding organization.

New Hope Group Online
http://www.newhope.com/
The official website of New Hope Communications, a health-food trade organization. It contains the journal *Nutrition Science News,* which has articles on sports-nutrition topics, mainly sports-supplement topics.

Nutrition Science News Online
www.nutritionsciencenews.com
The website of *Nutrition Science News,* a monthly trade magazine written by health professionals. Its purpose is to educate consumers about natural products and to provide the latest, in-depth information on nutrition.

Olympics
http://www.olympic.org/
The official website of the International Olympic Committee.

Bill Pearl
http://www.billpearl.com
Legendary bodybuilder Bill Pearl's personal website. It offers strength-training programs for twenty-one different sports in the off-season, preseason, and in-season. Bodybuilding and general conditioning programs are also included. A great site to learn how to personalize your weight training.

Physician and Sportsmedicine
http://www.physsportsmed.com/
The Physician and Sportsmedicine online. It offers articles on sports-medicine topics.

PowerBar Inc
2150 Shattuck Avenue
Berkeley, CA 94704
510–704–7228
http://www.powerbar.com
The home website of PowerBar Inc., the leading energy-nutrition bar. Included among its offerings is news of PowerBar-sponsored events, as well as information on nutrition and nutrition products.

Powerhouse Gym
24385 Halsted Road
Suite 2000
Farmington Hills, MI 48335
248–476–2888
http://www.powerhousegyms.com
A national chain of gyms. Its website includes information on gym locations and bodybuilding events, and even explains how to open a Powerhouse Gym.

Prime Health & Fitness Magazine
Weider Publications, Inc.
21100 Erwin Street
Woodland Hills, CA 91367
http://www.getbig.com/magazine/prime/prime.htm
Another magazine published by the Weider empire. This one is dedicated to the confident, active man over thirty-five years old, and its website is packed with information on health, fitness, job stress, sexuality, graying hair, marriage, parenting, and nutrition.

Runner's World Magazine
http://www.runnersworld.com/
Home site of *Runner's World* magazine. It's loaded with information on training, nutrition, events, and equipment for runners.

Sports Illustrated Magazine
http://www.cnnsi.com/
Sports Illustrated online, brought to you by CNN. The site gives you access to selected power-packed stories from *Sports Illustrated*; information on professional and college sporting events; and special features such as "Mean Streak," "Tips From Coach K!," "Inside Game Gang," "She Got Game," and the swimsuit articles. You can also sign up for free for CNN/SI's online calendar.

SUPPLEMENTFACTS International
http://www.supplementfacts.net
A website offering up-to-date information on dietary supplements, sports nutrition, weight loss, health, and fitness. It bridges the gap between scientific discoveries and human application.

Town Sports International
888 Seventh Avenue
New York, NY 10106
http://www.nysc.com/
A chain of high-quality fitness centers, including the New York Sports Club, Washington Sports Club, Philadelphia Sports Club, and Boston Sports Club. The website is packed with useful information on fitness and nutrition, as well as information on Sports Club locations, personal-trainer services, membership, class schedules, special fitness classes and programs, and employment.

Twin Laboratories, Inc.
2120 Smithtown Avenue
Ronkonkoma, NY 11779
http://www.twinlab.com
A leading supplement manufacturer. Its website includes information on the company, products, and sports nutrition.

VERIS Web Resources Link
http://www.veris-online.org/weblink2.htm
A site that links helpful nutrition-information resources on the Web.

David Waterman
4 Sunnybrook Lane
Utica, NY 13502
Powerlifting champion.

Weider Nutrition International

2002 South 5070 West
Salt Lake City, UT 84104
801–975–5000

http://www.weider.com/

A leading sports-nutrition company. Its website includes information on products and sports nutrition, and corporate information for investors.

Windmill Consumer Products

8 Henderson Drive
West Caldwell, NJ 07006

http://www.windmillvitamins.com

A pioneering supplement company that offers top-quality products through pharmacies. It recently launched a line of high-quality sports-nutrition products, for sale through gyms and health and fitness clubs, under the NutritionWORKS brand name.

World Gym

2210 Main Street
Santa Monica, CA 90405
310–450–0080

http://www.worldgym.com/

A national chain of gyms. Its website offers gym locations and health and fitness tips.

DICTIONARY OF TRAINING AND HEALTH TERMS

Following are key training and health terms as they apply to sports nutrition. Knowing the meanings of these terms will help you better understand the various topics discussed in this book.

acetylcholine. A neurotransmitter that is critical for optimum nervous-system functioning.

acid–base balance. The condition in which the pH of the blood is at a constant level of 7.35 to 7.45.

adaptive overload stress. A training method in which the body must adjust to increasingly greater amounts of resistance.

adenosine triphosphate (ATP). A compound that, when broken down, produces the energy that enables the muscles and other organs to function.

adipose tissue. The anatomical fat found in between the skin and muscle.

aerobic. With oxygen.

aerobic activity. A low-intensity, high-endurance activity that requires oxygen for endurance.

aerobic endurance. The ability to maintain aerobic muscle output over long periods of time.

alpha–linolenic acid. An essential fatty acid.

amine. A nitrogen-containing compound in which at least one hydrogen atom has been replaced with a hydrocarbon radical.

ammonia. A toxic metabolic waste product.

anabolism. The biochemical process in which different molecules combine to form larger, more complex molecules.

anaerobic. Without oxygen.

anaerobic activity. A high-intensity, low-endurance activity that requires bursts of energy for power or speed.

anaerobic power-endurance. The ability to exert maximum muscular effort time after time with no appreciable decline in force output.

anemia. A condition in which the oxygen-carrying capacity of the blood is reduced. It is the most common symptom of iron deficiency.

anticatabolic. Describing a substance that prevents catabolism.

antioxidant. A nutrient that has been found to seek out and neutralize free radicals in the body and to stimulate the body to recover more quickly from free-radical damage.

arachidonic acid. A fatty acid that becomes essential when a linoleic-acid deficiency exists.

arteriosclerosis. Hardening of the arteries.

assimilation. Conversion into living tissue.

atherosclerosis. A degenerative illness that causes hardening of the arteries.

beta oxidation. The metabolic process in which fatty acids are used to regenerate adenosine-triphosphate molecules; an oxidative energy system.

betaine. An alkaloid used to treat muscular degeneration.

bile. A substance secreted by the liver that is essential for the digestion and absorption of fats and for the assimilation of calcium.

bioavailability. The ability of an ingested nutrient to cross from the digestive tract into the bloodstream and then from the bloodstream into the cells in which it will be utilized.

biological value (BV). Both the biological efficiency of a protein and any of a number of methods used to measure a protein's biological efficiency.

blood buffer. A substance that helps maintain the pH balance in the blood.

blood plasma. The liquid part of the blood; the substance in the blood that carries the red blood cells.

blood pressure. The pressure of the blood against the walls of the arteries.

blood-brain barrier. A semipermeable membrane that keeps the blood that is circulating in the brain away from the tissue fluids surrounding the brain cells.

calorie. A unit of measurement used to express the energy value of food.

cannibalization. The breakdown of muscle tissue by the body for the purpose of obtaining amino acids for other metabolic purposes.

capillary. A tiny blood vessel through which nutrients and waste products travel between the bloodstream and the body's cells.

carbohydrate drink. A sports beverage designed to replenish the glycogen (energy) stores.

carbon dioxide. A metabolic waste product.

carcinogen. A substance that is either proven or suspected to cause cancer in humans or laboratory animals.

catabolism. The biochemical process in which complex molecules are broken down for energy production, recycling of their components, or excretion.

catalyze. To initiate.

catecholamine. One of the substances that function, primarily as neurotransmitters, in the sympathetic and central nervous systems. The substances include dopamine, epinephrine, and norepinephrine.

cell membrane. The outer boundary of a cell. Also called the *plasma membrane.*

cellular replication. The process in which a cell is duplicated for the purpose of creating a new cell.

cellular uptake. Absorption by the cells.

chromosome. A unit, located within the cell nucleus, that contains all of a person's genetic information, in the form of genes.

coenzyme. An enzyme cofactor.

cofactor. A substance that must be present for another substance to be able to perform a certain function.

collagen. A simple protein that is the chief component of connective tissue.

complete protein. A protein that contains the essential amino acids in amounts that are sufficient for the maintenance of normal growth rate and body weight.

connective tissue. Tissue that either supports other tissue or joins tissue to tissue, muscle to bone, or bone to bone. It includes cartilage, bone, tendons, ligaments, reticular tissue, areolar tissue, adipose tissue, blood, bone marrow, and lymph.

contraction. The development of tension within a muscle. The two kinds are isotonic, in which the muscle shortens as it becomes tense, and isometric, in which the muscle does not shorten as it becomes tense.

cortisol. A hormone secreted by the adrenal glands that stimulates catabolism.

creatine phosphate. A compound produced in the body, stored in the muscle fibers, and broken down by enzymes to quickly replenish the adenosine-triphosphate stores.

creatinine. A waste product of creatine metabolism.

cross-link. An undesirable bond between molecules that is induced by free radicals and results in deformed molecules that cannot function properly.

cytoplasm. The liquid between the cell membrane and nuclear membrane of a cell. Also called the *cytosol*.

degenerative illness. An illness that causes the body to deteriorate. Examples are cancer and arthritis.

deoxyribonucleic acid (DNA). The substance in the cell nucleus that contains the cell's genetic blueprint and determines the type of life form into which the cell will develop.

depletion. Draining.

dermatitis. A skin condition.

detoxifying agent. A substance that helps rid the body of carcinogens and dangerous chemicals.

diabetes. Diabetes mellitus. A condition in which the body does not properly metabolize carbohydrates due to a lack of or resistance against insulin.

digestive enzyme. An enzyme that acts as a catalyst for the breakdown of a food component.

di-peptide. Two amino acids linked together.

disaccharide. A simple carbohydrate composed of two sugar molecules.

diuretic. A substance that increases urination.

docosahexaenoic acid (DHA). An omega-3 fatty acid.

dopamine. A catecholamine that often functions as a neurotransmitter.

ectomorph. The slim, linear body type.

eicosanoid. One of a group of substances that help regulate a wide diversity of physiological processes.

eicosapentaenoic acid (EPA). An omega-3 fatty acid.

electrolyte balance. The ratio of chloride, potassium, sodium, and the other electrolytes in the body.

electron transport system. The metabolic process in which electrons are passed between certain protein molecules, releasing energy that is used to regenerate adenosine-triphosphate molecules.

emulsifier. A substance that, during digestion, helps disperse fats in water mediums.

endomorph. The fat, round body type.

endurance. The ability to continue performing without undue discomfort.

endurance sport. A sport that requires the ability to perform for long periods of time at low intensities, such as marathon running and cross-country skiing.

energy metabolism. A series of chemical reactions that break down foodstuffs and thereby produce energy.

energy supplement. A supplement designed to enhance the mental or physical energy levels.

energy system. A sequence of metabolic reactions that produces energy.

enteric coating. A coating on tablets that delays digestion of the tablets until they pass from the stomach into the intestines.

enzyme. One of a group of protein catalysts that initiate or speed chemical reactions in the body without being consumed.

ephedra. A plant that contains ephedrine and pseudoephedrine and is therefore banned by a number of sports governing organizations.

ephedrine. A drug that constricts the blood vessels and widens the bronchial passages.

epinephrine. A hormone secreted by the adrenal gland that prepares the body for the fight-or-flight reaction.

ergogenic. A catchall term that describes anything that can be used to enhance athletic performance. Ergogenic aids can be dietary or nondietary and include dietary supplements, special training techniques, and mental strategies.

essential nutrient. A nutrient that the body cannot produce itself or that it cannot produce in sufficient amounts to maintain good health.

excitatory neurotransmitter. A neurotransmitter that acts as a stimulant to the brain.

extracellular. Outside the cell.

fast-twitch muscle fibers. Muscle fibers that contract quickly, providing short bursts of energy, and therefore are used when strength and power are needed.

fat cell. A cell that stores fatty acids for energy.

fat metabolism. The process by which fat is changed to make new tissue.

fat soluble. Capable of being dissolved in lipid and organic solvents.

free radical. One of the highly reactive molecules that are known to injure cell membranes, cause defects in the deoxyribonucleic acid (DNA), and contribute to the aging process and a number of degenerative illnesses. Free radicals are byproducts of normal chemical reactions in the body that involve oxygen.

free-form amino acids. Amino acids that are in their free state, or single.

fructose. A simple carbohydrate that is a monosaccharide. It is absorbed and utilized by the body much slower than glucose and has therefore become the preferred form of sugar in health foods. Also called *levulose* or *fruit sugar.*

full profile. Containing all the nonessential as well as essential nutrients. For example, a full-profile amino-acid supplement contains all the nonessential amino acids as well as the essential amino acids. Also called *full spectrum.*

gluconeogenesis. The metabolic process in which glucose is synthesized from noncarbohydrate sources.

glucose. A simple carbohydrate that is a monosaccharide. Also called *dextrose* or *grape sugar.*

glucose polymer. A processed form of polysaccharides, or complex carbohydrates.

glucose tolerance factor. A substance that helps lower the blood-sugar level.

glucose-alanine cycle. An important biochemical process that occurs during exercise to produce energy. Glycogen is broken down to glucose and then to pyruvate, some of which is used directly for energy and the remainder of which is converted to alanine. The alanine is returned to the liver and stored as glycogen, then once again broken down to glucose and then to pyruvate.

glycogen. A complex carbohydrate that occurs only in animals; the form in which glucose is stored in the body.

glycogen depletion. The draining of the body's glycogen stores.

glycogen replenishment. The refilling of the body's glycogen stores.

glycogen sparing. The saving of glycogen by the body for other functions.

glycogen-bound water. The water that is stored in the muscles along with glycogen. About 3 ounces of water must be stored with every 1 ounce of glycogen.

glycogenolysis. The metabolic process in which glycogen is broken down.

glycolysis. The metabolic process in which glucose is converted to lactic acid.

glycolytic energy systems. The energy systems that produce energy through glycolysis. They include nonoxidative glycolysis and oxidative glycolysis.

glycoprotein. A conjugated protein found in blood.

glycosaminoglycans (GAGs). Long chains of modified sugars that are the main component of proteoglycan.

gram. A measurement of weight equal to approximately $\frac{1}{28}$ ounce.

guarana. A plant that contains caffeine and is therefore banned by a number of sports governing organizations.

hard gainer. A person who has trouble gaining weight.

heart rate. The rate at which the heart pumps the blood through the body.

hemoglobin. The oxygen carrier in red blood cells.

hemolytic anemia. A condition in which the hemoglobin becomes separated from the red blood cells.

hemorrhage. Bleed excessively.

herbal bitter. A liquor prepared with bitter herbs and used for various therapeutic purposes.

high–density lipoproteins (HDLs). The good lipoproteins that help prevent cholesterol buildup in the arteries.

hitting the wall. The sensation felt by marathon runners when they deplete their body's glycogen stores and begin running primarily on stored body fat.

homeostasis. The tendency of the body to maintain an internal equilibrium.

hormone. One of the numerous substances produced by the endocrine glands that regulate bodily functions.

hyaluronic acid. The principal glycosaminoglycan in proteoglycan.

hydrochloric acid. A stomach secretion that functions in protein metabolism, helps keep the stomach relatively bacteria-free, and assists in the maintenance of a low pH balance in the stomach.

hydrogenation. The process in which unsaturated fatty acids are saturated with hydrogen atoms to make them more solid.

hydrolysis. The breakdown of a substance through the use of water.

hydrolyzed protein. A protein that has already been broken down, usually by enzymes, and is a mixture of free-form, di-peptide, and tri-peptide amino acids.

hydrostatic weighing. A method for determining body composition that involves weighing the body under water.

hypertension. High blood pressure.

hypervitaminosis. *See* **vitamin toxicity.**

hypoglycemia. Low blood sugar.

immediate energy systems. The nonoxidative energy systems that supply immediate energy for bursts of power through the use of adenosine triphosphate and creatine phosphate.

immunoglobulin. A protein that functions as an antibody in the body's immune system.

incomplete protein. A protein that is usually deficient in one or more of the essential amino acids. Most plant proteins are incomplete.

inhibitory neurotransmitter. A neurotransmitter that is calming to the brain.

inorganic. Referring to something that is not biologically produced and that does not contain any living material.

insulin resistance. A condition in which the body is resistant against the effects of insulin.

insulin-like growth factors (IGFs). Substances that promote growth in the muscles. The two kinds are insulin-like growth factor I (IGF-I) and insulin-like growth factor II (IGF-II).

intermediary. A substance that plays a role in the middle of a process.

international unit (IU). A measure of potency based on an accepted international standard. It is usually used with beta-carotene and vitamins A, D, and E. Because it is a measure of potency, not weight or volume, the number of milligrams in an IU varies, depending on the substance being measured.

interstitial spaces. The tiny spaces between tissues or organ parts.

intracellular. Inside the cell.

involuntary muscle. A muscle that acts independently of the will.

ionic form. In the form of ions, which are atoms or groups of atoms that have either a positive or negative charge from having lost or gained one or more electrons.

ketone. An acidic substance produced during the incomplete metabolism of fatty acids. It can upset the physiology.

Krebs cycle. The metabolic process in which energy is released from glucose, fatty-acid, or protein molecules and used to regenerate adenosine-triphosphate molecules.

lactic acid. A byproduct of glycolysis.

lean body mass. All of a body's tissues apart from the body fat—the bones, muscles, organs, blood, and water. Also called *fat-free mass.*

limiting nutrient. A nutrient that has the ability, through its absence or presence, to restrict the utilization of other nutrients or the functioning of the body.

linoleic acid. An essential fatty acid.

lipolysis. The process in which lipids are broken down into their constituent fatty acids.

lipoprotein. A conjugated protein that transports cholesterol and fats in the blood.

lipotropic agent. A substance that prevents fatty buildup in the liver and helps the body metabolize fat more efficiently.

long-chain fatty acid. A fatty acid with a chain of thirteen to nineteen carbon atoms.

lymphatic fluid. A clear fluid derived from blood plasma that circulates throughout the body to nourish tissue cells and to return waste matter to the bloodstream.

lymphatic system. The system of vessels that carries the lymphatic fluid through the body.

macronutrient. One of the nutrients that are required daily in large amounts and that are thought of in quantities of ounces and grams. They include carbohydrates, protein, lipids, and water.

macronutrient modulation. The practice of varying the ratio of the macronutrients in the diet to meet specific metabolic needs to enhance performance. Also called *macronutrient manipulation*.

malabsorption. Incorrect absorption.

meal-replacement drink. A nutrient drink that is low in calories and designed to replace meals for weight-loss purposes.

medium-chain fatty acid. A fatty acid with a chain of six to twelve carbon atoms.

megadose. An extremely large dose.

mesomorph. The muscular body type.

metabolic booster. A substance whose digestion causes the body to produce more than the normal amount of energy. Also called *thermogenic aid*.

metabolic pathway. A sequence of metabolic reactions.

metabolic rate. The body's total daily caloric expenditure.

metabolic water. The water that is produced in the body as a result of energy production.

metalloenzyme. A mineral-containing enzyme.

metaloprotein. A conjugated protein found in blood.

microgram. A measurement of weight equal to 1/1000 milligram.

micronutrient. One of the nutrients present in the diet and the body in small amounts. Micronutrients are measured in milligrams and micrograms. They include the vitamins, minerals, metabolites, and herbs.

microtrauma. Small but widespread tears in the muscle cells from training stress.

milligram. A measurement of weight equal to 1/1000 gram.

mineralization. Hardening.

mitochondrion. The organelle that produces the cellular energy required for metabolism.

monosaccharide. A simple carbohydrate composed of one sugar molecule, such as glucose and fructose.

monounsaturated fatty acid. A fatty acid that has one unsaturated carbon molecule.

muscle fiber. A long muscle cell.

muscle mass. Muscle tissue.

muscle tissue. Tissue that has the ability to contract, either voluntarily or involuntarily. It can be striated or smooth. The three kinds are skeletal muscle tissue, cardiac muscle tissue, and smooth muscle tissue.

neurotransmitter. A chemical substance that helps transmit nerve impulses.

nonessential nutrient. A nutrient that is not considered essential—that is, a nutrient that the body does make in sufficient amounts to maintain good health.

nonoxidative energy systems. The systems that supply energy for high-intensity, low-endurance activities lasting up to several minutes, such as powerlifting and sprinting. They include the immediate energy systems and nonoxidative glycolysis.

nonoxidative glycolysis. The metabolic process in which a glucose molecule is split in half to regenerate adenosine diphosphate back into adenosine triphosphate; a nonoxidative energy system that is the major contributor of energy during near-maximum efforts lasting up to about one and a half minutes.

norepinephrine. A hormone secreted by the adrenal glands for a number of purposes and also released by the sympathetic nerve endings as a neurotransmitter.

nuclear membrane. The membrane surrounding the cell nucleus.

nucleic acid. A conjugated protein found in chromosomes.

nucleoplasm. The liquid within the cell nucleus in which the chromosomes are suspended.

nucleus. The control center of the cell.

organelle. One of the variety of components that make up a cell. The organelles include the cell membrane, nucleus, ribosome, endoplasmic reticulum, Golgi apparatus, lysosome, and mitochondrion.

organic. Biologically produced and containing carbon atoms as part of its structure.

osteoporosis. A condition in which the bones are very porous and can break very easily.

oxidation. A chemical reaction in which an atom or molecule loses electrons or hydrogen atoms.

oxidation–reduction reaction. A chemical reaction in which one substance loses electrons or hydrogen atoms while, at the same time, another substance gains electrons or hydrogen atoms.

oxidative energy systems. The systems that supply energy for low-intensity, high-duration activities lasting more than approximately three or four minutes, such as marathon running and aerobic dance. They include oxidative glycolysis and beta oxidation.

oxidative glycolysis. The metabolic process in which a glucose molecule is split in half to form pyruvate to regenerate adenosine triphosphate; an oxidative energy system that is a major contributor of energy during near-maximum efforts lasting up to about three or four minutes.

peptide-bonded amino acids. Amino acids that are linked together.

peroxidation. The formation of a peroxide compound.

pH. Potential of hydrogen. A measure of the concentration of hydrogen ions in a solution.

phosphoinositide. An inositol-containing phospholipid that has a profound effect on cellular functioning and on metabolism, particularly the metabolism of fats.

phosphoprotein. A conjugated protein found in casein, or milk protein.

polypeptide. Four or more amino acids linked together.

polysaccharide. A complex carbohydrate.

polyunsaturated fatty acid. A fatty acid that has more than one unsaturated carbon molecule. Polyunsaturated fatty acids tend to be liquid at room temperature.

potentiator. A substance that helps another substance perform its function.

power. Strength combined with speed.

power sport. A sport that requires the ability to perform at high intensities for short periods of time, such as powerlifting and golf.

precursor. An intermediate substance in the body's production of another substance.

prostaglandin. A hormone important in metabolism.

prostanoid. A derivative of prostaglandin.

protected nutrient. A nutrient that the body reserves (protects against being used) for a certain function.

protein supplement. A supplement that supplies extra protein.

pseudoephedrine. A decongestant; a drug that reduces nasal congestion.

pyruvate. A compound that is produced during the glucose-alanine cycle. Some of the pyruvate that is produced is used directly for energy, while the remainder is converted back to alanine, which is eventually converted into glucose and used for energy.

quick-release tablet. A tablet that releases its contents quickly.

red blood cell. The cell that carries the hemoglobin in blood.

renal. Pertaining to the kidneys.

replenishment. Refilling.

ribonucleic acid (RNA). The substance that carries the coded genetic information from the deoxyribonucleic acid (DNA), in the cell nucleus, to the ribosomes, where the instructions are translated into the form of protein molecules.

saturated fatty acid. A fatty acid that has the maximum number of hydrogen atoms that it can hold, with no unsaturated carbon molecules. Saturated fatty acids tend to be solid at room temperature.

series-1 prostaglandins. A group of hormones that regulate many cellular activities.

serotonin. A neurotransmitter that helps control the sleep cycle.

short-chain fatty acid. A fatty acid with a chain of four to five carbon atoms.

skeletal muscle. One of the muscles that work in conjunction with the skeletal system to create motion.

skin-fold calipers. The specialized calipers used to measure the thickness of skin folds.

skin-fold measurement. A method for determining body composition that involves measuring the thickness of selected folds of skin using special calipers.

slow-twitch muscle fibers. Muscle fibers that produce a steady, low-intensity, repetitive contraction and therefore are used when endurance is needed.

sodium bicarbonate. A bicarbonate that boosts performance in power sports.

somatotropin. Growth hormone.

somatotype. Body type.

sports rehydration drink. A drink that replaces water, glucose, and the electrolytes after exercising.

sports supplement. A dietary supplement with ergogenic benefits.

sports-nutrition drink. A beverage formulated to fulfill special athletic needs by providing specific nutrients.

starch. A complex carbohydrate that occurs only in plants.

strength. Force output.

strength-power. *See* **power.**

striated muscle. A muscle that has a grainy appearance.

sulfur. An acid-forming mineral that is part of the chemical structure of several amino acids. Because of its ability to protect against the harmful effects of radiation and pollution, it slows down the aging process.

superoxide dismutase (SOD). An antioxidant.

sustained power. The ability to maintain power output over long periods of time.

sustained-release tablet. A tablet that releases its contents slowly and continuously over an extended period of time.

synthesis. Formation.

thermogenesis. The process by which the body generates heat, or energy, by increasing the metabolic rate above normal.

thermogenic response. The rise in the metabolic rate. Also known as the *thermogenic effect* or *specific dynamic action (SDA)*.

timed-release tablet. A tablet that releases its contents in spurts over several hours.

tissue metabolism. The process by which foodstuffs are changed to make new tissues.

transamination reaction. The process in which an amino group is transferred from an amino acid to a molecule, usually to produce another amino acid.

transmethylation. The metabolic process in which an amino acid donates a methyl group to another compound.

triiodothyronine. A thyroid hormone.

tri-peptide. Three amino acids linked together.

ultra-endurance event. An event lasting longer than two hours.

urea cycle. The metabolic process in which ammonia is converted to the waste product urea, which is then excreted from the body.

uric acid. A toxic metabolic waste product.

vascularization. The creation of new blood vessels in the tissues.

vasodilator. A substance that increases blood flow.

very long chain fatty acid. A fatty acid with a chain of twenty or more carbon atoms.

vitamin toxicity. Vitamin poisoning.

VO$_2$ max. The maximum rate at which oxygen can be consumed.

voluntary muscle. A muscle that responds to an act of the will.

water soluble. Capable of being dissolved in water.

whole food. Food that is in its natural, complete state; unprocessed food.

BOOKS AND SOFTWARE

16

BOOKS

There are three major physical variables in athletic performance—genetics, training, and nutrition. Nothing can be done about the first. Hundreds of books are available on the second. The third, nutrition, is probably the most important variable and, as we have seen in the previous chapters of this book, the least understood of all. For people who exercise at any level, there are good books on the market that can serve as resources for additional information on diet, menus, supplements, and exercise physiology. However, there are only a few that are written for active individuals who do not possess a PhD in nutrition. Following are a few favorites.

Applegate, Liz, PhD. *Power Foods*. Emmaus, PA: Rodale Press, 1991.

Not just for athletes, *Power Foods* is an excellent guide to good nutrition for everyone. Chock full of information on how to incorporate healthy eating into any lifestyle, it provides useful tips on how to gauge the impact of your vitamin and mineral levels on your everyday performance. You'll also find out how to feast on fast foods—and still save on calories and fat. *Power Foods* features scores of quick reference charts and lists that spotlight the nutritionally best snacks, beverages, breakfast cereals, fast foods, and even sweets.

Berning, Jacqueline, and Suzanne Nelson Steen. *Nutrition for Sport and Exercise*. Gaithersburg, MD: Aspen Publishers, 1998.

Nutrition for Sport and Exercise provides an accurate and effective discussion of the major nutrients, along with in-depth looks at antioxidants, energy balance, eating disorders, nutrition for child athletes, and eating on the road. Each chapter is written by an expert involved in the care of athletes who is also conducting research in the field. Setting the book apart are a number of outstanding case studies, which are helpful not only to nutritionists who work with athletes, but also to athletes and serious exercisers who want to know how to apply sports nutrition to their personal programs.

Bucci, Luke. *Nutrients as Ergogenic Aids for Sports and Exercise.*
Boca Raton, FL: CRC Press, 1993.

Nutrients as Ergogenic Aids for Sports and Exercise focuses on the application of nutrients to enhance performance, rather than the interaction of nutrition and exercise. To this end, it discusses primarily the results of human studies, relying only minimally on animal data. Real-life situations are given consideration and, whenever possible, guidelines for safe usage are presented. Readers are urged to examine carefully the applicability of these guidelines to their individual purposes. To spur interest in applied research, speculative guidelines are also presented.

Bucci, Luke. *Nutrition Applied to Injury Rehabilitation and Sports Medicine.*
Boca Raton, FL: CRC Press, 1995.

Rehabilitation is concerned with the restoration of a body with a damaged musculoskeletal system to its maximum potential. Nutritional rehabilitation is the enhancement of this recovery and return to optimum physical function through the modulation of nutrient intake. In *Nutrition Applied to Injury Rehabilitation and Sports Medicine,* the focus is on the readily available choices of dietary supplements, since no current book combines the present knowledge of dietary supplements and injury rehabilitation into one source. Since the research is scattered into several nonoverlapping areas of interest, much of the material in the book may seem new to readers. Whenever possible, guidelines for nutritional programs for specific conditions are given, so that the results of the enormous amount of research presented in the book can be appropriately applied.

Burke, Edmund R., PhD. *Optimal Muscle Recovery.* **Garden City Park, NY: Avery Publishing Group, 1999.**

Optimal Muscle Recovery is based on the cutting edge research that led to the development of the R^4 System of muscle recovery, which established a new model explaining how the interaction of key physiological and nutritional factors enables muscles to operate at peak levels. The R^4 System is based on four simple, practical principles that all athletes can incorporate into their daily training to optimize their recovery and achieve their full muscle potential. *Optimal Muscle Recovery* shows you how to improve your peak muscle performance and extend your endurance; produce a faster recovery from exercise by rapidly replenishing your depleted muscle glycogen stores; reduce muscle stress and protect your muscles from the buildup of free radicals, thereby reducing postexercise muscle soreness; and rebuild and repair damaged muscle tissue.

Clark, Nancy, MS, RD. *Nancy Clark's Sports Nutrition Guidebook.*
Champaign, IL: Leisure Press, 1997.

Nancy Clark's Sports Nutrition Guidebook will help you create a winning diet for high energy and lifelong health. But you won't have to spend hours in the kitchen, give up eating out, or totally avoid fast food! Nancy Clark offers over 100 fast, practical, and nutritious recipes that are ideal for athletes, as well as information on pregame meals, protein needs, and weight loss or gain during training.

Coleman, Ellen, and Suzanne Nelson Steen. *The Ultimate Sports Nutrition Book.* **Palo Alto, CA: Bull Publishing Company, 1996.**

Ellen Coleman and Suzanne Nelson Steen address the everyday needs of people who exercise for health or just to improve their body image, as well as the special needs of elite athletes who want to shave minutes or seconds off their competitive times. *The Ultimate Sports Nutrition Book* is designed to help all people who exercise to excel, stay healthy, and enjoy their athletic performance.

Colgan, Michael. *Optimal Sports Nutrition.* **New York: Advanced Research Press, 1993.**

Get a helping hand with training and performance from *Optimal Sports Nutrition.* Dr. Michael Colgan explains how to maximize your athletic potential by going beyond sports nutrition but still playing by the rules of legal sports supplementation. Many people realize that no matter how hard they train, their work in the gym will be for naught without proper nutrition. *Optimal Sports Nutrition* covers all the nutritional theories and techniques and their relationship to the development of peak muscular performance. Presented are effective ways to supplement the diet with vitamins, minerals, and protein, as well as how to battle water retention and excess body fat. Special chapters present information on nutritional anabolics, supplements to increase the energy level, drugs to avoid, and how to design your own personal sports-nutrition program.

Cooper, Kenneth. *Antioxidant Revolution.* **Nashville, TN: Thomas Nelson, Inc., 1994.**

Dr. Kenneth Cooper has been the groundbreaker in preventive medicine for the past three decades. He is the father of the worldwide aerobics movement, and he showed millions how to control cholesterol and hypertension. Now, in *Antioxidant Revolution,* he takes the latest antioxidant research from around the world and creates a simple, four-step life plan designed to build up your personal defense system for a longer and healthier life.

Gastelu, Daniel, and Dr. Fred Hatfield. *Dynamic Nutrition for Maximum Performance.* **Garden City Park, NY: Avery Publishing Group, 1997.**

Designed for professional and amateur athletes, fitness exercisers, trainers, coaches, and nutritionists, *Dynamic Nutrition for Maximum Performance* is a complete, easy-to-use guide to today's sports nutrition. It is intended to help you achieve and maintain maximum levels of fitness and performance through sport-specific dietary intake and nutritional supplementation. Written by two highly qualified specialists in performance nutrition and fitness science, the book blends the latest in scientific research with time-tested techniques. It explains the basic elements of sports nutrition in plain language, and then helps you use that information to develop an effective customized performance-nutrition program.

Kies, Constance, and Judy Driskell. *Sports Nutrition: Minerals and Electrolytes.* **Boca Raton, FL: CRC Press, 1995.**

Sports Nutrition: Minerals and Electrolytes addresses the relationships of mineral and electrolyte needs and interactions to sports and exercise. The book is composed of chapters written by experts in several academic disciplines, some of whom have a long history of research in the area of mineral nutrition as it relates to sports and exercise. Some of the chapters describe specific research projects, while others are literature reviews. *Sports Nutrition* offers convincing evidence that exercise and sport activities do affect your mineral status.

Kleiner, Susan. *High Performance Nutrition.* **New York: John Wiley and Sons, 1996.**

If you exercise, you need to understand diet and nutrition to get the best results. Whether you want to achieve peak performance, improve your energy, increase your endurance, lose fat, tone muscle, increase your body's natural ability to fight disease, or slow the aging process, *High-Performance Nutrition* shows you how to eat to get more value from any type of exercise—aerobics, strength training, endurance training, cross training, or recreational sports. Included in the book are a proven nutritional formula for a fast increase in muscle tone and strength, and an easy-to-follow 30-Day Menu Plan, including shopping tips and meal preparation strategies.

Kleiner, Susan M. *Power Eating.* **Champaign, IL: Human Kinetics Publishers, 1998.**

Building muscle takes more than just long hours in the gym. What you eat, how much you eat, and when you eat also has a big impact on how strong, lean, and powerful you can be. *Power Eating* provides proven, research-based guidelines from a leading nutritionist for bodybuilders and power athletes. It includes advice on thirty-six supplements, herbs, and hormones, including a powerful technique to boost creatine absorption by 60 percent; optimal protein intake formulas; tips for eating at fast-food restaurants; advice for vegetarians; healthy alternatives to steroids; and eight complete eating plans to cut weight and add or maintain muscle.

Rudd, Jaime. *Nutrition and the Female Athlete.* **Boca Raton, FL: CRC Press, 1996.**

Nutrition and the Female Athlete focuses on sports nutrition as it specifically relates to women. It addresses topics of major importance to female athletes and their coaches, trainers, nutritionists, and physicians. Among the subjects covered are carbohydrates, proteins, fats, vitamins, and minerals; the role of water and electrolytes; body weight and composition; energy balance; and eating disorders.

Sahelian, Ray, MD, and Dave Tuttle. *Creatine: Nature's Muscle Builder.* **Garden City Park, NY: Avery Publishing Group, 1997.**

Creatine: Nature's Muscle Builder explains this nutrient popular among athletes in a clear and easy-to-understand manner. The topics include how creatine works, selecting the best dosage, and the benefits of use for both weekend and professional athletes. Also discussed are the lastest scientific studies showing creatine's potency, as well as the results of the first survey of long-term creatine users.

Smith, Nathan J., and Bonnie Worthington-Roberts. *Food for Sport.* **Palo Alto, CA: Bull Publishing Company, 1989.**

Food for Sport is about food—what it is, what it does, and how to use it to maximize physical performance. Written for the casual sports participant, the highly skilled athlete, and everyone in between, it provides basic information that will enhance your understanding of the nutritional needs of various sports to help you achieve a better level of athletic performance, as well as lifelong health.

Tribole, Evelyn, MS, RD. *Eating on the Run.* **Champaign, IL: Leisure Press, 1992.**

Eating on the Run provides the nutritional information needed to make healthy eating choices and still beat the clock. It includes forty mini-meals that take just one minute to fix; advice for coping with power meals and happy hour; snacks for the gym bag; and detailed nutritional information on more than 400 fast foods.

Wolinsky, Ira, and James Hickson. *Nutrition in Exercise and Sport,* **third edition. Boca Raton, FL: CRC Press, 1998.**

Nutrition in Exercise and Sport has been updated and expanded in this third edition to include the latest developments in the field. It now discusses the role of exercise and nutrition in both wellness and disease prevention. In addition, new chapters on the history of sports nutrition, antioxidants, vegetarianism, the young athlete, the older athlete, the diabetic athlete, the physically disabled athlete, sport-specific nutrient requirements, and body-composition changes have been added. *Nutrition in Exercise and Sport* was written as a college textbook, so it may be too advanced for persons who do not have a strong science or health background.

Wolinsky, Ira, and Judy Driskell. *Sports Nutrition: Vitamins and Trace Elements.* **Boca Raton, FL: CRC Press, 1996.**

Sports Nutrition: Vitamins and Trace Elements addresses the relationship of vitamin and trace-mineral needs and interactions to sports and exercise. It reviews the research claims regarding the effects of the vitamins and trace minerals on performance. Controversial studies reporting that megadoses of vitamins and trace minerals improve physical performance are discussed and evaluated. Every chapter of the book is devoted to one or more specific vitamins or trace minerals, providing a complete profile of the particular nutrient and the role it plays. Scientists from a variety of disciplines contributed their expertise to the various chapters.

SOFTWARE

Do you like to keep track of your calories and protein but hate having to figure out how many grams of protein, carbohydrate, and fat are in every portion of food you eat? If so, you might want to invest in nutrition software for your computer. The better nutrition programs are easy to install, easy to use, and surprisingly affordable. And once you are up to speed on them, you will find that they are a lot of fun and provide valuable information for your training log.

No matter what type of nutritional software you use, you must have the appropriate hardware. Different software programs require different amounts of memory, and some are not made for the Macintosh. When shopping for a software program, make sure you read the package and sales information, as each program has different requirements.

The only problem with comparing computerized nutrition programs is that it is a lot like comparing apples and oranges—both are fruits, high in simple sugars, and low in fat, but come in very different packages. Likewise, the different nutrition programs are similar in many ways, but the way they report information and the way they present it sometimes vary.

The following software programs were judged on what information they provide in their manuals, how well they provide the information, and how easy the programs are to use on a home computer. With these caveats in mind, however, you should find nutritional software to be a worthwhile investment of your time and money if you are serious about proper nutrition and its effects on your performance.

Home Software for Personal Use

The Diet Balancer. $59.95. Nutridata Software Corporation, PO Box 769, 1215 Route 9, Suite F, Wappingers Falls, NY 12590; 800–922–2988.

The Diet Balancer ranks foods as "low" or "high" according to their nutrient content. It also allows you to include your vitamin supplements in your daily calculations (most programs do not have this feature), plots your weight for up to two months, and charts your weekly and monthly nutrient averages. However, a few important food items are omitted, some foods are listed in grams rather than ounces, and no data is included for either beta-carotene or chromium.

DINE Healthy 3. $159.00. DINE Systems, Inc., 586 North French Road, Suite 2, Amherst, NY, 14228; 800–688–1848.

DINE Healthy's user-expandable database contains over 7,000 foods, analyzed for 26 nutrients. These foods can be looked up by their common name, brand name, and nickname. They can also be sorted by nutrient. DINE Healthy 3 highlights potential diet problems for quick and easy food exchanges. It can help you design a weight-control program appropriate for you, then can assist you in tracking your progress on a daily, weekly, and monthly basis.

Nutrition Pro. $29, home version; $79, professional version. ESHA Research, PO Box 13028, Salem, OR 97309; 503–585–6242.

Nutrition Pro is a very complete and comprehensive program. Its database contains 2,000 foods, with room to add up to 50 additional foods. It records personal statistics, exercise activities, and foods consumed. It calculates individual daily requirements based on the RDAs, analyzes dietary intake, and identifies deficiencies and excesses. It has the capacity to store data for up to ten persons. The portion sizes that Nutrition Pro uses are realistic, and it can assist you in designing a daily menu to meet your nutrient and caloric needs. However, the program analyzes the diet for only 16 nutrients, omitting nutrients such as chromium, folic acid, and zinc.

Perfect Diet. $49.00. Perfect Software, 1142 Old Boalsburg Road, State College, PA 16801; 800–852–8446.

Perfect Diet can help you design a realistic weight-loss program, then can assist you in charting your progress for up to six months. It analyzes the diet for 27 nutrients and tracks nutrient intake by the day, week, month, and quarter. Both individual foods and complete recipes can be analyzed and added to the database. Perfect Diet offers a large number of options to individualize the program for your needs. However, some people find that the large number of options make the program cumbersome to use. Perfect Diet can track up to nine individuals at once.

Advanced Software for Team Use

Food Processor. $295, Basic version; $495, Plus version. ESHA Research, PO Box 13028, Salem, OR 97309; 503–585–6242.

The big brother of Nutrition Pro, Food Processor does just about everything. It even plans menus and helps you reach your fat and caloric goals. Food Processor has a database of over 3,000 foods and analyzes the diet for 49 nutrients. The advanced version, called Food Processor Plus, analyzes the diet for 105 nutrients. Food Processor features seventy-five functions for nutrient analysis and menu planning, including individual nutrition information, single nutrient analysis, and average analysis over time. It will even supply an analysis of the amino-acid content of foods.

Nutritionist Five—Nutrition Analysis Software. $595. N-Squared Computing, First DataBank Division, The Hearst Corp., 1111 Bayhill Drive, Suite 270, San Bruno, CA 94066; 800–289–1701.

An extremely complete and comprehensive program, Nutritionist Five analyzes the diet for more than 75 nutrients and tells you what percentage of your goal you have consumed, based upon a questionnaire you fill out when you first use the program. The database has more than 12,000 different foods, including brand-name products, fast foods, and ethnic foods. The method for entering the food and diet information is very easy, and the program also has the ability to generate weight-loss and weight-gain profiles, including diet and exercise information and activity schedules.

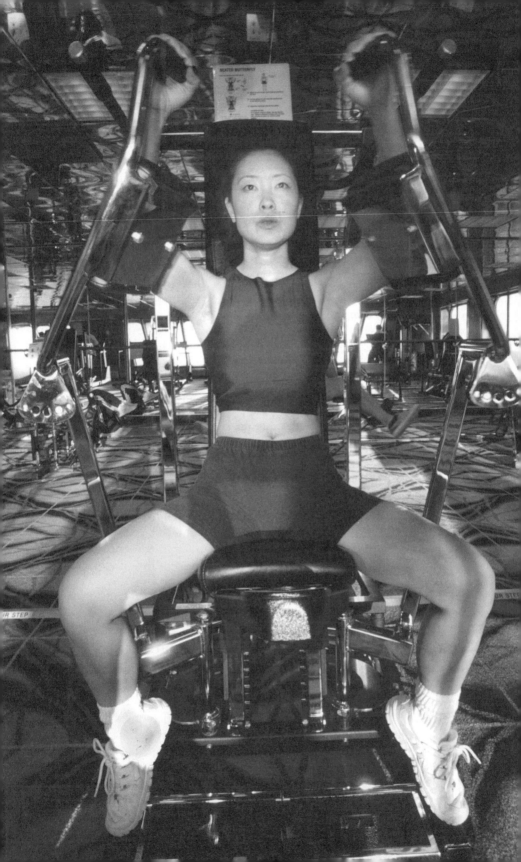

REFERENCE SOURCES

17

The following reference sources were used in the creation of the *Avery Sports Nutrition Almanac.*

A Handbook of the Composition and Pharmacology of Common Chinese Drugs. Beijing: Chinese Medical Technology Press, 1994.

Abassi, R., M. Herron, C. Weeks, and H. Lardy. "Dehydroepiandrosterone and 7-Keto DHEA Augment Interleukin 2 (IL2) Production by Human Lymphocytes In Vitro." Paper presented at the 5th Conference on Retroviruses and Opportunistic Infections, 1998.

Abumrad, N., and P. Flakoll. "The Efficacy and Safety of CaBHBM (Beta-Hydroxy Beta-Methylbutyrate) in Humans." *Vanderbilt University Medical Center Annual Report* (1991).

Adams, R. *The Big Family Guide to All the Vitamins.* New Canaan, CT: Keats Publishing, 1995.

Alberts, B., D. Bray, et al. *Energy Conversion: Mitochondria and Chloroplasts: Molecular Biology of the Cell,* 3rd Edition. New York: Garland Publishing, 1994.

Allen, Markku, Matti Reinla, and Reijo Vihko. "Response of Serum Hormones to Androgen Administration in Power Athletes." *Medicine and Science in Sports and Exercise,* Vol. 17 (1985), pp. 354–359.

Almada, A., et al. "Effects of B-BHBM Supplementation With and Without Creatine During Training on Strength and Sprint Capacity." *Federation of American Societies of Experimental Biology Journal,* Vol. 11 (1997), pg. A374.

Anderson, Helen L., Mary Belle Heindel, and Hellen Linkswiler. "Effect on Nitrogen Balance of Adult Man of Varying Source of Nitrogen and Level of Calorie Intake." *Journal of Nutrition* (1969), pp. 82–90.

Anderson, M., et al. "Pre-Exercise Meal Affects Ride Time to Fatigue in Trained Cyclists." *Journal of the American Dietetic Association,* Vol. 94 (1994), pp. 1152–1153.

Apfelbaum, Marian, Jacques Fricker, and Lawrence Igoin-Apfelbaum. "Low and

Very Low Calorie Diets." *American Journal of Clinical Nutrition,* Vol. 45 (1987), pp. 1126–1134.

Armstrong, R. B. "Mechanisms of Exercise-Induced Delayed Onset Muscular Soreness: A Brief Review." *Medicine and Science in Sports and Exercise,* Vol. 16 (1984), No. 6, pp. 529–538.

Armstrong, R. B. "Muscle Damage and Endurance Events." *Sports Medicine,* Vol. 3 (1986), pp. 370–381.

Bagchi, D., and J. Barilla. *Huperzine A: Boost Your Brain Power.* New Canaan, CT: Keats Publishing, 1998.

Baker, O., et al. "Absorption and Excretion of L-Carnitine During Single or Multiple Dosings in Humans." *International Journal of Vitamin and Nutrition Research,* Vol. 63 (1993), pp. 22–26.

Balch, James F., and Phyllis A. Balch. *Prescription for Nutritional Healing.* Garden City Park, NY: Avery Publishing Group, 1997.

Ball, T., et al. "Periodic Carbohydrate Replacement During 50 Minutes of High-Intensity Cycling Improves Subsequent Sprint Performance." *International Journal of Sport Science* (1995), pp. 151–158.

Bamman, M. M., et al. "Changes in Body Composition, Diet, and Strength of Bodybuilders During the 12 Weeks Prior to Competition." *Journal of Sports Medicine and Physical Fitness,* Vol. 33 (1993), pg. 383.

Beam, W. C. "The Effect of Chronic Ascorbic Acid Supplementation on Strength Following Isotonic Strength Training." *Medicine and Science in Sports and Exercise,* Vol. 30 (1998), pg. S219.

Belanger, A. Y., and A. J. McComas. "A Comparison of Contractile Properties in Human Arm and Leg Muscles." *European Journal of Applied Physiology,* Vol. 54 (1985), pp. 26–33.

Bell, D. G., et al. "Effects of Caffeine, Ephedrine and the Combination on Time to Exhaustion During High-Intensity Exercise." *European Journal of Applied Physiology,* Vol. 77 (1998), pp. 427–433.

Bell, R. D., J. D. MacDougall, R. Billeter, and H. Howald. "Muscle Fiber Types and Morphometric Analysis of Skeletal Muscle in Six-Year-Old Children." *Medicine and Science in Sports and Exercise,* Vol. 12 (1980), No. 1, pp. 28–31.

Bergstrom, Jonas, and Eric Hultman. "Nutrition for Maximal Sports Performance." *Journal of the American Medical Association,* Vol. 221 (1972), No. 9, pp. 999–1004.

Berning, J. R. "The Role of Medium-Chain Triglycerides in Exercise." *International Journal of Sport Nutrition,* Vol. 6 (1996), No. 3, pp. 121–133.

Bier, Dennis M., and Vernon R. Young. "Exercise and Blood Pressure: Nutritional Considerations." *Annals of Internal Medicine,* Part 2 (1983), pp. 864–869.

Birkmayer, G. D. *Energy for Life: NADH: The Energizing Coenzyme.* New York: MEMUCO Corp., 1996.

Birkmayer, G. D., and P. Vank. "Reduced Coenzyme 1 (NADH) Improves Pyschomotoric and Physical Performance in Athletes." White Paper Report. New York: MENUCO Corp., 1996.

Birkmayer, J.G.D. "Coenzyme Nicotinamide Adenine Dinucleotide: New Therapeutic Approach for Improving Dementia of the Alzheimer Type." Annals of Clinical and Laboratory Science, Vol. 26 (1996), No. 1, pp. 1–9.

Birkmayer, J.G.D., and W. Birkmayer. "The Coenzyme Nicotinamide Adenine Dinucleotide (NADH) as Biological Antidepressive Agent Experience With 205 Patients." In *New Trends in Clinical Neuropharmacology* (N.p., n.d.).

Birkmayer, J.G.D., C. Vrecko, et al. "Nicotinamide Adenine Dinucleotide (NADH)—A New Therapeutic Approach to Parkinson's Disease: Comparison of Oral and Parenteral Application." *Acta Neurologica Scandinavica,* Vol. 87 (1993), supplement, pp. 32–35.

Bonde-Petersen, Flemming, Howard G. Knuttgen, and Jan Henriksson. "Muscle Metabolism During Exercise With Concentric and Eccentric Contractions." *Journal of Applied Physiology,* Vol. 33 (1972), pp. 792–795.

Bonke, D., and B. Nickel. "Improvement of Fine Motoric Movement Control by Elevated Dosages of Vitamin B_1, B_6 and B_{12} in Target Shooting." *International Journal of Vitamin and Nutrition Research,* Vol. 30 (1989), pg. 198.

Borum, Peggy R. "Carnitine." *Annual Reviews of Nutrition,* Vol. 3 (1983), pp. 233–259.

Boyne, P. S., and H. Medhurst. "Oral Anti-inflammatory Enzyme Therapy in Injuries in Professional Footballers." *The Practitioner,* Vol. 198 (April 1967), pp. 543–546.

Brilla, L. R., and T. E. Landerholm. "Effect of Fish Oil Supplementation and Exercise on Serum Lipids and Aerobic Fitness." *Journal of Sports Medicine and Physical Fitness,* Vol. 30 (1990), No. 2, pp. 173–180.

Brodan, V., E. Kuhn, J. Pechar, Z. Placer, and Z. Slabochova. "Effects of Sodium Glutamate Infusion on Ammonia Formation During Intense Physical Exercise in Man." *Nutrition Reports International,* Vol. 9 (1974), No. 3, pp. 223–232.

"Bromelain and Musculoskeletal Injuries." *Research Reviews,* Herbal Gram No. 39 (1997), pg. 17.

Brown, C. Harmon, and Jack H. Wilmore. "The Effects of Maximal Resistance Training on the Strength and Body Composition of Women Athletes." *Medicine and Science in Sports,* Vol. 6 (1974), No. 3, pp. 174–177.

Bucci, L. *Nutrients as Ergogenic Aids for Sports and Exercise.* Boca Raton, FL: CRC Press, 1993.

Bucci, L. *Nutrition Applied to Injury Rehabilitation and Sports Medicine.* Boca Raton, FL: CRC Press, 1995.

Buono, Michael J., Thomas R. Clancy, and Jeff R. Cook. "Blood Lactate and Ammonium Ion Accumulation During Graded Exercise in Humans." *The American Physiological Society* (1984), pp. 135–139.

Burke, E. R. *Pyruvate: 40.* New Canaan, CT: Keats Publishing, 1997.

Burke, Edmond R., Frank Cerny, David Costill, and William Fink. "Characteristics of Skeletal Muscle in Competitive Cyclists." *Medicine and Science in Sports,* Vol. 9 (1977), No. 2, pp. 109–112.

Burke, L. M., and S. D. Read. "Dietary Supplements in Sport." *Sports Medicine,* Vol. 15 (1993), pp. 43–65.

Buskirk, Elsworth R., and José Mendez. "Sports Science and Body Composition Analysis: Emphasis on Cell and Muscle Mass." *Medicine and Science in Sports and Exercise,* Vol. 16 (1984), No. 6, pp. 584–593.

Butterfield, G. "Ergogenic Aids: Evaluating Sport Nutrition Products." *International Journal of Sport Nutrition,* Vol. 6 (1996), No. 3, pp. 191–197.

Butterfield, Gail E., and Doris H. Calloway. "Physical Activity Improves Protein Utilization in Young Men." *British Journal of Nutrition,* Vol. 51 (1984), pp. 171–184.

Calles-Escandon, Jorge, John J. Cunningham, Peter Snyder, Ralph Jacob, Gabor Huszar, Jacob Loke, and Philip Felig. "Influence of Exercise on Urea, Creatinine, and 3-Methylhistidine Excretion in Normal Human Subjects." *The American Physiological Society* (1984), pp. E334–E338.

Campbell, C. J., A. Bonen, R. L. Kirby, and A. N. Belcastro. "Muscle Fiber Composition and Performance Capacities of Women." *Medicine and Science in Sports,* Vol. 11 (1979), pp. 260–265.

Campbell, M. J., A. J. McComas, and F. Petitio. "Physiological Changes in Aging Muscles." *Journal of Neurology, Neurosurgery, and Psychiatry,* Vol. 36 (1973), pp. 174–182.

Carlson, Bruce M., and John A. Faulkner. "The Regeneration of Skeletal Muscle Fibers Following Injury: A Review." *Medicine and Science in Sports and Exercise,* Vol. 15 (1983), No. 3, pp. 187–198.

Carter, J. E. Lindsay, and William H. Phillips. "Structural Changes in Exercising Middle-Aged Males During a 2-Year Period." *Journal of Applied Physiology,* Vol. 27 (1969), pp. 787–794.

Casanueva, F. F., L. Villanueva, J. A. Cabranes, J. Cabezas-Cerrato, and A. Fernandez-Cruz. "Cholinergic Mediation of Growth Hormone Secretion Elicited by Arginine, Clonidine, and Physical Exercise in Man." *Journal of Clinical Endocrinology and Metabolism,* Vol. 59 (1984), No. 3, pp. 526–530.

Celejowa, I., and M. Homa. "Food Intake, Nitrogen and Energy Balance in Polish

Weight Lifters, During Training Camp." *Nutrition and Metabolism,* Vol. 12 (1970), pp. 259–274.

Chang, Tse Wen, and Alfred L. Goldberg. "The Metabolic Fates of Amino Acids and the Formation of Glutamine in Skeletal Muscle." *Journal of Biological Chemistry,* Vol. 253 (1978), No. 10, pp. 3685–3695.

Cheng, W., et al. "Beta-Hydroxy Beta-Methylbutyrate Increases Fatty Acid Oxidation by Muscle Cells." *Federation of American Societies of Experimental Biology Journal,* Vol. 11 (1997): pg. A381.

Cheng, Y. S., C. Z. Lu, Z. L. Ying, W.Y. Ni, C. J. Zhang, and G. W. Sang. "128 Cases of Myasthenia Gravis Treated With Huperzine A." *New Drugs and Clinical Remedies,* Vol. 5 (1986), pp. 197–199.

Chin, S. "Dietary Sources of Conjugated Dienoic Isomers of Linoleic Acid, a Newly Recognized Class of Anticarcinogens." *Journal of Food Composition and Analysis,* Vol. 5 (1992), pp. 185–195.

Chin, S., J. Storkron, K. Albright, M. Cook, and M. Pariza. "Conjugated Linoleic Acid is a Growth Factor for Rats as Shown by Enhanced Weight Gain and Improved Feed Efficiency." *Journal of Nutrition,* Vol. 124 (1994), pp. 2344–2349.

Christensen, H. "Muscle Activity and Fatigue in the Shoulder Muscles During Repetitive Work." *European Journal of Applied Physiology,* Vol. 54 (1986), pp. 596–601.

Cichoke, Anthony J. *The Complete Book of Enzyme Therapy.* Garden City Park, NY: Avery Publishing Group, 1999.

Clarkson, P., and E. Haymes. "Trace Mineral Requirements for Athletes." *International Journal of Sports Nutrition,* Vol. 4 (1994), pg. 104.

Clarkson, Priscilla M., Walter Kroll, and Thomas C. McBride. "Plantar Flexion Fatigue and Muscle Fiber Type in Power and Endurance Athletes." *Medicine and Science in Sports and Exercise,* Vol. 12 (1980), pp. 262–267.

Colgan, M. *Optimum Sports Nutrition.* Ronkonkoma, NY: Advanced Research Press, 1993.

Colker, C. M. "Immune Status of Elite Athletes: Role of Whey Protein Concentrate: A Review." *Medicine and Science in Sports and Exercise,* Vol. 30 (1998), pg. S17.

Conlay, L. A., R. J. Wurtman, J. K. Blusztajn, et al. "Decreased Plasma Choline Concentrations in Marathon Runners" (letter). *New England Journal of Medicine,* Vol. 175 (1986), pg. 892.

Conzolazio, C. Frank, Herman L. Johnson, Richard A. Nelson, Joseph G. Dramise, and James H. Skala. "Protein Metabolism During Intensive Physical Training in the Young Adult." *American Journal of Clinical Nutrition,* Vol. 28 (1975), pp. 29–35.

Cook, James D., and Elaine R. Monsen. "Vitamin C, the Common Cold, and Iron Absorption." *American Journal of Clinical Nutrition* (1977), pp. 235–241.

Cook, M. "Immune Modulation by Altered Nutrient Metabolism: Nutritional Control of Immune-Induced Growth Depression." *Poultry Science,* Vol. 72 (1993), pp. 1301–1305.

Cooper, K. H. *Advanced Nutritional Therapies.* Nashville, TN: Thomas Nelson Publishers, 1996.

Cooper, K. H. *Antioxidant Revolution.* Nashville, TN: Thomas Nelson Publishers, 1994.

Copinschi, Georges, Laurence C. Wegienka, Satoshi Hane, and Peter H. Forsham. "Effect of Arginine on Serum Levels of Insulin and Growth Hormone in Obese Subjects." *Metabolism,* Vol. 16 (1967), pp. 485–491.

Cossack, Zafrallah T., and Ananda Prasad. "Effect of Protein Source on the Bioavailability of Zinc in Human Subjects." *Nutrition Research,* Vol. 3 (1983), pp. 23–31.

Costill, D. L., A. Barnett, R. Sharp, W. J. Fink, and A. Katz. "Leg Muscle pH Following Sprint Running." *Medicine and Science in Sports and Exercise,* Vol. 15 (1983), pp. 325–329.

Costill, D. L., R. Bowers, et al. "Muscle Glycogen Utilization During Prolonged Exercise on Successive Days." *Journal of Applied Physiology,* Vol. 31 (1971), pp. 834–838.

Costill, D. L., and M. Hargreaves. "Carbohydrate Nutrition and Fatigue." *Sports Medicine,* Vol. 13 (1992), pg. 86.

Costill, D. L., W. M. Sherman, et al. "The Role of Dietary Carbohydrate in Muscle Glycogen Synthesis After Strenuous Running." *American Journal of Clinical Nutrition,* Vol. 34 (1981), pp. 1831–1836.

Costill, David L., Michael G. Flynn, John P. Kirwan, Joseph A. Houmard, Joel B. Mitchell, Robert Thomas, and Sung Han Park. "Effects of Repeated Days of Intensified Training on Muscle Glycogen and Swimming Performance." *Medicine and Science in Sports and Exercise,* Vol. 20 (1987), No. 3, pp. 249–254.

Coyle, Edward F., and Andrew R. Coggan. "Effectiveness of Carbohydrate Feeding in Delaying Fatigue During Prolonged Exercise." *Sports Medicine* (1984), pp. 446–458.

Craig, B. "The Influence of Fructose on Physical Performance." *American Journal of Clinical Nutrition,* Vol. 58 (1993), pg. S819.

Davidson, M.H., C.E. Weeks, H. Lardy, et al. "Safety and Endocrine Effects of 3-Acetyl-7-Oxo DHEA (7-Keto DHEA)." Paper presented at the Experimental Biology National Meetings, 1998.

Davies, Kelvin J. A., Alexandre T. Quintanilha, George A. Brooks, and Lester Packer. "Free Radicals and Tissue Damage Produced by Exercise." *Biochemical and Biophysical Research Communications,* Vol. 107 (1982), No. 4, pp. 1198–1205.

Davis, Teresa A., Irene E. Karl, Elise D. Tegtmeyer, Dale F. Osborne, Saulo Klahr, and Herschel R. Harter. "Muscle and Protein Turnover: Effects of Exercise Training and Renal Insufficiency." *The American Physiological Society* (1985), pp. E337–E345.

Despres, J. P., C. Bouchard, R. Savard, A. Tremblay, M. Marcotte, and G. Theriault. "Level of Physical Fitness and Adipocyte Lipolysis in Humans." *The American Physiological Society* (1984), pp.1157–1161.

Despres, J. P., C. Bouchard, A. Tremblay, R. Savard, and M. Marcotte. "Effects of Aerobic Training on Fat Distribution in Male Subjects." *Medicine and Science in Sports and Exercise,* Vol. 17 (1985), No. 1, pp. 113–118.

Devlin, T. M. *Biochemistry With Clinical Correlations,* 3rd Edition. New York: Wiley Liss, 1992.

DiPasquale, M. G. *The Bodybuilding Supplement Review.* N.p.: Optimum Training Systems, 1995.

DiPrampero, P. Enrico. "Energetics of Muscular Exercise." *Biochemical Pharmacology,* Vol. 89 (1981), pp. 143–209.

Dohm, G. Lynis, George J. Kasperek, Edward B. Tapscott, and Gary R. Beecher. "Effect of Exercise on Synthesis and Degradation of Muscle Protein." *Biochemical Journal,* Vol. 188 (1980), pp. 255–262.

Dray, F. "Role of Prostaglandins in Growth Hormone Secretion." *Advanced Prostaglandin and Thromboxane Research,* Vol. 8 (1980), pg. 1321.

Dyner, T., W. Lang, J. Geaga, et al. "An Open-Label Dose-Escalation Trial of Oral Dehydroepiandrosterone Tolerance and Pharmacokinetics in Patients With HIV Disease." *Journal of Immune Deficiency Syndromes,* Vol. 6 (1993), pp. 459–465.

"Effects of Branched Chain Amino Acid Supplementation Before and After Training." *Medicina Dello Sport,* Vol. 50 (1997), pp. 293–303.

Ehn, Lars, Bjorn Carlmark, and Sverker Hoglund. "Iron Status in Athletes Involved in Intense Physical Activity." *Medicine and Science in Sports and Exercise,* Vol. 12 (1980), No. 1, pp. 61–64.

Einzig, S., J. St. Cyr, R. Bianco, J. Schneider, E. Lorenz, and J. Foker. "Myocardial ATP Repletion With Ribose Infusion." *Pediatric Research,* Vol. 19 (1985), No. 4, pg. 127A.

Engelhandt, M., G. Neumann, A. Berbalk, et al. "Creatine Supplementation in Endurance Sports." *Medicine and Science in Sports and Exercise,* Vol. 30 (1998), pp. 1123–1129.

Erickson, Mark A., Robert J. Schwarzkopf, and Robert D. McKenzie. "Effects of Caffeine, Fructose, and Glucose Ingestion on Muscle Glycogen Utilization During Exercise." *Medicine and Science in Sports and Exercise,* Vol. 19 (1987), No. 6, pp. 579–583.

Erling, T. A "Pilot Study With the Aim of Studying the Efficacy and Tolerability of CLA (Tonalin) on the Body Composition in Humans." Medstat Research Ltd., Liilestrom, Norway, July 1997.

Essen, B. E., J. Jansson, J. Henriksson, A. W. Taylor, and B. Saltin. "Metabolic Characteristics of Fibre Types in Human Skeletal Muscle." *Acta Physiolgica Scandinavica,* Vol.19 (1975), pp.153–165.

Fahey, T.D., and M. Pearl. "Hormonal Effects of Phosphatidylserine During 2 Weeks of Intense Training." Abstract presented at the national meeting of the American College of Sports Medicine, June 1998.

Fahey, Thomas D., Lahsen Akka, and Richard Rolph. "Body Composition and VO_2 Max of Exceptional Weight-Trained Athletes." *Journal of Applied Physiology,* Vol. 19 (1975), No. 4, pp. 559–561.

"Fatigue and Underperformance in Athletes." *British Journal of Sports Nutrition,* Vol. 32 (1998), pp. 107–110.

Ferreira, M., R. Kreider, M. Wilson, and A. Almada. "Effects of Conjugated Linoleic Acid (CLA) Supplementation During Resistance Training on Body Composition and Strength." *Journal of Strength and Conditioning Research,* Vol. 11 (1997), pg. 280.

Food and Nutrition Board. *Recommended Dietary Allowances,* 9th Edition. Washington, DC: National Academy of Sciences, 1980.

Forbes, Gilbert B. "Body Composition as Affected by Physical Activity and Nutrition." *Metabolic and Nutritional Aspects of Physical Exercise: Federation Proceedings,* Vol. 44 (1985), No. 2., pp. 334–352.

Forbes, Gilbert B. "Growth of the Lean Body Mass in Man." *Growth,* Vol. 36 (1972), pp. 325–338.

Forbes, Richard M., and John W. Erdman, Jr. "Bioavailability of Trace Mineral Elements." *Annual Reviews of Nutrition,* Vol. 3 (1983), pp. 213–231.

Fournier, Mario, Joe Ricci, Albert W. Taylor, Ronald J. Ferguson, Richard R. Montpetit, and Bernard R. Chaitman. "Skeletal Muscle Adaptation in Adolescent Boys: Sprint and Endurance Training and Detraining." *Medicine and Science in Sports and Exercise,* Vol. 14 (1982), No. 6, pp. 453–456.

Fox, Edward L., Robert L. Bartels, James Klinzing, and Kerry Ragg. "Metabolic Responses to Interval Training Programs of High and Low Power Output." *Medicine and Science in Sports,* Vol. 9 (1977), No. 3, pp.191–196.

Franke, W. W, and B. Berendonk. "Hormonal Doping and Androgenization of Athletes: A Secret Program of the German Democratic Republic Government." *Clinical Chemistry,* Vol. 43 (1997), pp. 1262–1279.

Friedman, J. E., et al. "Regulation of Glycogen Resynthesis Following Exercise." *Sports Medicine,* Vol. 11 (1991), pg. 232.

Galton, David J., and George A. Bray. "Studies on Lipolysis in Human Adipose Cells." *Journal of Clinical Investigation,* Vol. 46 (1967), No. 4, pp. 621–629.

Gao, J. P., D. I. Costill, C. A. Horswill, and S. H. Park. "Sodium Bicarbonate Ingestion Improves Performance in Interval Swimming." *European Journal of Applied Physiology,* Vol. 58 (1988), pp. 171–174.

Gardier, A. M. "Effects of Acute and Chronic NADH Administration on Peripheral and Central Norepinephrine and Dopamine Synthesis in the Rat." Internal Lab Report No. 94070401, Birkmayer Institute for Parkinson Therapy, Vienna, Austria.

Garza, C., N. S. Scrimshaw, and V. R. Young. "Human Protein Requirements: The Effect of Variations in Energy Intake Within the Maintenance Range." *American Journal of Clinical Nutrition,* Vol. 29 (1976), pp. 280–287.

Gastelu, D. L. "Developing State-of-the-Art Amino Acids." *Muscle Magazine International,* May 1989, pp. 58–64.

Gastelu, Daniel, and Fred Hatfield. *Dynamic Nutrition for Maximum Performance.* Garden City Park, NY: Avery Publishing Group, 1997.

Gleeson, M., et al. "Effect of Low- and High-Carbohydrate Diets on the Plasma Glutamine and Circulating Leukocyte Responses to Exercise." *International Journal of Sports Nutrition,* Vol. 8 (1998), pp. 49–59.

Goldberg, Alfred L., Joseph D. Etlinger, David F. Goldspink, and Charles Jablecki. "Mechanism of Work-Induced Hypertrophy of Skeletal Muscle." *Medicine and Science in Sports,* Vol. 7 (1975), No. 3, pp.185–198.

Goldspink, David F. "The Influence of Activity on Muscle Size and Protein Turnover." *Journal of Physiology,* Vol. 264 (1976), pp. 283–296.

Gollnick, P. D., R. B. Armstrong, B. Saltin, C. W. Saubert IV, W. L. Sembrowich, and R. E. Shepherd. "Effect of Training on Enzyme Activity and Fiber Composition of Human Skeletal Muscle." *Journal of Applied Physiology,* Vol. 34 (1973), No. 1, pp. 107–111.

Gollnick, Philip D. "Metabolism of Substrates: Energy Substrate Metabolism During Exercise and as Modified by Training." *Metabolic and Nutritional Aspects of Physical Exercise: Federation Proceedings,* Vol. 44 (1985), No. 2, pp. 353–368.

Gontzea, I., P. Sutzescu, and S. Dumitrache. "The Influence of Muscular Activity on Nitrogen Balance and on the Need of Man for Proteins." *Nutrition Reports International,* Vol.10 (1974), pp. 35–43.

Green, Jerry Franklin, and Alan P. Jackman. "Peripheral Limitations to Exercise." *Medicine and Science in Sports and Exercise,* Vol. 16 (1984), No. 3, pp. 299–305.

Greenhaff, P., et al. "Effect of Oral Creatine Supplementation on Skeletal Muscle Phosphocreatine Resynthesis." *American Journal of Physiology,* Vol. 266 (1994), pp. E725–E730.

Gross, M., R. Kormann, and N. Zollner. "Ribose Administration During Exercise: Effects on Substrates and Products of Energy Metabolism in Healthy Subjects and a Patient With Myoadenylate Deaminase Deficiency." *Klinische Wochenschrift,* Vol. 69 (1991), pp. 151–155.

Haralambie, G., and A. Berg. "Serum Urea and Amino Nitrogen Changes With Exercise Duration." *European Journal of Applied Physiology* (1976), pp. 39–48.

Hargreaves, M., David L. Costill, A. Katz, and W. J. Fink. "Effect of Fructose Ingestion on Muscle Glycogen Usage During Exercise." *Medicine and Science in Sports and Exercise,* Vol. 17 (1985), pp. 360–363.

Harmsen, Eef, Peter P. DeTombe, Jan Willem DeJong, and Peter W. Achterberg. "Enhanced ATP and GTP Synthesis From Hypoxanthine or Inosine After Myocardial Ischemia." *The American Physiological Society* (1984), pp. H37–H43.

Harper, M.J.K. "Effects of Androstenedione on Pre-implantation Stages of Pregnancy in Rats." *Endocrinology,* Vol. 81 (1967), pp. 1091–1098.

Hartog, M., R. J. Havel, G. Copinschi, J. M. Earll, and B. C. Ritchie. "The Relationship Between Changes in Serum Levels of Growth Hormone and Mobilization of Fat During Exercise in Man." *Quarterly Journal of Experimental Physiology,* Vol. 52 (1967), pp. 86–96.

Hatfield, F. C. *Fitness: The Complete Guide,* 3rd Edition. Santa Barbara, CA: International Sports Sciences Association, 1996.

Hatfield, F. C. *Hardcore Bodybuilding: A Scientific Approach.* Chicago: Contemporary Books, 1993.

Hatfield, F. C., and M. Krotee. *Personalized Weight Training for Fitness and Athletics: From Theory to Practice.* Dubuque, IA: Kendall/Hunt Publishing Co., 1978.

Heeker, A. L., and K. B. Wheeler. "Protein: A Misunderstood Nutrient for the Athlete." *National Strength and Conditioning Association Journal,* Vol. 7 (1985), pp. 28–29.

Heilongjiang Institute of Traditional Chinese Medicine and Materia Medica. *Journal of Chinese Herbs and Medicine Research,* Vol. 1 (1973), pg. 1.

Helie, R., J.-M. Lavoie, and D. Cousineau. "Effects of a 24-Hour Carbohydrate-Poor Diet on Metabolic and Hormonal Responses During Glucose-Infused Leg Exercise." *European Journal of Applied Physiology,* Vol. 54 (1985), pp. 420–426.

Hellsten-Westling, Y., B. Norman, P. Balsom, and B. Sjodin. "Decreased Resting Levels of Adenine Nucleotides in Human Skeletal Muscle After High-Intensity Training." *Journal of Applied Physiology,* Vol. 74 (1993), No. 5, pp. 2523–2528.

Henneman, Dorothy, and Philip H. Henneman. "Effects of Human Growth Hormone on Levels of Blood and Urinary Carbohydrate and Fat Metabolites in Man." *Journal of Clinical Investigation,* Vol. 39 (1960), pp. 1239–1245.

Herbert, Victor, Elizabeth Jacob, and Kit-Tai Judy Wong. "Destruction of Vitamin

B$_{12}$ by Vitamin C." *American Journal of Clinical Nutrition,* Vol. 30 (1976), pp. 297–303.

Hermansen, Lars, Eric Hultman, and Bengt Saltin. "Muscle Glycogen During Prolonged Severe Exercise." *Acta Physiolgica Scandinavica,* Vol. 71 (1967), pp. 129–139.

Heymsfield, Steven B., Carlos Arteaga, Clifford McManus, Janet Smith, and Steven Moffitt. "Measurement of Muscle Mass in Humans: Validity of the 24-Hour Urinary Creatinine Method." *American Journal of Clinical Nutrition,* Vol. 37 (1983), pp. 478–494.

Hickson, James F., Jr., and Klaus Hinkelmann. "Exercise and Protein Intake Effects on Urinary 3-Methylhistidine Excretion." *American Journal of Clinical Nutrition,* Vol. 41 (1985), pp. 32–45.

Hickson, Robert C., and Maureen A. Rosenkoetter. "Reduced Training Frequencies and Maintenance of Increased Aerobic Power." *Medicine and Science in Sports and Exercise,* Vol. 13, No. 1 (1981), pp. 13–16.

Hill, J. O., and R. Commerford. "Physical Activity, Fat Balance, and Energy Balance." *International Journal of Sport Nutrition,* Vol. 6 (1996), No. 3, pp. 80–92.

Him-Che Yeung. *Handbook of Chinese Herbs and Formulas.* Beijing: Institute of Chinese Medicine, 1983.

Hobbs, C. *Handbook of Herbal Healing.* Santa Cruz, CA: Botanica Press, 1990.

Hofman, Z., et al. "Glucose and Insulin Responses After Commonly Used Sport Feedings Before and After a 1-Hour Training Session." *International Journal of Sport Nutrition,* Vol. 5 (1995), pp. 194–205.

Holloszy, John O. "Adaptation of Skeletal Muscle to Endurance Exercise." *Medicine and Science in Sports,* Vol. 7 (1975), No. 3, pp. 155–164.

Holloszy, John O. "Exercise, Health, and Aging: A Need for More Information." *Medicine and Science in Sports and Exercise,* Vol.15 (1983), No. 1, pp. 1–5.

Holt, Henry T. "Carica Paypaya as Ancillary Therapy for Athletic Injuries." *Current Therapeutic Research,* Vol. 11 (October 1969), pp. 621–624.

Hong-yen Hsu. *Chemical Constituents of Oriental Herbs.* N.p.: Oriental Healing Arts Institute, 1985.

Horn, M. E. "Improved Sprint Cycle Performance Following Consumption of a Chromium-Carbohydrate Beverage During Prolonged Exercise." *Medicine and Science in Sports and Exercise,* Vol. 30 (1998), pg. S288.

Horton, E., and R. Terjung. *Exercise, Nutrition, and Energy Metabolism.* New York: Macmillan Publishing Company, 1988.

Horton, Edward S. "Metabolic Aspects of Exercise and Weight Reduction." *Medicine and Science in Sports and Exercise,* Vol. 18 (1986), pg. 10.

Ip, C. "Potential of Food Modification in Cancer Prevention." *Cancer Research,* Vol. 54 (1994), pp. 1957s–1959s.

Ivy, J. L., R. T. Withers, P. J. Van Handel, D.L.L. Elger, and D. L. Costill. "Muscle Respiratory Capacity and Fiber Type as Determinants of the Lactate Threshold." *American Physiological Society* (1980), pp. 523–527.

Jacobs, Ira, Mona Esbjornsson, Christer Sylven, Ingemar Holm, and Eva Jansson. "Sprint Training Effects on Muscle Myoglobin, Enzymes, Fiber Types, and Blood Lactate." *Medicine and Science in Sports and Exercise,* Vol. 19 (1987), No. 4, pp. 369–374.

Jakeman, P., and S. Maxwell. "Effect of Antioxidant Vitamin Supplementation on Muscle Function After Eccentric Exercise." *European Journal of Applied Physiology,* Vol. 67 (1993), pg. 426.

Jayaram, S., et al. *Indian Drugs,* Vol. 30 (1993), No. 10, pp. 498–500.

Jezova, D., M. Vigas, P. Tatar, R. Kvetnansky, K. Nazar, H. Kaciuba-Uscilko, and S. Kozlowski. "Plasma Testosterone and Catecholamine Responses to Physical Exercise of Different Intensities in Men." *European Journal of Applied Physiology,* Vol. 54 (1985), pp. 62–66.

Jones, K. *Reishe: Ancient Herb for Modern Times.* Seattle: Sylvan Press, 1992.

Jones, K. *Shiitake: The Healing Mushroom.* Rochester, VT: Healing Arts Press, 1995.

Journal of Applied Physiology, Vol. 83 (1998), pp. 1159–1163.

Journal of the American Medical Association, Vol. 279 (1998), pp. 1383–1391.

Kaats, G. R., D. Blum, D. Pullin, et al. "A Randomized, Double Blind, Placebo Controlled Study of the Effects of Chromium Picolinate Supplementation on Body Composition: A Replication and Extension of a Previous Study." *Current Therapy Research,* Vol. 59 (1998), pp. 379–388.

Kaman, R. *Endurox: A Novel Agent That Increases Workout Performance.* Woodbridge, NJ: PacificHealth Laboratories, Inc., 1997.

Kanter, M. "Free Radicals, Exercise, and Antioxidant Supplementation." *International Journal of Sports Nutrition,* Vol. 4 (1994), pg. 205.

Karagiorgos, Athanase, Joseph F. Garcia, and George A. Brooks. "Growth Hormone Response to Continuous and Intermittent Exercise." *Medicine and Science in Sports,* Vol. 11 (1979), No. 3, pp. 302–307.

Karlsson, Jan, Lars-Olof Nordesjo, and Bengt Saltin. "Muscle Glycogen Utilization During Exercise After Physical Training." *Acta Physiolgica Scandinavica,* Vol. 90 (1974), pp. 210–217.

Karlsson, Jan, and Bengt Saltin. "Diet, Muscle Glycogen, and Endurance Performance." *Journal of Applied Physiology,* Vol. 31 (1971), No. 2, pp. 203–206.

Karlsson, Jan, and Bengt Saltin. "Lactate, ATP, and CP in Working Muscles During Exhaustive Exercise in Man." *Journal of Applied Physiology,* Vol. 29 (1970), No. 5, pp. 598–602.

Kasai, Kikuo, Masami Kobayashi, and Shin-Ichi Shimoda. "Stimulatory Effect of Glycine on Human Growth Hormone Secretion." *Metabolism,* Vol. 27 (1978), pp. 201–208.

Kasai, Kikuo, Hitoshi Suzuki, Tsutomu Nakamura, Hiroaki Shiina, and Shin-Ichi Shimoda. "Glycine Stimulates Growth Hormone Release in Man." *Acta Endocronologica,* Vol. 90 (1980), pp. 283–286.

Kasperek, George J., and Rebecca D. Snider. "Increased Protein Degradation After Eccentric Exercise." *European Journal of Applied Physiology,* Vol. 54 (1985), pp. 30–34.

Katch, F. "U.S. Government Raises Serious Questions About Reliability of U.S. Department of Agriculture's Food Composition Database." *International Journal of Sport Nutrition,* Vol. 5 (1995), pp. 62–67.

Katch, Victor L., Frank I. Katch, Robert Moffatt, and Michael Gittleson. "Muscular Development and Lean Body Weight in Body Builders and Weight Lifters." *Medicine and Science in Sports and Exercise,* Vol. 12 (1980), No. 5, pp. 340–344.

Kellis, J.T., and L. E. Vickery. "Inhibition of Estrogen Synthetase (Aromatase) by Flavones." *Science,* Vol. 225 (1984), pp. 1032–1033.

Kelly, V. G., and D. G. Jenkins. "Effect of Oral Creatine Supplementation on Near-Maximal Strength and Repeated Sets of High-Intensity Bench Press Exercise." *Journal of Strength and Conditioning Research,* Vol. 12 (1998), pp. 109-115.

Keville, K. *Ginseng.* New Canaan, CT: Keats Publishing, 1996.

Keville, K. *Herbs for Health and Healing.* Emmaus, PA: Rodale Press, 1996.

Kidd, P. M. *Phosphatidylserine.* New Canaan, CT: Keats Publishing, 1998.

Kidd, P. M. *Phosphatidylserine (PS): A Remarkable Brain Cell Nutrient.* Decatur, IL: Lucas Meyer, 1995.

Kies, C.V., and J. A. Driskell. *Sports Nutrition: Minerals and Electrolytes.* Boca Raton, FL: CRC Press, 1995.

Killingsworth, R., et al. "Hyperthermia and Dehydration-Related Deaths Associated With Intentional Rapid Weight Loss in Three Collegiate Wrestlers." *Morbidity and Mortality Weekly Report,* Vol. 47 (1998), pp. 105–108.

Kirkendall, D. "Effect of Nutrition on Performance in Soccer." *Medicine and Science in Sports and Exercise,* Vol. 25 (1993), pp. 1370.

Kirwan, John P., David L. Costill, Michael G. Flynn, Joel B. Mitchell, William J. Fink, P. Darrell Neufer, and Joseph A. Houmard. "Physiological Responses to Successive Days of Intense Training in Competitive Swimmers." *Medicine and Science in Sports and Exercise,* Vol. 20 (1988), No. 3, pp. 255–259.

Klissouras, Vassilis, Freddy Pirnay, and Jean-Marie Petit. "Adaptation to Maximal Effort: Genetics and Age." *Journal of Applied Physiology,* Vol. 35 (1973), No. 2, pp. 288–293.

Knopf, R. F., J. W. Conn, S. S. Fajans, J. C. Floyd, E. M. Guntsche, and J. A. Rull. "Plasma Growth Hormone Response to Intravenous Administration of Amino Acids." *Journal of Clinical Endocrinology,* Vol. 25 (1965), pp. 1140–1144.

Koeslag, J. H. "Post-Exercise Ketosis and the Hormone Response to Exercise: A Review." *Medicine and Science in Sports and Exercise,* Vol. 14 (1982), No. 5, pp. 327–334.

Kreider, R., et al. "Effects of B-BHBM Supplemetation With and Without Creatine During Training on Body Composition Alterations." *Federation of American Societies of Experimental Biology Journal,* Vol. 11 (1997), pg. A374.

Kreider, R. B., et al. "Effects of Creatine Supplementation on Body Composition, Strength, and Sprint Performance." *Medicine and Science in Sports and Exercise,* Vol. 30 (1998), pp. 73–82.

Kurkin, V. A., and G. G. Zapesochnaya. "Chemical Composition and Pharmacological Properties of Rhodiola Rosea." *Chemical-Pharmaceutical Journal,* Vol. 20 (1986), No. 10, pp. 1231–1244.

Kurzman, I. D., D. L. Panciera, J. B. Miller, et al. "The Effect of Dehydro-epiandrosterone Combined With a Low-Fat Diet in Spontaneously Obese Dogs: A Clinical Trial." *Obesity Research,* Vol. 6 (1998), No. 1, pp. 20–28.

Lander, Jeffrey E., Barry T. Bates, James A. Sawhill, and Joseph Hamill. "A Comparison Between Free-Weight and Isokinetic Bench Pressing." *Medicine and Science in Sports and Exercise,* Vol. 17 (1985), No. 3, pg. 344.

Lardy, H. A., N. Kneer, M. Bellei, et al. "Induction of Thermogenic Enzymes by DHEA and Its Metabolites." *Annals of the New York Academy of Sciences,* Vol. 774 (1995), pp. 171–179.

Lee, H., R. Graeff, and T. Walseth. "Cyclic ADP—Ribose and Its Metabolic Enzymes." *Biochimie,* Vol. 77 (1995), pp. 345–355.

Lehninger, A. L. *Vitamins and Coenzymes: Biochemistry,* 2nd Edition. New York: Worth Publishers, 1975.

Lemon, P. W. R., et al. "Protein Requirements and Muscle Mass/Strength Changes During Intensive Training in Novice Bodybuilders." *Journal of Applied Physiology,* Vol. 73 (1992), pp. 767–775.

Lemon, P.W.R., and J. P. Mullin. "Effect of Initial Muscle Glycogen Levels on Protein Catabolism During Exercise." *The American Physiological Society* (1980), pp. 624–629.

Lemon, P. W. R., and F. J. Nagle. "Effects of Exercise on Protein and Amino Acid Metabolism." *Medicine and Science in Sports and Exercise,* Vol. 13 (1981), No. 3, pp. 141–149.

Lemon, P.W.R., and D. Proctor. "Protein Intake and Athletic Performance." *Sports Medicine,* Vol. 12 (1991), No. 5, pg. 313.

Leung, A.Y., and S. Foster. *Encyclopedia of Common Natural Ingredients Used in Food, Drugs, and Cosmetics.* New York: John Wiley & Sons, 1996.

Lewis, Steven M. A., William L. Haskell, Peter D. Wood, Norman M. A. Manoogian, Judith E. Bailey, and MaryBeth B. A. Pereira. "Effects of Physical Activity on Weight Reduction in Obese Middle-Aged Women." *American Journal of Clincial Nutrition,* Vol. 29 (1976), pp. 151–156.

Lieberman, Shari, and Nancy Bruning. *The Real Vitamin and Mineral Book,* 2nd Edition. Garden City Park, NY: Avery Publishing Group, 1997.

Linderman, J., and T. D. Fahey. "Sodium Bicarbonate Ingestion and Exercise Performance." *Sports Medicine,* Vol. 11, No. 9, pg. 71.

Lucke, Christoph, and Seymour Glick. "Experimental Modification of the Sleep-Induced Peak of Growth Hormone Secretion." *Journal of Clinical Endocrinology and Metabolism,* Vol. 32 (1971), pp. 729–736.

MacDougall, J. D., D. G. Sale, S. E. Alway, and J. R. Sutton. "Muscle Fiber Number in Biceps Brachii in Bodybuilders and Control Subjects." *The American Physiological Society* (1984), pg. 1399.

MacDougall, J. D., D. G. Sale, G.C.B. Elder, and J. R. Sutton. "Muscle Ultrastructural Characteristics of Elite Powerlifters and Bodybuilders." *European Journal of Applied Physiology,* Vol. 48 (1982), pp. 117–126.

MacDougall, J. D., D. G. Sale, J. R. Moroz, G.C.B. Elder, J. R. Sutton, and H. Howald. "Mitochondrial Volume Density in Human Skeletal Muscle Following Heavy Resistance Training." *Medicine and Science in Sports and Exercise,* Vol. 11 (1979), No. 2, pp. 164–166.

Mackova, Eva V., Jan Melichna, Karel Vondra, Toivo Jurimae, Thomas Paul, and Jaroslav Novak. "The Relationship Between Anaerobic Performance and Muscle Metabolic Capacity and Fibre Distribution." *European Journal of Applied Physiology,* Vol. 54 (1985), pp. 413–415.

MacLean, William C., Jr., and George G. Graham. "The Effect of Level of Protein Intake in Isoenergetic Diets on Energy Utilization." *American Journal of Clinical Nutrition* (1979), pp. 1381–1387.

Mahesh, V. B., and R. B. Greenblatt. "The In Vivo Conversion of Dehydroepiandrosterone and Androstenedione to Testosterone in the Human." *Acta Endocrinology,* Vol. 41 (1962), pp. 400–406.

Malina, Robert M., William H. Mueller, Claude Bouchard, Richard F. Shoup, and Georges Lariviere. "Fatness and Fat Patterning Among Athletes at the Montreal Olympic Games, 1976." *Medicine and Science in Sports and Exercise,* Vol. 14 (1982), No. 6, pp. 445–452.

Manore, M. "Vitamin B_6 and Exercise." *International Journal of Sports Nutrition,* Vol. 4 (1994), pg. 89.

Marable, N. L., J. F. Hickson Jr., M. K. Korslund, W. G. Herbert, R. F. Desjardins, and F. W. Thye. "Urinary Nitrogen Excretion as Influenced by a Muscle-Building Exercise Program and Protein Intake Variation." *Nutrition Reports International,* Vol. 19 (1979), No. 6, pp. 795–805.

Maresh, C., et al. "Dietary Supplementation and Improved Anaerobic Performance." *International Journal of Sport Nutrition,* Vol. 4 (1994), pg. 387.

Marriott, B. *Food Components to Enhance Performance.* Washington, DC: National Academy Press, 1994.

Marsit, Joseph, et al. "Effects of Ascorbic Acid on Serum Cortisol and the Testosterone: Cortisol Ratio in Junior Elite Weightlifters." *Journal of Strength and Conditioning Research,* Vol. 12 (1998), pp. 179–184.

Maughan, Ronald. "Creatine Supplementation and Exercise Performance." *International Journal of Sport Nutrition* (1995), pp. 94–101.

Mayer, Jean, Roy Purnima, and Kamakhya Prasad Mitra. "Relation Between Caloric Intake, Body Weight, and Physical Work: Studies in an Industrial Male Population in West Bengal." *American Journal of Clinical Nutrition,* Vol. 4 (1956), No. 2, pp. 169–175.

McBride, J. M., et al. "Effect of Resistance Exercise on Free Radical Production." *Medicine and Science in Sports and Exercise,* Vol. 30 (1998), pp. 67–72.

Medicine and Science in Sports and Exercise, Vol. 30 (1998), pp. 587–595.

Merimee, T. J., D. Rabinowitz, and S. E. Fineberg. "Arginine-Initiated Release of Human Growth Hormone." *New England Journal of Medicine* (1969), pp. 1434–1438.

Merimee, Thomas J., David Rabinowitz, Lamar Riggs, John A. Burgess, David L. Rimoin, and Victor A. McKusick. "Plasma Growth Hormone After Arginine Infusion." *New England Journal of Medicine,* Vol. 23 (1967), pp. 434–438.

Mertz, Walter. "Assessment of the Trace Element Nutritional Status." *Nutrition Research* (1985), pp. 169–174.

Meydani, M., et al. "Protective Effect of Vitamin E on Exercise-Induced Oxidative Damage in Young and Older Adults." *American Journal of Physiology,* Vol. 264 (1993), pp. R992–R998.

Mikesell, Kevin A., and Gary A. Dudley. "Influence of Intense Endurance Training on Aerobic Power of Competitive Distance Runners." *Medicine and Science in Sports and Exercise,* Vol. 16 (1984), No. 4, pp. 371–375.

Mindell, E. *Earl Mindell's Vitamin Bible.* New York: Warner Books, 1991.

Mindell, E. L. *The MSM Miracle.* New Canaan, CT: Keats Publishing, 1997.

Mitchell, J. B., D. L. Costill, J. A. Houmard, M. G. Flynn, W. J. Fink, and J. D. Beltz. "Effects of Carbohydrate Ingestion on Gastric Emptying and Exercise Performance." *Medicine and Science in Sports and Exercise,* Vol. 20 (1988), No. 2, pp. 110–115.

Mittleman, K. D., M. R. Ricci, and S. P. Bailey. "Branched-Chain Amino Acids Prolong Exercise During Heat Stress in Men and Women." *Medicine and Science in Sports and Exercise,* Vol. 30 (1998), pp. 83–91.

Monteleone, P., L. Beinat, C. Tanzillo, M. Maj, and D. Kemali. "Effects of Phosphatidylserine on the Neuroendocrine Response to Physical Response in Humans." *Neuroendocrinology,* Vol. 52 (1990), pp. 243–248.

Monteleone, P., M. Maj, L. Beinat, M. Natale, and D. Kemali. "Blunting by Chronic Phosphatidylserine Administration of the Stress-Induced Activation of the Hypothalamo-Pituitary-Adrenal Axis in Healthy Men." *European Journal of Clinical Pharmacology,* Vol. 43 (1992), pp. 385–388.

Morgan, William P. "Affective Beneficence of Vigorous Physical Activity." *Medicine and Science in Sports and Exercise,* Vol. 17 (1985), No. 1, pp. 94–100.

Morrissey, S. "Evaluation of the Effects of a Complex Herbal Formulation on Lactate Metabolism." *Medicine and Science in Sports and Exercise,* Vol. 30 (1998), pg. S277.

Morrissey, S., R. Wang, and E. R. Burke. "Evaluation of the Effects of a Complex Herbal Formulation on Lactate Metabolism." Paper presented at the national meeting of the American College of Sports Medicine, Orlando, Florida, June 6, 1998.

Murphy, T., et al. "Performance Enhancing Ration Components Project: U.S. Army." Abstract presented at the 11th Annual Symposium of Sports and Cardiovascular Nutritionists, Atlanta, Georgia, 22–24 April 1994.

Murray, F. *The Big Family Guide to All the Minerals.* New Canaan, CT: Keats Publishing, 1995.

Murray, Robert; Dennis E. Eddy, Tami W. Murray, John G. Seifert, Gregory L. Paul, and George A. Halaby. "The Effect of Fluid and Carbohydrate Feedings During Intermittent Cycling Exercise." *Medicine and Science in Sports and Exercise,* Vol. 19 (1987), No. 6, pp. 597–604.

Mutch, B.J.C., and E. W. Banister. "Ammonia Metabolism in Exercise and Fatigue: A Review." *Medicine and Science in Sports and Exercise,* Vol. 15 (1983), No. 1, pp. 41–50.

Nishizawa, N., M. Shimbo, S. Hareyama, and R. Funabiki. "Fractional Catabolic Rates of Myosin and Actin Estimated by Urinary Excretion of N-Methylhistidine: The Effect of Dietary Protein Level on Catabolic Rates Under Conditions of Restricted Food Intake." *British Journal of Nutrition,* Vol. 37 (1976), pp. 345–421.

Nissen, S., et al. "Effect of Leucine Metabolite Beta-Hydroxy Beta-Methylbutyrate on Muscle Metabolism During Resistance Training." *Journal of Applied Physiology,* Vol. 81 (1996), pp. 2095–2104.

Nissen, S., et al. "Effects of Feeding Beta-Hydroxy Beta-Methylbutyrate (BHBM) on Body Composition in Women." *Federation of American Societies of Experimental Biology Journal,* Vol. 11 (1997), pg. A290.

"Nutrition, Exercise, and Bone Status in Youth." *International Journal of Sports Nutrition,* Vol. 8 (1998), pp. 124–142.

Okano, Goroh, Hidekatsu Takeda, Isao Morita, Mitsuru Katoh, Zuien Mu, and Shosuke Miyake. "Effect of Pre-Exercise Fructose Ingestion on Endurance Performance in Fed Men." *Medicine and Science in Sports and Exercise,* Vol. 20 (1987), No. 7, pp. 105–109.

Oscai, Lawrence B., and John O. Holloszy. "Effects of Weight Changes Produced by Exercise, Food Restriction, or Overeating on Body Composition." *Journal of Clinical Investigation,* Vol. 48 (1969), pp. 2124–2128.

Ostaszewski, P., et al. "The Effect of Leucine Metabolite Beta-Hydroxy Beta-Methylbutyrate (BHBM) on Muscle Protein Synthesis and Protein Breakdown in Chick and Rat Muscle," abstract. In *Journal of Animal Science* (1996).

Paddon-Jones, D. J., and D. Pearson. "Cost-Effectiveness of Pre-Exercise Carbohydrate Meals and Their Impact on Performance." *Journal of Conditioning Research,* Vol. 12 (1998), pp. 90–94.

Palmer, Warren K. "Introduction to Symposium: Cyclic AMP Regulation of Fuel Metabolism During Exercise." *Medicine and Science in Sports and Exercise,* Vol. 20 (1988), No. 6, pp. 523–524.

Pariza, M. "Mechanism of Body Fat Reduction by Conjugated Linoleic Acid." *Federation of American Societies of Experimental Biology Journal,* Vol. 11 (1997), pg. A139.

Pariza, M. U.S. Patent 5,385,616, "A Method of Enhancing Weight Gain and Feed Efficiency in an Animal Which Comprises Administering to the Animal a Safe and Effective Amount of a Conjugated Linoleic Acid."

Parkhouse, W. S., and D. C. McKenzie. "Possible Contribution of Skeletal Muscle Buffers to Enhanced Anaerobic Performance: A Brief Review." *Medicine and Science in Sports and Exercise,* Vol. 16 (1984), No. 4, pp. 328–338.

Passwater, R., and J. Fuller. *Building Muscle Mass, Performance and Health With BHBM.* New Canaan, CT: Keats Publishing, 1997.

Pavlou, Konstantin N., William P. Steffee, Robert H. Lerman, and Belton A. Burrows. "Effects of Dieting and Exercise on Lean Body Mass, Oxygen Uptake, and Strength." *Medicine and Science in Sports and Exercise,* Vol. 17 (1974), No. 4, pp. 466–471.

Penn State Sports Medicine Newsletter, Vol. 6 (1998), pg. 3

Phillips, B. *Sports Supplement Review.* Golden, CO: Mile High Publishing, 1997.

Piehl, Karin. "Time Course for Refilling of Glycogen Stores in Human Muscle Fibres Following Exercise-Induced Glycogen Depletion." *Acta Physiologica Scandinavica,* Vol. 90 (1974), pp. 297–302.

Pizza, F., et al. "A Carbohydrate Loading Regimen Improves High Intensity, Short Duration Exercise Performance." *International Journal of Sport Science* (1995), pp. 110–116.

Potischman, N., et al. "Case-Control Study of Endogenous Steroid Hormones and Endometrial Cancer." *Journal of the National Cancer Institute,* Vol. 88 (1996), pp. 1127–1135.

Prasad, Ananda S. "Role of Trace Elements in Growth and Development." *Nutrition Research* (1985), pp. 295–299.

Prud'homme, D. C. Bouchard, C. Leblanc, F. Landry, and E. Fontaine. "Sensitivity of Maximal Aerobic Power to Training Is Genotype-Dependent." *Medicine and Science in Sports and Exercise,* Vol. 16 (1984), No. 5, pp. 489–493.

Robertson, R. J., R. T. Stanko, F. L. Goss, et al. "Blood Glucose Extraction as a Mediator of Perceived Exertion During Prolonged Exercise." *European Journal of Applied Physiology,* Vol. 61 (1990), pp. 100–105.

Romieu, Isabelle, Walter C. Willett, Meir J. Stampfer, Graham A. Colditz, Laura Sampson, Bernard Rosner, Charles Hennekens, and Frank E. Speizer. "Energy Intake and Other Determinants of Relative Weight." *American Journal of Clinical Nutrition,* Vol. 47 (1988), pp. 406–412.

Rubin, M. A., et al. "Acute and Chronic Resistive Exercise Increase Urinary Chromium Excretion in Men as Measured With an Enriched Chromium Stable Isotope." *Journal of Nutrition,* Vol. 128 (1998), pp. 73–78.

Rudofsky, G. "The Effect of Intra-Arterial Infusion Treatment With Prostaglandin E_1 in a Model of Ischemia in Healthy Volunteers." In H. Sinzinger H, Ed., *Prostaglandin E_1 in Atherosclerosis.* New York: Springer Verlag, 1986, pg. 49.

Saitoh, Shin-ichi, Yutaka Yoshitake, and Masahige Suzuki. "Enhanced Glycogen Repletion in Liver and Skeletal Muscle With Citrate Orally Fed After Exhaustive Treadmill Running and Swimming." *Journal of Nutritional Science and Vitaminology,* Vol. 29 (1983), pp. 45–52.

Salleo, Alberto, Guiseppe Anastasi, Guiseppa LaSpada, Guiseppina Falzea, and Maria G. Denaro. "New Muscle Fiber Production During Compensatory Hypertrophy." *Medicine and Science in Sports and Exercise,* Vol. 12 (1980), No. 4, pp. 268–273.

Sandage, B. W., L. A. Sabounjian, R. White, et al. "Choline Citrate May Enhance Athletic Performance." *Physiologist,* Vol. 35 (1992), pg. 236a.

Saratikov, A. S., and E. A. Krasnov. *Rhodiola Rosea Is a Valuable Medicinal Plant (Golden Root)*. Tomsk, Russia: Tomsk University Publishers, 1987.

Satabin, Pascale, Pierre Portero, Gilles Defer, Jacques Bricout, and Charles-Yannick Guezennec. "Metabolic and Hormonal Responses to Lipid and Carbohydrate Diets During Exercise in Man." *Medicine and Science in Sports and Exercise,* Vol. 19 (1987), No. 3, pp. 218–223.

Saudek, Christopher D. "The Metabolic Events of Starvation." *American Journal of Medicine,* Vol. 60 (1976), pp. 117–126.

Schalch, Don S. "The Influence of Physical Stress and Exercise on Growth Hormone and Insulin Secretion in Man." *Journal of Laboratory and Clinical Medicine,* Vol. 69 (1967), No. 2, pp. 256–267.

Schauss, A. G. "Colloidal Minerals: Clinical Implicataions of Clay Suspension Products Sold as Dietary Supplements." *American Journal of Natural Medicine,* Vol. 4 (1997), pp. 5–10.

Schauss, A. G. *Trace Elements and Human Health,* 2nd Edition. Tacoma, WA: Life Sciences, 1996.

Sen, C., et al. "Oxidative Stress After Human Exercise: Effect of N-Acetylcysteine Supplementation." *Journal of Applied Physiology,* Vol. 76 (1994), pp. 2570–2577.

Shanghai Compilation of New Drugs Confirmed in 1976. Shanghai: Sci-Tech Literature Publishing House, 1976.

Sharp, R. "Less Pain, More Gain for Distance Runners on HMB." Presented at the national meeting of Experimental Biology, San Francisco, CA, 1998.

Shaw, P. C. "The Use of a Trypsin-Chymotrypsin Formulation in Fractures of the Hand." *The British Journal of Clinical Practice,* Vol. 23 (January 1969), pp. 25–26.

Shippen, E., and E. Fryer. *The Testosterone Syndrome.* New York: Evans and Company, Inc, 1998.

Short, S. "Dietary Surveys and Nutrition Knowledge." In Hickson, J. F., and I. W. Wolinsky, Eds., *Nutrition in Exercise and Sport.* Boca Raton, FL: CRC Press, 1989.

Simoneau, J.-A., G. Lortie, M. R. Boulay, M. Marcotte, M.-C. Thibault, and C. Bouchard. "Human Skeletal Muscle Fiber Type Alteration With High-Intensity Intermittent Training." *European Journal of Applied Physiology,* Vol. 54 (1985), pp. 250–253.

Simon-Schnass, I., and H. Pabst. "Influence of Vitamin E on Physical Performance." *International Journal of Vitamin Nutrition Research* (1987), pp. 49–54.

Skolnik, A. A. "Old Chinese Herbal Medicine Used for Fever Yields Possible New Alzheimer Disease Therapy." *Journal of the American Medical Association,* Vol. 277 (March 1997), No. 10, pg. 776.

Soares, M. J., et al. "The Effect of Exercise on Riboflavin Status of Adult Men." *British Journal of Nutrition,* Vol. 69 (1993), pp. 541–551.

Spector, S. A., M. R. Jackman, L. A. Sabounjian, et al. "Effects of Choline Supplementation on Fatigue in Training Cyclists." *Medicine and Science in Sports and Exercise,* Vol. 27 (1995), pp. 669–673.

Spiller, G. A., C. D. Jensen, T. S. Pattison, C. S. Chuck, J. H. Whittam, and J. Scala. "Effect of Protein Dose on Serum Glucose and Insulin Response to Sugars." *American Journal of Clinical Nutrition,* Vol. 46 (1987), pp. 474–480.

Sports Medicine, Vol. 25 (1998), pp. 7–23.

Stanko, R. T., A. Mitrakou, et al. "Effect of Dihydroxyacetone and Pyruvate on Plasma Glucose Concentration and Turnover in Noninsulin-Dependent Diabetes Mellitus." *Clinical Physiology and Biochemistry* (1990), pp. 283–288.

Stanko, R. T., H. Reiss Reynolds, et al. "Pyruvate Supplementation of a Low-Cholesterol, Low-Fat Diet: Effects on Plasma Lipid Concentrations and Body Composition in Hyperlipidemic Patients." *American Journal of Clinical Nutrition,* Vol. 59 (1994), pp. 423–427.

Stanko, R. T., R. J. Robertson, R. W. Galbreath, et al. "Enhanced Leg Exercise Endurance With a High Carbohydrate Diet and Dihydroxyacetone and Pyruvate." *Journal of Applied Physiology,* Vol. 69 (1990), pp. 1651–1656.

Stanko, R. T., R. J. Robertson, R. J. Spina, et al. "Enhancement of Arm Exercise Endurance Capacity With Dihydroxyacetone and pyruvate." *Journal of Applied Physiology,* Vol. 68 (1990), pp. 119–124.

Street, C., et al. "Androgen Use by Athletes: Reevaluation of the Health Risks." *Canadian Journal of Applied Physiology,* Vol. 21 (1996), pp. 421–440.

Tesch, Per, et al. "Skeletal Muscle Glycogen Loss Evoked by Resistance Exercise." *Journal of Strength and Conditioning Research,* Vol. 12 (1998), pp. 67–73.

Thomas, D., et al. "Plasma Glucose Levels After Prolonged Strenuous Exercise Correlate Inversely With Glycemic Response to Food Consumed Before Exercise." *International Journal of Sport Nutrition,* Vol. 4 (1994), pg. 361.

Thompson, Deborah A., Larry A. Wolfe, and Roelof Eikelboom. "Acute Effects of Exercise Intensity on Appetite in Young Men." *Medicine and Science in Sports and Exercise,* Vol. 20 (1988), No. 3, pp. 222–227.

Thorland, William G., Glen O. Johnson, Thomas G. Fagot, Gerald D. Tharp, and Richard W. Hammer. "Body Composition and Somatotype Characteristics of Junior Olympic Athletes." *Medicine and Science in Sports and Exercise,* Vol. 13 (1981), No. 5, pp. 332–338.

Todd, Karen S., Gail E. Butterfield, and Doris Howes Calloway. "Nitrogen Balance in Men With Adequate and Deficient Energy Intake at Three Levels of Work." *Journal of Nutrition,* Vol. 114 (1984), pp. 2107–2118.

Torun, B., N. S. Scrimshaw, and V. R. Young. "Effect of Isometric Exercises on Body Potassium and Dietary Protein Requirements of Young Men." *American Journal of Clinical Nutrition,* Vol. 30 (1977), pp. 1983–1993.

Training and Conditioning, June 1998.

"Tribulus Gold," report on tribulus terrestis. Visalia, CA: C.A.B. Enterprises, n.d.

Tric, I., and E. Haymes. "Effects of Caffeine Ingestion on Exercise-Induced Changes During High-Intensity, Intermittent Exercise." *International Journal of Sport Nutrition,* Vol. 5 (1995), pp. 37–44.

Trickett, P. "Proteolytic Enzymes in Treatment of Athletic Injuries." *Applied Therapeutics* (August 1964), pp. 647–652.

Tsomides, J., et al. "Controlled Evaluation of Oral Chymotrypsin-Trypsin Treatment of Injuires to the Head and Face." *Clinical Medicine* (November 1996), pp. 40–45.

Tullson, P., P. Arabadjis, K. Rundell, and R. Terjung. "IMP Reamination to AMP in Rat Skeletal Muscle Fiber Types." *American Journal of Physiology,* Vol. 270 (1996), pp. C1067–C1074.

Tullson, P., J. Bangsbo, Y. Hellsten, and E. Richter. "IMP Metabolism in Human Skeletal Muscle After Exhaustive Exercise." *Journal of Applied Physiology,* Vol. 78(1995), No. 1, pp. 146–152.

Tullson, P., and R. Terjung. "Adenine Nucleotide Synthesis in Exercising and Endurance-Trained Skeletal Muscle." *American Journal of Physiology,* Vol. 261 (1991), pp. C342–C347.

Tullson, P., D. Whitlock, and R. Terjung. "Adenine Nucleotide Degradation in Slow-Twitch Red Muscle." *American Journal of Physiology,* Vol. 258 (1990), pp. C258–C265.

Udischev, S. N., and K. V. Yaremenko. "The Use of the Characteristic of the Rhodiola Rosea Extract to Stimulate Regenerative Processes for an Increase in the Selectivity of the Cyclophoshamide Anti-Tumor Action." In *New Medicinal Preparations From Plants of Siberia and the Far East.* Tomsk, Russia: Tomsk University Publishers, 1968, pp. 151–152.

Ulene, A., and V. Ulene. *The Vitamin Strategy.* Berkeley, CA: Ulysses Press, 1994.

Valeriani, A. "The Need for Carbohydrate Intake During Endurance Exercise." *Sports Medicine,* Vol. 12 (1991), No. 6, pg. 349.

Van der Berg, J., N. Cook, and D. Tribble. "Reinvestigation of the Antioxidant Properties of Conjugated Linoleic Acid." *Lipids,* Vol. 73 (1995), pp. 595–598.

Van Erp-Baart, A. M., J., W.H.M. Saris, R. A. Binkhorst, J. A. Vos, and J.W.H. Elvers. "Nationwide Survey on the Nutritional Habits of Elite Athletes," part 1: "Energy, Carbohydrate, Protein, and Fat Intake." *International Journal of Sports Medicine,* Vol. 10 (1989), supplement, pp. S3–S10.

Viru, A. *Adaptation in Sports Training.* Boca Raton, FL: CRC Press, 1995.

Von Allworden, H. N., S. Horn, J. Kahl, et al. "The Influence of Lecithin on Plasma Choline Concentrations in Triathletes and Adolescent Runners During Exercise." *European Journal of Applied Physiology,* Vol. 67 (1983), pp. 87–91.

Walberg, Janet L., V. Karina Ruiz, Sandra L. Tarlton, Dennis E. Hinkle, and Forrest W. Thye. "Exercise Capacity and Nitrogen Loss During a High or Low Carbohydrate Diet." *Medicine and Science in Sports and Exercise,* Vol. 20 (1986), pp. 34–43.

Wang, R., and Q. Zheng. "Relationship Between Lactic Acid Metabolism and Exercise Performance Capacity Changes in Mice as a Result of Ingesting a Complex Herbal Formulation and Other Compounds." Report. Beijing: China Academy of Medical Sciences, 1997.

Ward, P. S., and D.C.L. Savage. "Growth Hormone Responses to Sleep, Insulin Hypoglycemia and Arginine Infusion." *Hormone Research,* Vol. 22 (1985), pp. 7–11.

Weeks, C., H. Lardy, and S. Henwood. "Preclinical Toxicology Evaluation of 3-Acetyl-7-Oxo-Dehydroepiandrosterone (7-Keto DHEA)." Paper presented at the Experimental Biology National Meetings, 1998.

Weil, Andrew. *Spontaneous Healing.* New York: Alfred E. Knopf, 1995.

Weir, Jane, Timothy D. Noakes, Kathryn Myburgh, and Brett Adams. "A High Carbohydrate Diet Negates the Metabolic Effects of Caffeine During Exercise." *Medicine and Science in Sports and Exercise,* Vol. 19 (1986), pp. 100–105.

Weltman, Arthur, Sharleen Matter, and Bryant A. Stamford. "Caloric Restriction and/or Mild Exercise: Effects on Serum Lipids and Body Composition." *American Journal of Clinical Nutrition,* Vol. 33 (1980), pp. 1002–1009.

West, D. "Reduced Body Fat With Conjugated Linoleic Acid Feeding in the Mouse." *Federation of American Societies of Experimental Biology Journal,* Vol. 11 (1997), pg. A599.

Wilcox, Anthony R. "The Effects of Caffeine and Exercise on Body Weight, Fat-Pad Weight, and Fat-Cell Size." *Medicine and Science in Sports and Exercise,* Vol. 14 (1981), pp. 317–321.

Williams, L. *C.L.A.* Pleasant Grove, UT: Woodland Publishing, 1997.

Williams, M. H. *Nutritional Aspects of Human Physical and Athletic Performance,* 2nd Edition. Springfield, IL: Charles C. Thomas, 1985.

Williams, M. H. "Vitamin Supplementation and Athletic Performance." *International Journal of Vitamin and Nutrition Research,* Vol. 30 (1989), pg. 163.

Wolinsky, I. *Nutrition in Exercise and Sport.* Boca Raton, FL: CRC Press, 1998.

Wolinsky, I., and J. A. Driskell. *Sports Nutrition.* Boca Raton, FL: CRC Press, 1997.

Wolinsky, I., and J. Hickson. *Nutrition in Exercise and Sport,* 2nd Edition. Boca Raton, FL: CRC Press, 1994.

Wright, J. "Tribulus: A Natural Wonder." *Muscle and Fitness,* September 1996, pp. 140–142, 224.

Wu, F. C. "Endocrine Aspects of Anabolic Steroids." *Clinical Chemistry,* Vol. 43 (1997), pp. 1289–1292.

Yan, W., et al. *Phytochemistry,* Vol. 42 (1996), No. 5, pp. 1417–22.

Yan, X. F., W. H. Lu, W. J. Lou, and X. C. Tang. "Effects of Huperzine A and B on Skeletal Muscle and Electroencephalogram." *Acta Pharmacologica Sinica,* Vol. 8, pp. 117–123.

Young, K., and C.T.M. Davies. "Effect of Diet on Human Muscle Weakness Following Prolonged Exercise." *European Journal of Applied Physiology,* Vol. 53 (1984), pp. 81–85.

Young, Vernon R., and Peter L. Pellett. "Protein Intake and Requirements With Reference to Diet and Health." *American Journal of Clinical Nutrition,* Vol. 45 (1987), pp. 1323–1343.

Zawadzki, K. M., B. B. Yaspelkis, and J. L. Ivy. "Carbohydrate-Protein Complex Increases the Rate of Muscle Glycogen Storage After Exercise." *Journal of Applied Physiology,* Vol. 72 (1992), pp. 1854–1859.

Zhang, S. L. "Therapeutic Effects of Huperzine A on the Aged With Memory Impairment." *New Drums Clinical Remedies,* Vol. 5 (1986), pp. 260–262.

INDEX

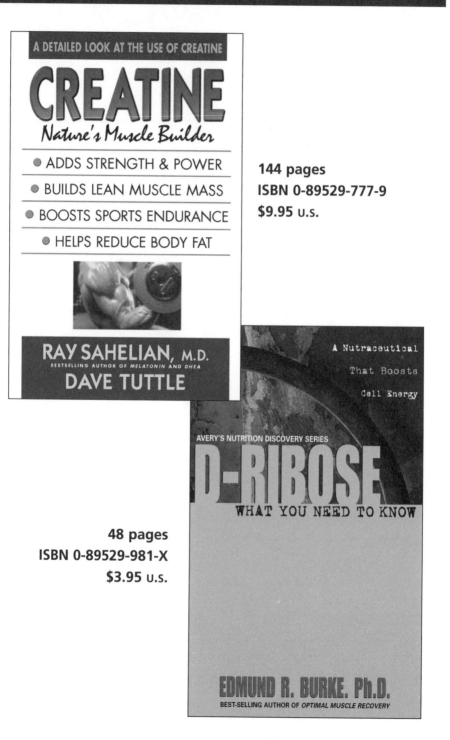

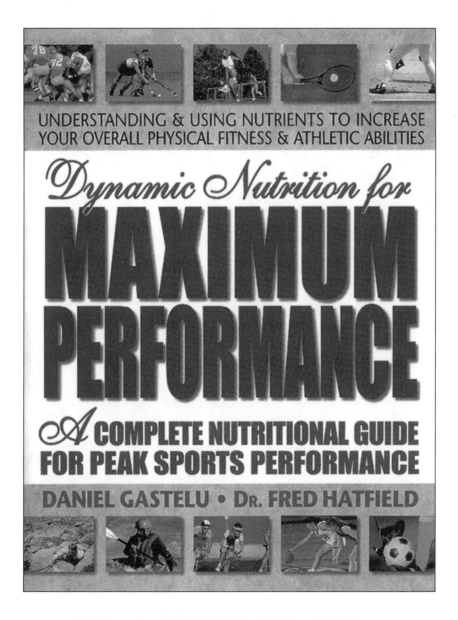

UNDERSTANDING & USING NUTRIENTS TO INCREASE
YOUR OVERALL PHYSICAL FITNESS & ATHLETIC ABILITIES

Dynamic Nutrition for

MAXIMUM PERFORMANCE

A COMPLETE NUTRITIONAL GUIDE
FOR PEAK SPORTS PERFORMANCE

DANIEL GASTELU • Dr. FRED HATFIELD

416 pages • ISBN 0-89529-756-6 • $19.95 U.S.

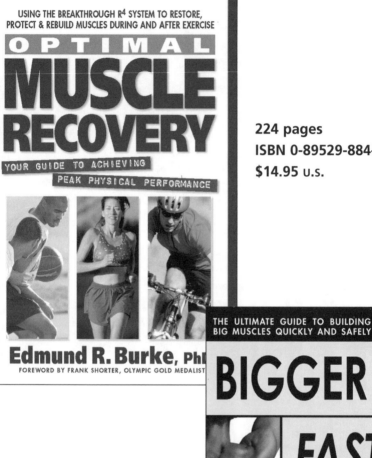

USING THE BREAKTHROUGH R⁴ SYSTEM TO RESTORE,
PROTECT & REBUILD MUSCLES DURING AND AFTER EXERCISE

OPTIMAL
MUSCLE
RECOVERY
YOUR GUIDE TO ACHIEVING
PEAK PHYSICAL PERFORMANCE

Edmund R. Burke, PhD
FOREWORD BY FRANK SHORTER, OLYMPIC GOLD MEDALIST

224 pages
ISBN 0-89529-884-8
$14.95 U.S.

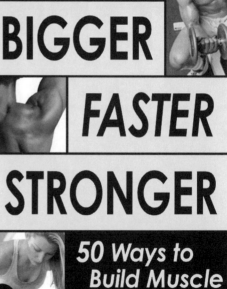

THE ULTIMATE GUIDE TO BUILDING
BIG MUSCLES QUICKLY AND SAFELY

BIGGER
FASTER
STRONGER
*50 Ways to
Build Muscle*
DAVE TUTTLE
FROM THE BEST-SELLING CO-AUTHOR OF *CREATINE*

160 pages
ISBN 0-89529-951-8
$9.95 U.S.

Healthy Habits

are easy to come by—

IF YOU KNOW WHERE TO LOOK!

Get the latest information on:

- **better health • diet & weight loss**
- **the latest nutritional supplements**
- **herbal healing • homeopathy and more**

HEALTH BOOK CATALOG

ACHIEVING HEALTH

AVERY PUBLISHING GROUP

1998

RECEIVE A FREE COPY OF AVERY'S HEALTH CATALOG

COMPLETE AND RETURN THIS CARD RIGHT AWAY!

Where did you purchase this book?

- ❑ bookstore
- ❑ health food store
- ❑ pharmacy
- ❑ supermarket
- ❑ other (please specify)_____

Name_____

Street Address_____

City_____State_____Zip_____

GIVE ONE TO A FRIEND ...

Healthy Habits

are easy to come by—

IF YOU KNOW WHERE TO LOOK!

Get the latest information on:

- **better health • diet & weight loss**
- **the latest nutritional supplements**
- **herbal healing • homeopathy and more**

HEALTH BOOK CATALOG

ACHIEVING HEALTH

AVERY PUBLISHING GROUP

1998

RECEIVE A FREE COPY OF AVERY'S HEALTH CATALOG

COMPLETE AND RETURN THIS CARD RIGHT AWAY!

Where did you purchase this book?

- ❑ bookstore
- ❑ health food store
- ❑ pharmacy
- ❑ supermarket
- ❑ other (please specify)_____

Name_____

Street Address_____

City_____State_____Zip_____

Avery Publishing Group
120 Old Broadway
Garden City Park, NY 11040

Avery Publishing Group
120 Old Broadway
Garden City Park, NY 11040